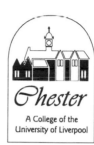
b

Diagnostic and Therapeutic Antibodies

METHODS IN MOLECULAR MEDICINE™

John M. Walker, SERIES EDITOR

METHODS IN MOLECULAR MEDICINE™

Diagnostic and Therapeutic Antibodies

Edited by

Andrew J. T. George

Department of Immunology, Imperial College School of Medicine,
Hammersmith Hospital, London, UK

and

Catherine E. Urch

Department of Pharmacology, University College, London, UK

Humana Press Totowa, New Jersey

The cover illustration shows a model of the entire human IgG$_1$ molecule. It was generated using the RasMol program (1) from a composite model generated by Dr. Eduardo Padlan of the National Institutes of Health, Bethesda, MD, using coordinates for F(ab')$_2$ and Fc fragments and theoretical modeling of the hinge region. The model is described in Padlan (2). The PDB file is available from http://www.umass.edu/microbio/rasmol/padlan.htm.

1. Sayle, R. A. and Milner, W.-E. J. (1995) RasMol: biomolecular graphics for all. *Trends Biochem. Sci.* **20**, 374.
2. Padlan, E. A. (1994) Anatomy of the antibody molecule. *Mol. Immunol.* **31**, 169–217.

For additional copies, pricing for bulk purchases, and/or information about other Humana titles, contact Humana at the above address or at any of the following numbers: Tel.: 973-256-1699; Fax: 973-256-8341; E-mail: humana@humanapr.com

Photocopy Authorization Policy:

Printed in the United States of America. 10 9 8 7 6 5 4 3 2 1

Library of Congress Cataloging in Publication Data

Main entry under title:

Methods in molecular medicine™.

Diagnostic and therapeutic antibodies / edited by Andrew J. T. George and Catherine E. Urch.
        p.   cm. -- (Methods in molecular medicine™)
     Includes index.
     ISBN 0-89603-798-3 (alk. paper)
        1. Monoclonal antibodies—Therapeutic use. 2. Immunoglobulins—Therapeutic use. 3. Immunotherapy. 4. Monoclonal antibodies—Diagnostic use. I. George, Andrew J. T. II. Urch, Catherine E. III. Series.
        [DNLM: 1. Antibodies, Monoclonal—diagnostic use. 2. Antibodies, Monoclonal—Therapeutic use. 3. Immunotherapy—methods.
     QW 575.5.A6 D536 2000]
     RM282.M65D53   2000

Preface

Soon after the first description of monoclonal antibodies in 1976, there was enormous interest in the clinical application of antibodies, especially in the context of cancer. Antibodies appeared to offer the "magic bullet" that would allow the specific destruction of neoplastic cells. However, many years' effort resulted in very few cases of successful immunotherapy with antibodies. As a result there was a major backlash against antibody therapy, and the field lost a considerable amount of popularity.

Fashion, in science as well as in other things, tends to be cyclical. Antibody-based therapy is once again attracting scientists and clinicians. There are several reasons for the renewed optimism; certainly the experience of the last two decades has provided a wealth of information about problems associated with antibody therapy, and possible solutions to these problems. Recombinant antibody engineering has rejuvenated the field, allowing both the modification of antibodies to improve their in vivo properties and the isolation of novel antibody molecules by such techniques as phage display. The results of recent clinical trials have demonstrated unequivocally the benefit of antibody therapy in a number of settings, and, finally, more careful consideration has been taken of the types of disease best treated using this approach.

The result is a more realistic climate of opinion, one in which antibody therapies are seen to have a role to play in the clinical management of patients, but are not seen as the panacea for all disease. *Diagnostic and Therapeutic Antibodies* is, therefore, especially timely, and is aimed at a new generation of clinicians and scientists who are entering the field and need to know both the background to the subject and also gain real competence in the basic techniques that they will be using. The book covers both theoretical and practical aspects of the clinical use of antibodies. It also looks at the in vitro diagnostic application of antibodies, an area where the impact of monoclonal antibodies has been enormous and consistent.

To that end the book is divided into four sections. The first acts as a short introduction to the basic science of the antibody molecule, including its structure and how to generate antibodies. The second section is a series of reviews looking at different applications of antibodies in the clinic (including clinical laboratories). Such a section might seem unusual for a book in the *Methods in Molecular Medicine* series, but as every reader will have in mind a different in vivo application, this will allow them to get a picture of how antibodies can be used in varied clinical settings. It will also allow a certain degree of cross fertilization between different clinical disciplines. The third section covers the interaction between industry and the basic scientist. Such interaction is vital for the scientist to understand; if researchers have any ambitions to see their antibody in wide-scale clinical use, they will need to involve pharmaceutical and/or biotechnology companies. If they are to do this, then the nature of the intellectual property and the practicalities of its management need to be considered. This section consists of two chapters, one outlining the essentials of intellectual property and the second giving the case history of one antibody, CAMPATH-1, and the disasters and triumphs that accompanied its progress to the marketplace.

The final section contains a series of protocols that will be of use to people new to the field. The first set gives methods for producing and purifying antibodies, as well as the quality control procedures that are needed in preparing material for the clinic. The second set describes how to modify antibodies for clinical application, and how to measure the affinity and immunoreactivity of the molecules. The use of antibodies in a variety of in vitro assays and staining procedures is then given. Finally, a pair of chapters outline basic protocols for the early stages in antibody engineering.

The antibody is an extremely versatile molecule, with a myriad of potential applications. We trust that in *Diagnostic and Therapeutic Antibodies* we have collected together a series of chapters that will both inspire readers to explore some of the possibilities, and give them the basic theoretical and practical tools to start this task. We are extremely grateful to all the authors who have given their time, expertise, and energy to this project.

Finally, we would like to dedicate this book to Philippa, who was born as we started this project and without whom it would have been completed much sooner.

Andrew J. T. George
Catherine E. Urch

Contents

Contributors

CEZMI A. AKDIŞ • *Swiss Institute of Allergy and Asthma Research, Davos, Switzerland*

ABDULHAMID A. AL-TUBULY • *Department of Immunology and Medical Microbiology, Alfatah University for Medical Sciences, Tripoli, Libya*

SARAH M. ANDREW • *Department of Biology, Chester College of Higher Education, Chester, UK*

KULDIP BHAMRA • *Therapeutic Antibody Centre, Oxford, UK*

PRU BIRD • *Therapeutic Antibody Centre, Oxford, UK*

EKATERINI BOLETI • *Department of Clinical Oncology, The Royal London Hospital, London, UK*

WILLIAM M. BROWN • *Taro Pharmaceuticals USA Inc., Hawthorne, NY*

DENISE L. FAUSTMAN • *Massachusetts General Hospital and Harvard Medical School, Boston, Massachusetts General Hospital, Charlestown, MA*

RUTH R. FRENCH • *Lymphoma Research Unit, Tenovus Research Laboratories, Southampton General Hospital, Southampton, UK*

JÓNA FREYSDÓTTIR • *Department of Oral Medicine, Leeds Dental Institute, Leeds, UK*

ANDREW J. T. GEORGE • *Department of Immunology, Imperial College School of Medicine, London, UK*

MARTIN J. GLENNIE • *Lymphoma Research Unit, Tenovus Research Laboratories, Southampton General Hospital, Southampton, UK*

CALVIN S. R. GOODEN • *SmithKline Beecham Pharmaceuticals, Essex, UK*

GEOFF HALE • *Sir William Dunn School of Pathology, Oxford University, Oxford, UK*

PATRICK HARRISON • *Therapeutic Antibody Centre, Oxford, UK*

BRIDGET HEELAN • *Department of Immunology, Imperial College School of Medicine, London, UK*

JAMIE HONEYCHURCH • *Lymphoma Research Unit, Tenovus Research Laboratories, Southampton General Hospital, Southampton, UK*

MICHAEL JOHNS • *Department of Immunology, Imperial College School of*

Medicine, London, UK

BILL JORDAN • *Department of Immunology, Imperial College School of Medicine, London, UK*

IAN T. W. MATTHEWS • *ChemOvation Ltd., Horsham, UK*

PAUL F. MCKAY • *Department of Viral Pathogenesis, Beth Israel Deaconess Medical Center and Department of Medicine, Harvard Medical School, Boston, MA*

DAVID J. NEWMAN • *South West Thames Institute for Renal Research, Surrey, UK*

STEVE NICOLSON • *Department of Oncology, St. George's Hospital, Tooting, UK*

H. BARBAROS ORAL • *Immunology Unit, Department of Microbiology, School of Medicine, Uludag University, Bursa, Turkey*

DONALD B. PALMER • *Department of Immunology, Imperial College School of Medicine, London, UK*

A. MICHAEL PETERS • *Department of Nuclear Medicine, New Addenbrookes Hospital, Cambridge, UK*

JENNY PHILLIPS • *Therapeutic Antibody Centre, Oxford, UK*

MAUREEN POWER • *Lymphoma Research Unit, Tenovus Research Laboratories, Southampton General Hospital, Southampton, UK*

MARY A. RITTER • *Department of Immunology, Imperial College School of Medicine, London, UK*

GAIL ROWLINSON-BUSZA • *Antisoma Research Laboratories, St. George's Hospital Medical School, London, UK*

CATHERINE E. SARRAF • *Department of Histology, Imperial College School of Medicine, London, UK*

RICHARD SMITH • *Academic Renal Unit, Southmead Hospital, Bristol, UK*

PETER C. TAYLOR • *The Mathilda and Terence Kennedy Institute of Rheumatology, Hammersmith Hospital, London, UK*

ALISON L. TUTT • *Lymphoma Research Unit, Tenovus Research Laboratories, Southampton General Hospital, Southampton, UK*

CATHERINE E. URCH • *Department of Pharmacology, University College, London, UK*

SUSAN VAN NOORDEN • *Department of Histochemistry, Division of Diagnostic Sciences, Imperial College School of Medicine, London, UK*

RAKESH VERMA • *Department of Immunology, Imperial College School of Medicine, London, UK*

HERMAN WALDMANN • *Sir William Dunn School of Pathology, Oxford University, Oxford, UK*

I

INTRODUCTION

1

The Antibody Molecule

Andrew J. T. George

1. Introduction

The importance of antibody molecules was first recognized in the 1890s, when it was shown that immunity to tetanus and diphtheria was caused by antibodies against the bacterial exotoxins (*1*). Around the same time, it was shown that antisera against cholera vibrios could transfer immunity to naïve animals, and also kill the bacteria in vitro (*1*). However, although antitoxin antibodies rapidly found clinical application, there was little understanding regarding the nature of the antibody molecule. Indeed, the earliest theories suggested that the antitoxins were derived by modification of the toxin—intriguingly similar "antigen incorporation" theories were propounded as late as 1930 (*1*).

In more recent times, thanks to the efforts of both cellular and molecular immunologists, we have a more complete understanding of the structure, genetics, and function of an antibody molecule. As is discussed in the rest of this volume, this knowledge has allowed the design of improved molecules for clinical application.

2. Structure of the Antibody Molecule

The basic structure of an antibody (immunoglobin G [IgG]) molecule is shown in **Fig. 1**, and is reviewed in detail in **ref. 2**. It consists of four chains: two identical heavy (H) and two identical light (L) chains. The heavy chains vary between different classes and subclasses of antibody (e.g., ε heavy chains are found in IgE, μ in IgM, γ1 in IgG1, and so forth). These different classes and subclasses have specialized roles in immunity. There are two types of light chains, κ and λ. These do not have different functions, but represent alternatives that help increase the diversity of immune recognition by antibod

From: *Methods in Molecular Medicine, Vol. 40: Diagnostic and Therapeutic Antibodies*
Edited by: A. J. T. George and C. E. Urch © Humana Press Inc., Totowa, NJ

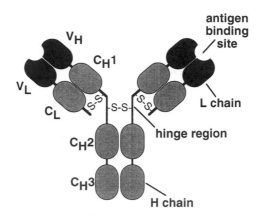

Fig. 1. The antibody molecule. The structure of IgG is shown, with the domains represented by separate blocks. The hinge region contains multiple disulfide bonds; one is shown for convenience.

ies. The four chains are held together by both noncovalent interactions and disulfide bonds, as shown in **Fig. 1**.

The H and L chains are made up of a number of domains of approx 110 amino acids arranged as two layers of antiparallel β-sheets held together by a conserved disulfide bond. These Ig domains, which fold independently, provide a modular structure to the antibody molecule, which has been exploited in antibody engineering studies (*see* Chapter 3). These domains are the archetype of those found in members of the immunoglobulin superfamily. In addition to the Ig domains, there is a hinge region, which has an extended structure that provides flexibility for the molecule.

A comparison of the sequence similarity between the domains of the antibody molecule shows that the majority of the domains have the same sequence between antibody molecules of the same subclass, and so are termed constant (C) domains (C_H1, C_H2, and so forth on the H chain, and C_L on the L chain). However, one domain in each chain has a variable sequence, and so is termed the variable (V) domain (V_H and V_L). Comparison of the sequence between different V regions shows that most of the variability is confined to three parts of the molecule, termed the complementarity-determining regions (CDRs), which come together in three-dimensional space when the molecule is folded to form the antigen-binding site (containing six CDR regions, three from the V_H domain and three from the V_L domain).

The structure of the antibody molecule was determined, in part, by the use of enzymes that cut the molecule into distinct fragments. Thus, papain cleaves the molecule N terminal to the disulfide bonds in the hinge region to yield the

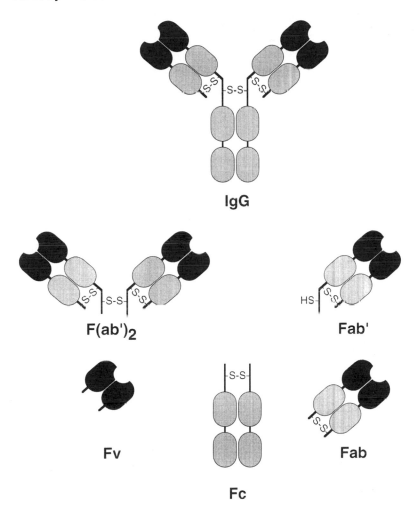

Fig. 2. Fragments of antibody molecule. The major fragments of an IgG molecule are represented here, with the antigen-binding Fv (~25 kDa in size), the Fab and Fab' (~50 kDa), and the F(ab')$_2$ (~100 kDa) compared to the intact IgG (~150 kDa) and the Fc region.

Fab (fraction antigen binding) and Fc part of the molecule. Pepsin cuts the C terminal of the cysteines to produce a F(ab')$_2$ fragment. This can be mildly reduced to produce the Fab' fragment (*see* **Fig. 2**). Other fragments that can be produced by proteolytic cleavage include the Fv (V$_H$ and V$_L$ domains). The production of these fragments was instrumental in our understanding of the structure–function relationship of the immunoglobulin molecule: thus the antigen-binding property of the molecule was shown to reside in the Fab fragment, with the Fab and Fab′ being monovalent and the $F(ab')_2$ being bivalent. However, none of these parts of the molecule are capable of recruiting effector function. That property resides in the Fc portion.

3. Functions of the Antibody Molecule

The antibody molecule has two major functions. The first is to act as the antigen receptor for B cells. Thus, binding of antigen by surface immunoglobulin on a B cell is a vital step in the triggering of the cell for activation (and in delivering antigen to the MHC class II processing pathway). The second function is to act as the antigen-specific soluble effector molecule in the humoral arm of the immune response. It is this function that is the topic of this volume. Antibodies can exert their effector functions in one of three ways. The first is to simply bind to their target antigen and neutralize it. Thus, antiviral antibodies can bind to molecules on the virus surface that are essential for binding to and infection of target cells; this can result in steric blocking of these molecules and so prevent infection. Similarly, antitoxin antibodies can act in a similar manner. The other two ways in which antibodies can work rely on the molecule-recruiting effector functions, either as complement or cells bearing receptors for the Fc part of the molecule.

3.1. Complement

The complement system consists of a series of proteins arranged in a series of pathways. In terms of antibodies there are three pathways of importance: the classical pathway, the alternative pathway, and the lytic pathway. The classical pathway is initiated by the binding of the first component of the pathway, C1, to the Fc of antibody molecules that have bound their antigen. This causes activation of C1, which can then activate the next component of the pathway, C4, by chopping it up into the fragments C4a and C4b. C4b can associate with C2, which is then cleaved by C1 into C2a and C2b. The complex formed of C4bC2b is then capable of proteolytic cleavage of C3 into C3a and C3b.

The alternative pathway similarly serves to cleave C3 into C3a and C3b. This pathway can be activated in several ways. However, in the context of antibody-mediated activation, it serves as an amplification pathway. This is because the pathway is initiated by C3b. Thus, once C3b is generated by the classical pathway, it activates the alternative pathway, which then cleaves C3 to produce more C3b, thus providing a positive feed-forward pathway.

The lytic pathway is also initiated by C3b. This activates C5 by cleavage into C5a and C5b. The membrane attack complex ($C5b678(C9)n$) is then assembled. This forms a pore in membranes, and can lead to death of targeted cells by osmotic lysis.

Table 1
FcγR

Name	CD	Distribution	Affinity	Specificity
FcγR1	CD64	Monocytes	High ($10^{-8}M$)	IgG1 = IgG3 > IgG4
FcγRII	CD32	Monocytes, neutrophils, eosinophils, platelets, B cells	Low ($\sim 10^{-6}$ M)	IgG1 = IgG3 > IgG2,IgG4
FcγRIII	CD16	Neutrophils, eosinophils, macrophages, NK cells	Low ($\sim 10^{-6}$ M)	IgG1 = IgG3

The effector functions of the complement system include lysis via the membrane attack complex, opsonization (through receptors for C3b and C4b on leukocytes) and the proinflammatory effects of anaphylotoxins (C5a, C3a, C4a), which are chemotactic and also cause the release of vasoactive molecules by mast cells and basophils.

3.2. Binding to FcR⁺ Cells

Many cell types express receptors for different classes of immunoglobulin. These recognize determinants on the Fc part of the molecule. In the case of IgG there are three major types of FcR on human leukocytes, as shown in **Table 1**. The function of these molecules depends on the cell type expressing them, and other features of the interaction, such as the affinity of the interaction. Thus, CD16 (FcγRIII), when expressed on natural killer (NK) cells, directs antibody-dependent cellular cytotoxicity (ADCC) against antibody-coated target cells. The same molecule on monocytes promotes phagocytosis. In addition to promoting phagocytosis, FcRs are involved in clearance of immune complexes and antibody-coated debris by the reticuloendothelial system, and in the release of mediators by basophils and mast cells (which bind IgE by high-affinity FcεR). They can also have a role in antigen presentation and activation of B cells.

3.3. Classes and Subclasses of Antibodies

As we discussed, antibodies can have different Fc regions depending on their class or subclass. Different classes and subclasses have different functions in immunity, as they show different abilities to recruit effector mechanisms. In addition, some antibody classes have specialized functions, e.g., IgA

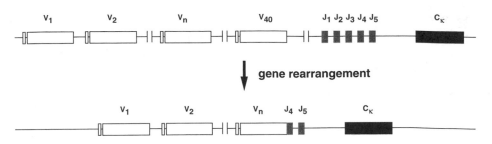

Fig. 3. Human κ gene locus. The κ gene locus consists of 40 V gene segments, (although there is some variation in the population regarding the exact number), 4 J segments, and a constant segment. During rearrangement one of the V segments is recombined with one of the J segments at random. The figure is diagrammatic. In reality the gene segments are more widely separated by introns. For an accurate map *see* **ref. 3**.

molecules can be dimerized to form $(IgA)_2$, which are secreted onto mucosal surfaces and are an important component of host defenses at these sites. IgM molecules are produced early in the immune response, before affinity maturation (*see* **Subheading 4.**) has occurred. In order to compensate for the low affinity of primary antibodies, IgM is found as a pentamer, with five components similar to the archetypal Y-shaped IgG joined by disulfide bonds and an additional J chain. This structure increases the valency of the molecule (from 2 to 10 antigen-binding sites) and so increases the avidity of its interaction with antigen.

4. Genetics of Antibodies

In order to produce an antibody molecule with its variable domains and constant domains, the B cell has to undergo complex DNA rearrangements. These allow the vast diversity of antibody specificities to be produced, while retaining constant regions capable of recruiting effectors. Mice and humans have three immunoglobulin loci; the heavy chain, κ light-chain, and λ light-chain loci. Each locus has a number of different gene segments. We first consider the κ locus. This consists of a number of V-region gene segments (in the human 40), J gene segments (5 in the human), and a single constant-gene segment (*see* **Fig. 3**) *(3)*. During B-cell development, the V and J gene segments recombine at random, such that one V segment is juxtaposed to one J segment, with the intervening DNA being lost. This recombinatorial diversity means that 200 (40 × 5) different combinations of V and J segments can be obtained in the human κ chain.

A similar arrangement is seen in the human λ locus with 30 V and 4 J segments (although the mouse λ locus has very little diversity, with just 2 V

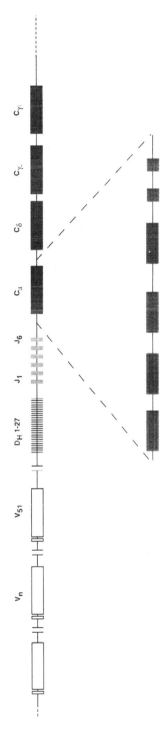

Fig. 4. **Heavy-chain locus.** The heavy-chain locus differs from the κ locus by having additional D segments that are rearranged with the V and J segments. It also has multiple genes encoding different constant regions, corresponding to the different classes and subclasses of immunoglobulin. These are rearranged during the process of class switching. Each of the genes for the constant region contains multiple exons, as illustrated for μ in the expanded section at the bottom of the figure, rather than the one shown. For more detailed maps *see* **ref. 3**.

segments). The heavy-chain locus has an additional source of diversity in the D segments (27 in humans), which are between the V (51 in humans) and J (6 in humans) (**Fig. 4**) *(3–5)*. The heavy chain needs to undergo V-D-J recombination. The potential number of V(D)J recombinations in the human is therefore 8262 for the H chain locus, 200 for κ, and 120 for λ. This then allows for combinatorial diversity, because any H chain can be paired with any light chain, giving 1,652,400 possible different H-κ and 991,440 H-λ pairings.

Additional diversity can still be obtained by the imprecise nature of the joining process between the gene segments, resulting from both untemplated nucleotide addition, which adds random coding sequences at the junction of the segments, and by variations in the exact site of splicing of the DNA.

The diversity seen in the naïve B-cell repertoire is, therefore, largely the result of recombinatorial diversity (using different V[D]J segments), combinatorial diversity (different H and L chains), and junctional diversity. This diversity is sufficient to allow the selection of the low-affinity antibodies during the primary immune response. However, to obtain high-affinity antibodies seen during the secondary immune response a further process occurs, that of somatic mutation. This is seen in the germinal centers of lymph nodes and involves essentially random mutation of the V(D)J gene segments that encode the variable domains of the antibody. Some of these mutations lead to antibodies that have a higher affinity for the antigen than the parental molecules; these are selected. As a result of this process of random mutation, followed by selection, affinity maturation of the antibody response occurs.

The final process that we need to consider is class switching; the process by which an antibody of one class changes to a different class or subclass. This event involves the heavy-chain locus. Downstream of the V, D, and J gene segments are a number of genes encoding for the constant regions of the different antibody classes and subclasses (**Fig. 4**). Thus in mouse, the heavy-chain genes are in the order μ-δ-γ_3-γ_1-γ_{2b}-γ_{2a}-ϵ-α. Naïve B cells express IgM and IgD, using a process of differential splicing of the primary RNA transcript so that in the mRNA the recombined V(D)J sequence is spliced to either the μ or δ genes. When class switching occurs there is a recombination event whereby the gene encoding for the new antibody isotype is spliced into the position previously occupied by the μ gene, losing all the intermediate DNA.

5. Antibody–Antigen Interactions

5.1. Affinity

The interaction between an antibody and antigen is formed by noncovalent interactions; ionic bonds, hydrogen bonds, van der Waal's forces, and hydrophobic interactions (for reviews *see* **refs. *6–8***). One important consequence of this is that the interaction is reversible and can be represented by the equilibrium interaction:

$$A + B \underset{\longleftarrow}{\overset{\longrightarrow}{}} C \tag{1}$$

where A is the antigen, B is the antibody, and C the complex of antibody and antigen (for simplicity we will assume a monovalent interaction, in which one molecule of A interacts with one molecule of B, as would be seen if B were a Fab fragment).

If, therefore, one mixes antigen and antibody together, the reaction will initially go with a relatively fast rate from left to right. As the reactants (A and B) are consumed the reaction will slow down. At the same time, as the concentration of the produce (C) builds up the reaction from right to left increases. Eventually equilibrium is reached, i.e., the reaction from left to right is proceeding at the same rate as the reaction from right to left. At this time the concentrations of A, B, and C remain constant. However, it is important to realize that the association of A and B to form C is continuing, as is the dissociation of C to form A and B. While the reaction is in equilibrium, any one molecule of antibody (or antigen) may find itself changing from the free state to being bound in the complex and back again.

The affinity of an antibody for its antigen is a measure in which the equilibrium of the reaction shown in **Eq. 1** lies. For a high-affinity interaction the equilibrium is further over to the right than a low-affinity interaction. This can be expressed by the concentration of A, B, and C at equilibrium:

$$\frac{[C]}{[A][B]} = K_a \tag{2}$$

Note that [A] and [B] are the concentrations of free antigen and antibody at equilibrium, not the starting concentrations. The term K_a is the association equilibrium constant, and has terms M^{-1}. The higher K_a, the higher the concentration of C at equilibrium and the higher the affinity of the interaction.

Immunologists often prefer to think of affinity in terms of the dissociation equilibrium constant (K_d). This is the reciprocal of K_a:

$$K_d = \frac{1}{K_a} = \frac{[A][B]}{[C]} \tag{3}$$

The K_d has units M; the higher the affinity the lower K_d. The K_d is useful because it gives the concentration of free antibody at which half the antigen is bound in a complex (in other words when [A] = [C]; substituting one for the other in **Eq. 3** gives $K_d = [B]$). As in many cases, we use vast excess of anti-

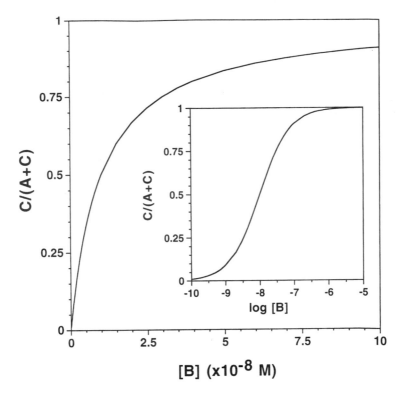

Fig. 5. Binding of antigen by an antibody. Shown here is the proportion of antigen (C/(A+C)) bound by a Fab fragment of an antibody that has an affinity (K_d) of 10^{-8} M for the antigen. The concentration of free Fab ([B]) is shown both on a linear and a log (inset) scale. Fifty percent saturation is achieved when [B] = 10^{-8} M.

body so only a very small proportion of the antibody is bound up in an immune complex. The K_d of an antibody–antigen interaction gives useful information regarding the concentration of antibody needed to get half maximal binding to the antigen.

The importance of the affinity of an antibody–antigen interaction is that it tells one how much antibody is needed to get binding to an antigen. This can be obtained from **Eq. 4**, and is shown in graphical form in **Fig. 5**.

$$\frac{C}{A + C} = \frac{B}{B + K_d} \tag{4}$$

The left-hand term corresponds to the degree of saturation of the antigen, i.e., the proportion of antigen bound by antibody. In the context of antibody-based assays (such as enzyme-linked immunosorbent assay [ELISA], cell, or tissue staining) the goal is to use the minimum concentration of antibody needed to get close to maximal staining (= saturation). In the in vivo clinical setting it tells one what concentrations of antibody need to be achieved to obtain maximal binding to the target antigen (remembering that other parameters, such as tissue penetrance, will be important in vivo). A higher affinity antibody can be used at a lower concentration than a low-affinity antibody to obtain the same degree of saturation of the target antigen.

It is clearly important to use enough antibody to obtain the degree of binding of the target antigen. What is not always so appreciated is that it is important not to use too much antibody. The most obvious (and not trivial!) reason for this is economy. However, there are also good scientific reasons. In the in vivo situation, if the antibody is conjugated to a toxic moiety (e.g., a radioisotope) then administration of too high a dose of antibody will result in excess radiolabel staying in the circulation, resulting in nonspecific toxicity. In addition, high concentrations of antibody run the risk of nonspecific interactions, for example via the Fc region. The final reason relates to the specificity of the antibody. Such terms as "exquisite specificity" are often used in the context of antibody interactions. Unfortunately, these convey the false impression that antibodies are uniquely specific for their antigen, and so will bind to only that antigen. However, immunological specificity is not absolute. Antibodies will bind to antigens other than the antigen for which they are "specific", but they will do so with a lower affinity. Because the degree of saturation of the antigen is a product of both the affinity and the concentration of the antibody for its antigen, such low-affinity interactions will occur if the antibody concentration is high enough. This is illustrated in **Fig. 6**, which shows the affinity of a monoclonal antibody (mAb) (40-50) raised against the cardiac glycoside digoxin *(9)*. The affinity of the antibody for three other representative glycosides is shown. These molecules vary in structure from digoxin in one of three positions, as shown in the table. As can be seen, an mAb affinity of 40-50 antibody has an affinity for digoxin that is nearly 10,000 times higher than that for one of the analogs, oleandrigenin. As a result, it can be a very specific reagent that can be used to distinguish between these two molecules. At a concentration of free-antigen binding sites of 10^{-8} M (750 ng/mL free IgG, assuming two antigen-binding sites/molecule) 95.9% of digoxin molecules are bound by the antibody, with only 0.3% of the oleandrigenin—truly exquisite specificity. But, if a higher concentration of antibody is used (10^{-4} M antigen-binding sites, equivalent to 7.5 mg/mL), then 96.4% of the oleandrigenin molecules are also bound—showing no specificity. As is illustrated by the binding curves for the other analogs, which have intermediate affinities for the antibody, the fine specificity of 40-50 for the different molecules is very dependent on the concentration.

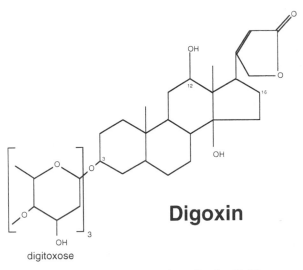

Digoxin

digitoxose

Specificity of binding of antibody 40-50 to digoxin and gitoxin analogues

Glycoside	3β	12β	16β	K_d (M)
Digoxin	Tridigitoxose	-OH		4.3×10^{-10}
Gitoxin	Tridigitoxose		-OH	7.0×10^{-9}
Oleandrin	Oleandrose		-OCOCH$_3$	8.6×10^{-8}
Oleandrigenin	-OH		-OCOCH$_3$	3.7×10^{-6}

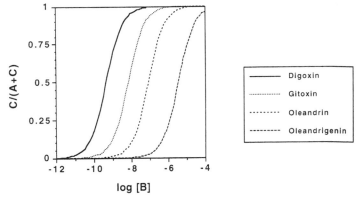

Fig. 6. Specificity of 40-50 antibody for digoxin and related glycosides. The table shows the affinity of interaction between 40-50 and four glycosides (taken from a larger panel). These molecules differ from each other in one of three positions on the backbone of the molecule (the structure of digoxin is shown, with the relevant positions marked). The expected binding curves for 40-50 and the four molecules is shown at the bottom of the figure, where [B] is the concentration of free antigen-binding sites and C/(A+C) the proportion of the antigen bound by the molecule. As can be seen at low concentrations 40–50 binds preferentially to digoxin. As the concentration of antibody is increased this specificity is lost.

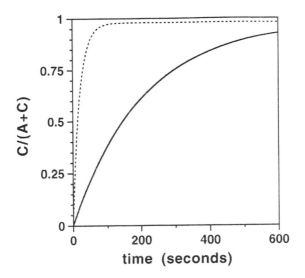

Fig. 7. Association rate constant. This graph models the interaction of two antibodies with an antigen over time. The two molecules have the same affinity for the antigen, although one (broken line) has a 10-fold higher k_{ass} (and a 10-fold higher k_{diss}). When added to the antigen the two antibodies will reach the same equilibrium, because they have the same affinity. However, the "fast-on fast-off" reaches equilibrium faster than the "slow-on slow-off."

5.2. Rate Constants

Subheading 5.1. dealt with the situation at equilibrium. However, the speed of the reactions is also important. These are given by the association and dissociation equilibrium constants (k_{ass} and k_{diss}).

$$A + B \underset{k_{diss}}{\overset{k_{ass}}{\rightleftharpoons}} C \tag{5}$$

These are obviously related to the equilibrium constants

$$K_a = \frac{k_{diss}}{k_{ass}} \tag{6}$$

However, it is possible for there to be two antibody–antigen interactions with the same affinity but different kinetics. One could have relatively high k_{ass} and k_{diss}, the other a lower k_{ass} and k_{diss}. If one mixes the antibodies with their antigens, the antibody with the high k_{ass} and k_{diss} will reach equilibrium more rapidly than the one with the low k_{ass} and k_{diss} (**Fig. 7**). The equilibrium will be the

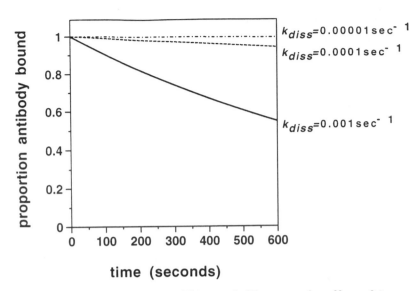

Fig. 8. Dissociation rate constant. This graph illustrates the effect of k_{diss} on the interaction of antibodies with their antigen. Three antibodies are shown, with different values for k_{diss} (right). The graph shows the dissociation of the complex between antigen and antibody over time in the absence of free antibody. This is the situation seen when free antibody is removed from the system; for example, following washing of an ELISA plate or tissue section. As can be seen, after 10 min nearly half of the antibody with a high k_{diss} has dissociated, whereas very little of that with a 100-fold lower k_{diss} has dissociated.

same. However, the complex formed by the low k_{ass} and k_{diss} reaction will be more stable. If one removes all the free antibody from the system then one can follow the dissociation of the complex (**Fig. 8**).

This has obvious implications for therapy. The k_{ass} and k_{diss} of the interaction will give information regarding how fast the antibody will bind to its target antigen and, once bound, how stable that interaction will be. An antibody with a high k_{diss} will not be appropriate if it is necessary for the antibody to remain bound to its target for a long time. Similar considerations apply for in vitro assays, in which an antibody with a low k_{ass} and k_{diss} will take longer to bind its target antigen than an antibody with equivalent affinity (necessitating longer than normal incubation times), but will be more stable once bound (allowing more stringent washing procedures).

5.3. Avidity

An important component of the antibody–antigen interaction is the avidity of the interaction. The affinity of an interaction is determined in part by the rate at which the complex C dissociates into A and B. If B is the Fab fragment of an

Table 2
Problems Associated with Antibody Therapy

- Immunogenicity of rodent antibodies
- Poor penetration of solid tissue
- Slow clearance of unbound material
- Nonspecific localization via Fc region
- Inadequate cytotoxicity
- Insufficient specificity
- Modulation of surface antigen
- Heterogeneous or low expression of surface antigen
- Mutation of surface antigen

antibody, then it needs just one antibody–antigen bond to dissociate for the complex to fall apart. However, if B is an IgG molecule with two antigen-binding sites (and assuming that A has multiple epitopes that B can bind to) it would require both antigen-binding sites to dissociate for the complex to fall apart. Because this is less likely to occur than a single dissociation event, the rate at which C dissociates into A and B is reduced, and the affinity of the reaction is increased.

This increase in affinity consequent on multivalent binding is termed the avidity of the interaction. It is very important in the case of IgM, in which there are 10 antigen-binding sites available for interacting with antigen. This compensates for the relatively low affinity of IgM antibodies produced during the primary immune response.

It should be noted that the avidity advantage only occurs if the antigen and antibody are multivalent. If the antigen has only one epitope recognized by the antibody then only a single dissociation event is required for the complex to fall apart. Thus, IgM antibodies sometimes are very good at recognizing antigens on the surface of cells or on ELISA plates (where the antigen is multivalent) but cannot immunoprecipitate the antigen from solution (where the antigen is monovalent).

6. Modification of the Structure of Antibody Molecules

As will be discussed extensively in Chapters 5–12 and 16 in this volume, antibodies have been applied to many clinical situations. However, many problems have to be faced with the clinical application of antibodies (**Table 2**). Some of these are associated with the choice of the antigen being targeted (e.g., mutation of target antigen, low or heterogeneous expression of antigen), and can be remedied by choosing antibodies with an alternative specificity. However, others problems have been addressed by altering the structure of the antibody molecule (*10*).

6.1. Immunogenicity

One of the major problems faced with using mAbs in the clinic has been that the vast majority of such molecules are made from mice or rats. As a result, they are immunogenic in humans, and elicit a Human Anti-Mouse Antibody (HAMA) response. The generation of antibodies that recognize the therapeutic antibody block the antibody molecule from reaching its target, and also can lead to serum sickness (type III hypersensitivity reactions). Several solutions for this problem. One solution is to make mAbs from human B cells. This is not easily done using hybridoma technology because good fusion partners for human cells are not plentiful, and the resulting hybridomas tend to be unstable and secrete only low levels of antibody. Increasingly, phage-display technology (Chapter 4) is being used; this can also lead to antibodies that recognize self epitopes because the library is not subject to in vivo negative selection, unlike the B-cell repertoire. An alternative approach is to modify the existing rodent hybridoma, using genetic approaches, to reduce its immunogenicity (Chapter 3). This can be done by chimerization (where the constant domains of the rodent antibody are replaced by those of human origin) or humanization (where the CDR regions of the antibody are sewn onto a human framework).

6.2. Pharmacokinetic Problems

The antibody molecule also has a number of pharmacokinetic problems. These include the difficulty that the molecule has in penetrating solid tissue, the slow clearance of unbound material from the circulation, and nonspecific localization to FcR^+ cells of the reticuloendothelial system. This causes both nonspecific toxicity (or in imaging applications an excessive background) and inadequate localization to the target cells. These problems can be solved by making smaller versions of antibodies, using either genetic (Chapter 3) or chemical approaches. Thus, the antigen-binding fragments shown in **Fig. 2** are all smaller than the whole IgG molecule, and so show better penetration of solid tissue. They also lack the Fc region. In some cases they are smaller than the glomerular filtration cutoff and so are rapidly cleared through the kidneys, shortening the half-life of the unbound material. These antibody fragments are either monovalent or bivalent; bivalency leads to an increase in the avidity of binding, as discussed in **Subheading 5.3.**

6.3. Improving the Cytotoxicity of Antibody Molecules

Antibodies are in many cases used "naked"; that is, as an unmodified molecule. For therapy this approach relies on the ability of the molecule to recruit natural effector functions (such as complement or ADCC) or act by signaling to the cell. However, in many cases this is not sufficient. In particular, murine antibodies are poor at recruiting human effectors (although humanization or

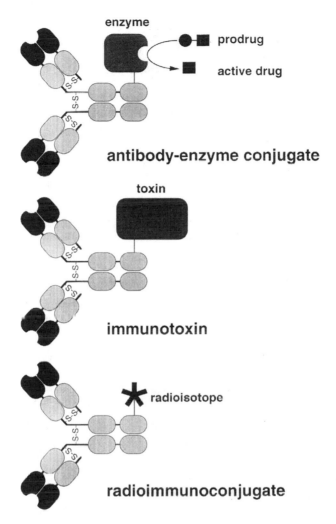

Fig. 9. Immunoconjugates. Three typical immunoconjugates are illustrated:
between an antibody and an enzyme (capable of activating a prodrug), an antibody and
a toxin, and an antibody and a radioisotope.

chimerization of the molecule gives it a human Fc region). One strategy to
overcome this is to use the antibody molecule to target an artificial effector
molecule to the cell. Typically this is done by making a conjugate between
the antibody and the effector molecule, using either chemical or genetic
approaches. The effector molecules can include drugs, toxins, radioisotopes
(also used in imaging), and enzymes capable of converting nontoxic prodrugs
to cytotoxic drugs (**Fig. 9**).

These targeting strategies have several features. Some of them rely on the toxic agent binding directly to the target cell. Thus, immunotoxins work by internalization of the toxic element into the cell, causing its death. Neighboring cells are not destroyed. This has the clear advantage of specificity; only cells recognized by the antibody are killed. However, in many cases it is problematic to target every cell with antibody, both because the expression of the relevant antigen may be heterogeneous and because the cell may be buried deep in a tumor mass. Other strategies, such as targeting radioisotopes with radioimmunoconjugates, will not have the same degree of specificity, because the radiation can kill neighboring cells and so will have a greater degree of nonspecific killing (which can be advantageous if not all the target cells have bound antibody).

Other features of the different strategies are also important. Thus, in the case of immunotoxins, which use plant- or bacterially derived toxin molecules, the toxin molecule is so potent that only one molecule is needed to kill a cell. However, that molecule must be in the cytosol to have an effect. To get to the cytosol it has to cross a membrane (either the plasma membrane or that of a vesicle that has been internalized by the cell). This is an inefficient process, and so many molecules of immunotoxin need to be bound to the surface of a cell for that cell to be killed. One of the attractions of targeting enzymes to the cell is that a single enzyme may convert thousands of molecules of a prodrug into an active drug, thus achieving an amplification. In addition, because all the components of the system are nontoxic (antibody–enzyme conjugate and prodrug), and can be given separately (i.e, the antibody–enzyme is administered first and allowed to localize to the target so that only when unbound conjugate has cleared from the system is the prodrug given), there is little systemic toxicity.

An alternative to conjugates are bispecific antibodies, in which the molecule has two specificities (**Fig. 10**) *(11)*. These can be created by chemical means (Chapter 26), recombinant technology, or fusing two hybridomas to make a hybrid hybridoma. Bispecific antibodies have been used in two approaches in the clinic. One is to target soluble effector molecules, such as those described earlier. In this case the bispecific antibody has specificity for both the target antigen and the effector molecule. The advantages of this approach are that there is no need to chemically conjugate the two molecules, and that it might be feasible to administer the bispecific antibodies and the effector molecules separately, thus increasing the specificity of targeting. Bispecific antibodies can also be used to target effector cells, such as T cells and NK cells. Such bispecific antibodies have specificity for the target antigen and a "trigger" molecule on the effector cell; typically CD3 for T cells and FcR

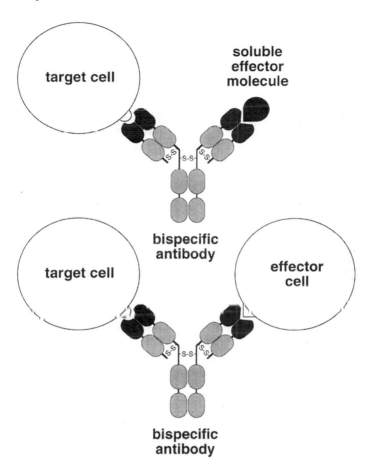

Fig. 10. Bispecific antibody. Bispecific antibodies contain two different antigen-binding sites, and can be used to target soluble effector molecules (such as toxins, drugs, or radiolabeled molecules) to cells bearing the appropriate antigen. Alternatively they can be used to redirect cytotoxic cells (e.g., T cells or NK cells), via appropriate trigger molecules, to kill target cells.

for NK cells. Because both T and NK cells are adapted to kill eukaryotic cells, this is a highly promising strategy for eliminating neoplastic and other unwanted cells *(11)*.

6.4. Which Molecule Should Be Used?

Clearly with such a plethora of different antibody molecules (IgG, fragments, human, rodent) and different effector functions (natural, toxins, prodrug, radioisotopes, bispecific, and so forth), it can be difficult to know which system to opt for. Unfortunately there is no universal answer! It will depend on the biology of the system, and you need to ask numerous questions. Is the target cell radiosensitive? Where is the target cell? Is it accessible to whole antibodies? Do I need rapid clearance of the antibody to reduce toxicity, or is prolonged circulation necessary to maximize binding to the target cell? Is my target antigen expressed on all cells, and throughout the cell cycle? Does my target antigen internalize into a pathway that facilitates toxin entry? Do I need to kill 100% of my target cells to achieve a therapeutic effect, or if I kill 90% will that be of benefit to the patient? Naturally the answer to many of these (and other!) questions may be unknown, and the final outcome may need to be a compromise.

7. Conclusion

The structure and genetics of the antibody molecule have given the immune system a means whereby it can target foreign antigens with a number of different effector mechanisms. The same system can also be readily adapted for clinical applications for targeting unwanted cells. In this volume a wide number of examples of such applications are given, involving both natural and artificial molecules and effector functions. However, the adaptability of the molecule, and the ingenuity of the scientists and clinicians who wish to exploit it, will ensure that over the years to come we will continue to be surprised by novel and exciting applications based on the antibody.

References

1. Silverstein, A. M. (1988) *A History of Immunology.* Academic Press, San Diego.
2. Padlan, E. A. (1994) Anatomy of the antibody molecule. *Mol. Immunol.* **31,** 169–217.
3. Tomlinson, I. M. (1997) The V BASE directory of human V gene sequences. MRC Centre for Protein Engineering, Hills Road, Cambridge CB2 2QH, UK. http://www.mrc-cpe.cam.ac.uk/imt-doc/public/INTRO.html.
4. Cook, G. P. and Tomlinson, I. M. (1995) The human immunoglobulin V_H repertoire. *Immunol. Today* **16,** 237–42.
5. Tomlinson, I. M., Cox, J. P. L., Gherardi, E., Lesk, A. M., and Chothia, C. (1995) The structural repertoire of the human V_K domain. *EMBO J.* **14,** 4628–4638.
6. Berzofsky, J. A., Berkower, I. J., and Epstein, S. L. (1993) Antigen-antibody interactions and monoclonal antibodies, in *Fundamental Immunology* (Paul, W. E., ed.), Raven, New York, 421–465.
7. George, A. J. T., Rashid, M., and Gallop, J. L. (1997) Kinetics of biomolecular interactions. *Expert Opin. Therapeutic Patents* **7,** 947–963.

8. Morris, R. J. (1995) Antigen–antibody interactions: how affinity and kinetics affect assay design and selection procedures, in *Monoclonal Antibodies. Production, Engineering and Clinical Application* (Ritter M.A. and Ladyman, H. M., eds.), Cambridge University Press, Cambridge, UK, 34–59.
9. Huston, J. S., Margolies, M. N., and Haber, E. (1996) Antibody binding sites. *Adv. Protein Chem.* **49,** 329–450.
10. George, A. J. T., Spooner, R. A., and Epenetos, A. A. (1994) Applications of monoclonal antibodies in clinical oncology. *Immunol. Today* **15,** 559–561.
11. George, A. J. T. and Huston, J. S. (1997) Bispecific antibody engineering, in *The Antibodies* (Zanetti, M. and Capra, J. D., eds.), Harwood Academic Publishers, Luxembourg, 99–141.

2

Polyclonal and Monoclonal Antibodies

Mary A. Ritter

1. Introduction

The breadth of repertoire yet beautiful specificity of the antibody response is the key to its physiological efficacy in vivo; it also underpins the attractiveness of antibodies as laboratory and clinical reagents. One aspect of the body's reaction to invasion by a microorganism is the activation and clonal expansion of antigen-reactive B lymphocytes. Once these have matured into plasma cells, each clone of cells will secrete its own unique specificity of antibody—thus, the invading pathogen will be met by a barrage of antibody molecules capable of binding to many different sites on its surface. Such a polyclonal response, whose range of specificities and affinities can shift with time, is ideal for combatting infection, and indeed for certain laboratory applications (such as secondary reagents for immunoassay); however, in many experimental and clinical situations the ability to have an unlimited supply of a single antibody that is clearly defined and of reproducible specificity and affinity is of greater value. To produce such a reagent it is necessary to isolate and culture a single clone of B lymphocytes secreting antibody of the appropriate characteristics—that is, to produce a monoclonal antibody (mAb).

2. Generation of an Immune Response
2.1. Selection of Animal for Immunization

The generation of an immune response to the antigen of interest is a necessary prerequisite to the production of both polyclonal and monoclonal antibodies; the major difference between the two systems lies mainly in the size of the animal to be immunized. Since polyclonal antibodies are collected from the serum of the immunized individual it is advisable to use as large an animal as

From: *Methods in Molecular Medicine, Vol. 40: Diagnostic and Therapeutic Antibodies*
Edited by: A. J. T. George and C. E. Urch © Humana Press Inc., Totowa, NJ

possible; for commercial reagents rabbit, goat, and sheep are the usual choices, although pig, donkey, horse, and kangaroo antibodies are also available. For a phylogenetically more distant view of a mammalian immunogen, the chicken can be very useful.

Two further factors affect the choice of animal. First, the greater the genetic disparity between donor antigen and recipient to be immunized, the greater the number of distinct epitopes to which the immune response can be directed. Thus, unless the target antigen is a defined alloantigen, the recipient should be as phylogenetically unrelated to the donor as possible. For polyclonal antibodies this is not a problem since the choice of recipient is a wide one. However, for mAbs, for which mouse, rat, and hamster are the best source of immune cells (*see* **Subheading 4.2.**), this can cause a problem for those working with rodent antigens.

Second, it is better to use female recipients since they, in general, mount a more effective immune response than their male counterparts—a characteristic that has as its downside an increased incidence of autoimmune disease. Additionally, the use of outbred or F1 hybrid animals will bring in a wider range of Major Histocompatibility Complex (MHC) molecules and hence potentially will increase the range of epitopes presented to T lymphocytes, thus enhancing the generation of T-cell help (*see* **Subheading 2.2.1.**).

2.2. Selection and Preparation of the Immunogen

2.2.1. Immunogenicity

Immunologists distinguish between the terms antigen and immunogen. Although at first sight this may seem a prime example of unecessary jargon, there is a very sound scientific basis for the distinction. Whereas an immunogen is any substance that can generate an immune response (such as the production of specific antibodies), an antigen is one that can be recognized by an ongoing response (e.g., by antibodies) but may be incapable of generating a response *de novo*. This difference reflects the requirement for T lymphocyte activation in the generation of most antibody responses—the so-called "T-dependent" antigens, in which T-cell–derived signals are needed for full B-cell activation and expansion (only molecules that are directly mitogenic or have a high crosslinking capacity can activate B cells in the absence of this T-cell "help"). For T-cell help to be effective, the epitope seen by the T cell and the epitope seen by the B cell that it is helping must be present on the same antigen (termed "linked recognition"), although these epitopes need not be identical *(1)*. Thus, when the antigen is a whole microorganism or complex macromolecule there is plenty of scope for the provision of both T- and B-cell epitopes and the antigen will be an effective immunogen. In contrast, where the antigen is a small chemical group, such as the "hapten" di- or trinitrophenyl (DNP, TNP) that cannot be presented to T cells, the antigen will be unable to generate an immune response unless coupled to a larger "carrier" protein macromolecule *(2)*. Similarly, a peptide antigen, unless it can by chance bind to one of the recipient's MHC molecules, will not be presented to T cells and so will require conjugation to a larger carrier molecule. In addition, carbohydrate antigens, although they may be large in size, cannot be presented to T cells via classical MHC molecules and so again will require a carrier if a good high-affinity antibody response is to be generated.

The practical implications of this are that if the antigen of interest is nonprotein (e.g., bacterial capsular polysaccharide) or is a small peptide, it should be coupled to a large protein molecule of known immunogenicity, such as bovine serum albumin (BSA) or keyhole limpet hemocyanin (KLH) *(3,4)*.

2.2.2. Choice of Immunogen Preparation

The preparation used for immunization is very much "project specific" and depends mainly on the purpose for which the antibody is being generated. Hence the immunogen could be: whole, killed, bacteria, or virus; a tissue homogenate; live whole cells in suspension (although after injection in vivo these will be neither alive nor whole for very long!); purified protein; or, as discussed in **Subheading 2.2.1.**, a hapten-carrier conjugate. In general, for polyclonal antibody production the immunogen should be as pure as possible so that only relevant B-cell clones are generated; for mAb generation purity at the immunogen stage is less crucial since a stringent screening procedure (*see* **Subheading 4.5.**) later in the technique will ensure that only the specific clones are selected.

2.2.3. Adjuvants

The immunogenicity of an immunogen can be enhanced by the coadministration of an adjuvant. These have two main modes of action: the provision of an in vivo depot from which antigen is slowly released, and the induction of an inflammatory response to enhance the overall immune responsiveness of the host animal in the vicinity of the injected immunogen. The most frequently used adjuvants are Freund's complete (FCA) and incomplete adjuvant (FIA). These comprise mineral oil, emulsifying agent, and, in the case of FCA, killed mycobacteria. Several commercial adjuvants with similar properties are also available.

Adjuvants should never be used with the iv route of immunization. FCA should be used at only the first immunization, with FIA used thereafter. The use of adjuvants is strictly regulated, and guidelines must be adhered to.

2.3. Immunization Schedule

Immunization schedules are based on both logic and empiricism. The former requires a basic knowledge of how an immune response is generated. For the latter, it is sufficient to say—if you have a system that is successful, do not change it!

The main points to consider are the isotype and the affinity of antibody that you require. IgM antibodies are produced predominantly during the early phase of an immune response, and if it is this isotype that you require you should immunize the recipient either once, or at the most twice. Conversely, if IgG antibodies are wanted, a minimum of three or four immunizations is advisable. The likelihood of producing high-affinity antibodies is increased by repeated immunization (affinity maturation occurs in germinal centers during development of memory B cells), and is also theoretically enhanced by increasing the time between immunizations to ≥4 wk, since as immunogen is cleared from the body only those B cells with high affinity receptors will be triggered by the low levels of immunogen remaining *(5)*.

2.4. Route of Immunization

The route by which an immunogen is administered is governed both by the species of recipient and by the immunogen itself. Soluble molecules and single cell suspensions can be injected intravenously, but all other preparations should be injected via a nonvascular route (intraperitoneal, intramuscular, intradermal, subcutaneous). Intraperitoneal immunization is good for small animals, such as mice and rats, but for larger recipients the intramuscular, subcutaneous, and intradermal methods are more appropriate.

For mAb production, for which a source of activated B lymphocytes is required, it is important to consider the route of immunization, since the site of antigen entry will affect the anatomical location of the immune response; in general iv entry will lead to an immune response in the spleen, whereas ip, id, im, and sc entry will focus immunity in the draining lymph node. The degree of such compartmentalization varies according to the species; thus for rats, ip immunization may give little response in the spleen and it is wise to use lymphocytes from the draining lymph nodes in addition to the spleen when performing the fusion. In contrast, in mice ip injection gives a good splenic response, which is fortunate given the small size of murine lymph nodes! A good compromise may be to use a non-intravenous site for all but the last immunization, and then to give a final boost, without adjuvant, intravenously to drive the immune response to the spleen *(6)*. For polyclonal antibodies the site of entry is less important since all will eventually give rise to antibodies in the circulation.

2.5. Assessment of Immunity

Before collecting blood for serum (polyclonal antibodies) or spleen/lymph node cells (mAbs), it is useful to take a small sample of blood from the immunized animal to test for antibody production. Different recipients may vary in both the quantity and speed of their immune response, and the number of immunizations can be adjusted accordingly.

3. Polyclonal Antibodies

Once the recipient is fully immunized and antibodies specific for the immunogen can be detected in the serum (e.g., effective in immunohistochemistry at <1:100), a larger sample of blood can be collected (volume determined by the species of the recipient). A good polyclonal antiserum should contain approx 1 mg/mL specific antibody, although the actual concentration will depend on both the purity and immunogenicity of the immunogen used. Where the immunogen is a purified molecule, it can then be used to affinity-purify the specific antibody from the serum (e.g., secondary, antimouse Ig antibodies for use in immunoassays). If this is not possible, the serum should be used with caution since it will contain many specificities of antibody other than those directed against the chosen target.

4. Monoclonal Antibodies

4.1. Overview

The technique of mAb production was first devised by Köhler and Milstein, as part of an investigation of antibody diversity and affinity maturation *(7,8)*. The technique has found an enormous range of laboratory, clinical, and industrial applications, and provides an excellent example of the crucial value of pure basic research to the more applied areas of science. The importance of their discovery was recognized by the award of the Nobel Prize in Medicine in 1984 *(9)*.

In theory, the production of a mAb is very simple; it requires the growth of a clone of B lymphocytes and collection of the antibody produced by these genetically identical cells. In practice, however, it is much more difficult since B lymphocytes are mortal and cannot live for long ex vivo. The major purpose of the technology that we use is therefore to confer immortality on these important cells. This is achieved by fusion of an antigen-specific B cell with a myeloma cell, such that the resulting hybridoma inherits the ability to secrete specific antibody from its B lymphocyte parent and the property of immortality from the myeloma parent. The fusion itself is both rapid and simple, but a considerable amount of labor-intensive work is subsequently required to isolate individual antigen-specific clones from the multitude of fused and nonfused cells that emerge from this initial step in the technique (for technical details *see* Freysdóttir; Chapter 17).

4.2. Myeloma Cells

Successful B cell hybridomas have been produced using myeloma cells of mouse and rat origin; several of these are available commercially. The two crucial features of these lines are that they have been genetically selected for an inability to produce their own immunoglobulin heavy and light chains, thus ensuring that the only antibody produced after fusion with a B cell is that encoded by the B cell's genome; and failure to survive in HAT (hypozanthine, aminopterin, thymidine) selection medium (**Subheading 4.4.**), thus providing a means by which nonfused myeloma cells can be removed from hybridoma cell cultures.

The choice of myeloma depends to some extent on the ease with which they can be cultured. The nonadherent mouse lines are easier to handle and divide more rapidly than the adherent rat cells lines, and although successful mAbs have been produced using the rat system, the majority have been generated using murine myeloma cells.

A second consideration in the selection of the myeloma line is the species in which the immunized B lymphocytes will be generated. For optimal hybridoma stability the B cells and the myeloma cells should be from the same species since "mouse × mouse" and "rat × rat" hybridomas are genetically more stable, losing fewer chromosomes during the early stages after fusion when compared to species-mismatched hybrids. However, fusions using cells from closely related species, such as "rat × mouse" and "hamster × mouse," are also relatively stable and have been very successfully used to generate a wide range of rat and hamster mAb. It is only with more phylogenetically distant fusions that the problems of chromosome instability pose a serious problem, as for example with "rabbit × mouse" or "sheep × mouse" *(6)*.

4.3. The Fusion

The original fusogen used by Köhler and Milstein was Sendai virus *(7)*; however the technology was soon simplified, with polyethylene glycol replacing the virus. The effect of the fusogen is to cause fusion of adjacent cells; initially only the outer cell membrane fuses, leading to the formation of large "cells" that contain two different nuclei, one derived from the myeloma and the other from the B-cell parent. After the first mitotic division the nuclear contents are also pooled and two daughter hybridoma cells are produced. It is at this and subsequent early cell divisions that chromosome loss is likely to occur.

4.4. Selection of Fused Cells

Once the fusion has been performed, two major problems must be addressed: first, not all cells will have fused with a partner cell (discussed in this section); second, of those cells that did enter into a fusion, many will have fused with an inappropriate cell type, such as a T lymphocyte or a macrophage. Others will have fused with a B lymphocyte of an irrelevant specificity (*see* **Subheadings 4.5.** and **4.6.**).

The first problem to be dealt with is the presence of unfused cells in the cultures. Spleen cells that have not entered into a fusion are in fact very easy to remove, since their mortality ensures that they will die within 1–2 wk in vitro. Unfused myeloma cells pose a much greater threat since they are immortal and if allowed to remain in the cultures will, with time, completely overgrow the slower-growing hybridoma cells.

The problem is overcome by the use of the selective medium HAT (Hypozanthine, Aminopterin, Thymidine). Aminopterin blocks the main biosynthetic pathways for DNA and RNA synthesis. Cells containing a normal genome (unfused spleen cells and "myeloma × spleen cell" hybrids) can switch to alternative "salvage" pathways providing they are also given a source of hypozanthine and thymidine for RNA and DNA synthesis, respectively. Utilization of these molecules for the salvage pathway requires the enzymes hypozanthinephosphoribosyl transferase (HPGRT) and thymidine kinase; these are present in all normal cells, but the myeloma cells have been selected for loss of expression of HPGRT, and thus cannot survive in HAT medium. Thus, after 2–3 wk in selective medium, all unfused myeloma cells will have died resulting from their lack of HPGRT and all unfused spleen cells will have died because of their lack of immortality.

4.5. Tracking the Antigen-Specific B-Cell Hybridomas

After HAT selection, the cultures will contain only hybrids; the next step is to locate those hybrids that are secreting antibody specific for the target antigen.

To track the relevant hybrids, a small sample of supernatant medium is removed from each tissue culture well and is tested for specific antibody activity. The assay selected for this testing will be depend very much on the final use for which the antibody is being prepared, and should be as close to this final use as possible since antibodies will perform with differing efficiencies in different assay systems. Nevertheless, certain characteristics are required of all assay systems: sensitivity (~1 μg/mL), reliability, speed, and ability to deal with multiple samples (you may have to test >100 samples/d). Suitable techniques include immunohistochemistry, flow cytometry, Western blotting, and enzyme-linked immunosorbent assay (ELISA). This is one of the most crucial steps in mAb production since an mAb is only as specific as the tests that you have put it through.

4.6. Ensuring Monoclonality

The next problem that must be solved is that of clonality. At the start of culture a large number of different cells is placed in each well, and even after HAT selection and antibody screening more than a single clone of cells will exist in each well. Although after screening you know which wells contain cells that are secreting antibody with specificity for the immunogen, other hybrids in the same well may be secreting antibody to an irrelevant antigen (e.g., pathogens previously encountered by the immunized animal), or that may produce no antibody at all (e.g., "T cell × myeloma").

The most popular method for establishing monoclonality of specific antibody-secreting cells is that of limiting dilution. Hybridomas from wells that contain specific antibody activity are transferred to 96-well tissue culture plates at very high dilution such that the average plating density is one cell per three wells, although the actual cell plating follows a Poisson distribution. Feeder cells are also added (e.g., peritoneal macrophages) to provide cell contact and cytokines. Once the plated hybridomas have grown, their supernatant medium is again tested for antibody activity, and the cells from positive wells are again cloned by limiting dilution. The antibody screening and recloning is then repeated once more to ensure monoclonality. In addition, if NSO murine myeloma cells were used for the initial fusion, the distinct compact colonies formed can readily be recognized, providing visual confirmation of the presence of a single clone. Alternatively, hybridomas can be cloned by flow cytometry or in semisolid agar.

4.7. Bulk Production

At this stage of the technique it is likely that the precious, specific antibody-secreting hybridomas comprise a maximum of one million cells in a volume of 200 µL of antibody. The next task is therefore to grow the cells up in bulk so that a large amount of antibody can be produced and cell samples can be frozen and stored for future use (*see* **Subheading 4.8.**). Hybridoma cells dislike sudden alterations in their lifestyle, so expansion of cell numbers should be carried out by gradually increasing the size of the container in which they are grown. Thus, they are transferred from small (200 µL) wells to larger (2 mL) wells and from there to small, medium, and then large flasks. After this, the hybridomas can be grown in a variety of in vitro culture systems designed for bulk production of mAb, ranging from large, but simple, culture flasks and bottles to the purpose-designed complex hollow fiber and other specialized equipment. Culture under standard conditions provides an antibody yield of 2–50 μg/mL, but much higher concentrations can be obtained with the specialized systems.

An alternative method that is now rarely used is the production of ascite mAb. Hybridoma cells can be grown as an ascitic tumor in genetically compatible, or immunoincompetent, hosts, and the antibody-containing ascitic fluid collected. The advantage of the method is that high concentrations of antibody can be produced (approx 10 mg/mL); the major disadvantage is that it requires the use of experimental animals. Given the efficiency with which mAb can be produced by in vitro methods, use of the ascites method cannot now be justified.

4.8. Paranoia

The production of a mAb is highly labor-intensive and will, on average, take approx 6 mo from initial immunization to the point at which you have sufficient mAb for use. Moreover, at many points along this route disasters can occur and annihilate all your hard work. For this reason it is entirely acceptable to indulge in a little paranoia!

A major threat is contamination of the cell cultures with bacteria, yeast, or fungi. All are serious, but by far the most devastating is mycoplasma since it is not visible by eye and its presence is frequently only appreciated when the infected cells exhibit poor growth and low yields of antibody. All cell lines should therefore be tested regularly for mycoplasma contamination, using one of the many kits that are available commercially. The most frequent source of mycoplasma contamination is via the introduction of a new cell line into your laboratory. The only effective policy is to test all new lines prior to admitting them into your main tissue-culture facility (keep them in "quarantine"). This may cause friction with the donor, who will state categorically that his or her cells are clean, but it is wise to be absolutely firm on this! Wherever possible, contaminated cultures should be rapidly disposed of. If the infected culture is very valuable, it can be treated with antibiotics or an antifungal agent, as appropriate, although the latter frequently causes death of the hybridoma cells as well.

As soon as you have sufficient cells, aliquots should be frozen and stored in liquid nitrogen. Batches should be frozen on different days, to provide insurance against contamination, and should be stored in more than one liquid nitrogen tank. This will protect you against the accidental drying out of the liquid nitrogen tank and the loss of your irreplaceable cells.

Finally, do treat your antibodies with respect. Individual antibodies have very different properties; some are stable for months and even years at +4°C, whereas others can survive at this temperature for only a few days. The majority are stable for long periods of time if stored at –20 or –80°C, preferably the latter. The preparation of the antibody also affects its storage properties. Tissue-culture supernatants store well, since the serum proteins present in the medium improve the stability of the low concentration of mAb (~10 µg/mL). Purified antibodies should be stored in neutral isotonic buffer (phosphate-buffered saline, Tris-buffered saline) at a concentration >500 µg/mL. Lower concentrations should be stored with a carrier protein (e.g., 0.1% BSA). Antibody activity is progressively destroyed by repeated freezing and thawing, so mAb should be stored in appropriately sized aliquots.

5. Polyclonal vs Monoclonal Antibodies: The Choice

Which is better, a monoclonal or a polyclonal antibody? The answer to this question depends on the use to which the reagent is to be put.

Polyclonal antibodies have been particularly useful in two situations: first, where it is beneficial for a reagent to recognize more than one epitope on a target molecule, and second, where the molecule of interest is highly conserved.

One of the most frequent and important applications of polyclonal antibodies for the detection of multiple epitopes is as secondary, conjugated, reagents for indirect immunoassays (e.g., ELISA, Western blotting, immunohistochemistry, flow cytometry; *see* Chapters 30, 32–35), where polyclonal binding to the primary layer antibody leads to considerable amplification of the signal.

Highly conserved molecules are in general poorly immunogenic, since they will closely resemble the recipient's own equivalent molecule, to which it will be tolerant. It has therefore proved useful to move away from mouse, rat, and hamster to genetically more distant mammals, such as rabbit and sheep, or even to birds, such as the chicken *(10,11)*; however, in these species polyclonal antibodies are the only feasible conventional option.

Despite these advantages, polyclonal antibodies have several disadvantages. A major problem is that of quantity, since a single animal is unlikely to produce sufficient reagent. This leads to a second, related problem: no two animals will produce an identical response to the same immunogen. Indeed, the same animal will respond differently to each dose of immunogen, as its immune response evolves. Polyclonal antibodies are therefore limited in the amount that can be produced and, once exhausted, can never be exactly reproduced since subsequent batches will contain a different range of specificities and affinities.

Monoclonal antibodies, in contrast, provide an unlimited source of antibody that is homogeneous and, once characterized, predictable in its behavior. mAbs have been invaluable in providing excellent primary reagents to molecules previously defined by less reliable polyclonal antibodies. However, their major impact has been in their use to discover and characterize the structure and function of novel molecules. For example, almost every molecule that we now know to be important in an immune response, with the exception of CD4 and CD8, owes its identification to the generation of specific mAb *(12)*. Once fully characterized, mAbs provide highly reproducible reagents for clinical diagnostic assays and, with modification to reduce their immunogenicity, they have potential for clinical therapy (*see* Chapters 3, 5–12, and 14).

The disadvantage of mAbs is that they cannot provide signal amplification (unless an artificial "polyclonal" antibody is made by mixing several mAbs); and since only rodent B cells have been really successful, there are epitopes to which these reagents cannot be generated. An important recent approach to this latter problem has been the use of phage display for selection of recombinant monoclonal antibodies, a technique that avoids the in vivo deletion of self-reactive specificities *(13,14)*; (Chapters 4 and 37).

Thus, each type of reagent has distinct advantages and disadvantages, and there is a clear need for both in the generation of antibodies for use in laboratory and clinic.

References

1. Parker, D. C. (1993) T cell-dependent B cell activation. *Ann. Rev. Immunol.* **11,** 331–340.
2. Michison, N. A. (1971) The carrier effect in the secondary response to hapten-protein conjugates. 3. The anatomical distribution of helper cells and antibody-forming cell precursors. *Eur. J. Immunol.* **1,** 63–65.
3. Dadi, H. K., Morris, R. J., Hulme, E. C., and Birdsell, N. J. M. (1984) Antibodies to a covalent agonist used to isolate the muscarinic cholinergic receptor from rat brain, in *Investigation of Membrane Located Receptors* (Reid, E., Cook, G. M. W. and Morre, D. J., eds.), Plenum, New York, pp. 425–428.
4. von Gaudecker, B., Kendall, M. D., and Ritter, M. A. (1997) Immuno-electron microscopy of the thymic epithelial microenvironment. *Microscopy Res. Technique* **38,** 237–249.
5. Klinman, N. (ed.) (1997) B-cell memory. *Sem. Immunol.* **9.**
6. Ritter, M. A. and Ladyman, H. M. (eds.) (1995) *Monoclonal Antibodies: Production, Engineering and Clinical Application.* Cambridge University Press, Cambridge, UK.
7. Köhler, G. and Milstein, C. (1975) Continuous cultures of fused cells producing antibodies of predefined specificity. *Nature* **256,** 495–497.
8. Galfre, G. and Milstein, C. (1981) Preparation of monoclonal antibodies: strategies and procedures. *Methods Enzymol.* **73B,** 3–46.
9. Milstein, C. (1985) From the structure of antibodies to the diversification of the immune response. *EMBO J.* **4,** 1083–1092.
10. Morris, R. J. and Wiiliams, A. F. (1975) Antigens of mouse and rat lymphocytes recognised by rabbit antiserum against rat brain: the quantitative analysis of a xenogeneic antiserum. *Eur. J. Immunol.* **5,** 274–281.

11. Wynick, D., Hammond, P. J., Akinanya, K. O., and Bloom, S. R. (1993) Galanin regulates basal and oestrogen-stimulated lactotroph function. *Nature* **364,** 529–532.
12. Barclay, A. N., Beyers, A. D., Birkeland, M. L., Brown, M. H., Davis, S. J., Somozo, C., and Williams, A. F. (1992) *The Leucocyte Antigen Facts Book.* Academic Press, London, UK.
13. Palmer, D. B., George, A. J. T., and Ritter, M. A. (1997) Selection of antibodies to cell surface determinants on mouse thymic epithelial cells using a phage display library. *Immunology* **91,** 473–478.
14. Ritter, M. A. and Palmer, D. B. (1998) The human thymic microenvironment. *Semin. Immunol.* **11,** 13–21.

3

Engineering Antibody Molecules

Rakesh Verma and Ekaterini Boleti

1. Cloning of V Region Genes

Advances in PCR techniques and the increase of the antibody V region sequences in the database have boosted developments in the field of antibody engineering. The V region genes can be amplified from hybridomas *(1)*, preimmunized donors *(2)*, naive donors *(3)*, or from the cells expressing antibodies.

A number of strategies have been used to amplify the V region sequences and a large number of primers have been described that amplify the V region of human and other species based on the database of V region sequences. The following types of primers are commonly used.

1. Primers specific for leader sequences and constant region of the gene.
2. Degenerate primers designed to complement the 5' and 3' ends of the conserved sequences of V region.
3. Panels of oligonucleotides specific for families of the V region genes.

2. Antibody Molecules

There are two main classes of recombinant antibodies. The first is based on the intact immunoglobulin molecule (**Fig. 1**) and is designed to reduce the immunogenicity of the murine molecule. Thus, both chimeric molecules, which consist of the murine V regions and human constant regions, have been developed *(4–7)* as well as humanized antibodies in which just the CDRs are of rodent origin *(8,9)*.

The second class of molecules consists of fragments of antibody molecules. These include fragments that are accessible through proteolysis, such as Fab, Fab', and F(ab')$_2$, as well as other fragments, such as Fv-based molecules (**Fig. 2**). These molecules include sFv (single-chain Fv) *(10,11)*, and the dsFv (disulfide-stabilized Fv) (**Fig. 3**) *(12)*.

From: *Methods in Molecular Medicine, Vol. 40: Diagnostic and Therapeutic Antibodies*
Edited by: A. J. T. George and C. E. Urch © Humana Press Inc., Totowa, NJ

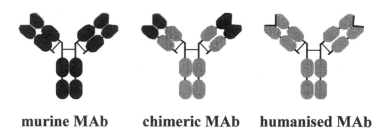

murine MAb   chimeric MAb   humanised MAb

Fig. 1. Reduction of immunogenicity. This illustrates the most commonly used strategies to make mAb that are less immunogenic in patients. Regions with murine sequences are shown in black, those with human in gray. On the left is the parental murine mAb. In chimeric mAb the variable domains are of murine origin, the rest is human. In humanized antibodies the entire sequence is human with the exception of the residues that constitute the antigen binding site (derived from the CDRs of the mAb).

2.1. Chimeric and Humanized Antibodies

The ability to clone V region genes has allowed generation of novel constructs based on the IgG molecule. The first class of such molecules was designed to reduce the immunogenicity of rodent antibodies in humans, thus preventing the induction of human antimouse antibody (HAMA), as described in Chapter 1. Other constructs have been designed to reduce the size of the molecule, remove the Fc portion, and add novel effector functions.

The first generation of antibody molecules designed to reduce the immunogenicity were chimeric molecules. These consist of the variable region domains (V_H and V_L) from the parental rodent mAb, but the constant region domains derived from the human sequence *(4,5)*. These molecules can be easily made by cloning the variable region genes from the antibody into constructs containing the exons encoding the constant domains of the human immunoglobulin. The resulting molecule is predominantly human in sequence, and has been shown in a number of trials to have reduced immunogenicity when compared to the parental murine antibody. In addition the procedure allows selection of the human constant region used, so that the antibody has an appropriate isotype for the functions required of it.

Chimeric antibodies still have V_H and V_L domains of rodent origin, which are potentially immunogenic. The use of human V_H and V_L domains, in which the CDR sequences are replaced with those of the rodent antibody, offers the potential to remove even this residual antigenic sequence *(8,13)*. The resulting antibodies are termed humanized. In the first report of this approach the CDRs of the V_H domain of an anti-NP antibody were grafted onto the V_H of the human antibody NEWM, in combination with a human IgE constant region

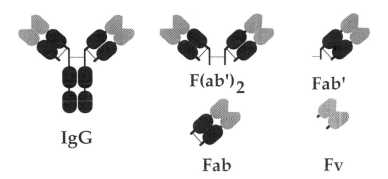

Fig. 2. Structure of the antibody molecule and its fragments. This figure shows the common antigen binding fragments of an IgG molecule. The IgG molecule is shown with the constant domains in dark shading and the variable domains of both the chains in lighter shading. The F(ab')₂ fragment can be made by pepsin digestion; following mild reduction this yields the Fab' molecule. Fab fragments can be made by papain digestion. In some molecules it is possible to generate Fv fragment by enzymatic approaches. Expression of the relevant gene segments also permits expression of recombinant versions of these molecules.

(8). Often the initial constructs have a reduced affinity for their antigen, and it can be necessary to alter some of the framework determinants to increase the affinity to that of the parental antibody *(14–16)*. This can be achieved either by modeling and design of the mutants, or by use of a phage display approach in which affinity techniques are used to select antibodies, sometimes with a higher affinity than the parental molecule *(17)*.

Although chimeric and humanized antibodies are considerably less immunogenic than the rodent molecule, the CDRs can themselves be immunogenic, eliciting an anti-idiotypic response. In addition, allotypic determinants on the constant domains can be immunogenic, although mutation of the appropriate residues has been shown to abolish this *(18)*.

In addition to humanization and chimerization, resurfacing or veneering of antibodies has been proposed as a mechanism to reduce immunogenicity *(19)*. This involves identifying amino-acid residues on the surface of the V_H and V_L domains that differ between mouse and human, and mutating just these to the human sequence. The result are domains that are human on the outside, but murine inside. This approach has been demonstrated with a number of antibodies *(20,21)*. However, although this approach should abolish the induction of antibodies capable of recognizing the surface of the veneered domains (with the exception of the idiotypic determinants), the remaining murine sequences may provide T cell epitopes that will help the induction of the anti-idiotypic immune responses.

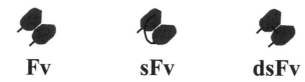

Fig. 3. Recombinant molecules based on the Fv fragment. The Fv fragment is the smallest antibody fragment that retains an intact antigen binding site. However it is unstable, as the V_H and V_L domains are free to dissociate. Two strategies have been adopted to overcome this. The first is to link the domains with a peptide to generate a single-chain Fv (sFV). The second is to introduce cysteine residues at the interface between the V_H and V_L domains, forming a disulphide bridge that holds them together (a disulfide-stabilized Fv [dsFv]). the location of the bond shown in the figure is for illustrative purposes only.

The next class of constructs is to reduce size and other factors. This was initially done by proteolysis.

2.2. Proteolytic Forms of Immunoglobulin

Classical limited proteolysis studies of rabbit IgG by Rodney Porter and coworkers gave insight into the structural features of antibodies *(22)*. Extended, flexible regions of polypeptide chains are more susceptible to peptide bond cleavage by limited enzymatic proteolysis than rod-like or globular domains of folded proteins. In the case of the IgG molecule the most susceptible part is the hinge region, located between C_{H1} and C_{H2} domains of heavy chain. Papain preferentially cleaves rabbit IgG into three fragments, two of which are identical and consist of intact light chain and the V_H-C_{H1} fragment of heavy chain (**Fig. 2**). These fragments retain antigen-binding ability, and are therefore called fragment, antigen binding (Fab). The third fragment is composed of the C_{H2} and C_{H3} domains and has a tendency to crystallize into a lattice, and is therefore called fragment, crystalline (Fc).

Inbar and colleagues, during the purification of MoPC-315 Fab by chromatography, observed that there is an active antibody fragment that is smaller than Fab *(23)*. When Fab was digested with pepsin at pH 3.6 and purified through a DNP-lysyl-sepharose column, the adsorbed material was almost half the size of Fab and retained antigen-binding activity. This fragment was named fragment variable (Fv) (**Fig. 2**) *(23,24)*.

The Fv fragment of anti-DNP myeloma antibody XRPC-25, which was prepared by trypsin digestion, was shown to have the same antigen-binding affinity as its parent mAb *(25)*. This led to the observation that Fv, which is approx 25 kDa in size, is almost as good as the intact antibody molecule in recognizing antigenic epitopes.

2.3. Structure of Fv Region

In the process of dissecting the "Y" shape structure of the immunoglobulin molecule by proteolysis or genetic manipulation the upper half of "Y" became the center of intense scientific investigation. The segments that form the contact with antigenic epitopes are in the variable domains of both the light and heavy chains. Kabat and colleagues have shown that variability is largely restricted to six of the segments in the two variable domains, called hypervariable regions or complementarity-determining residues (CDRs) *(26)*. The other parts of the variable region are called framework regions (FRs). The FRs show an average variability of about 5%, but they are important in bringing CDRs into a correct position and stabilizing the three-dimensional structure of the V region.

The variable domains are folded into two roughly parallel β-pleated sheets; one containing three strands and other containing four strands. Strands of the same sheet are connected by β-hairpin strands, whereas strands of adjacent sheets are connected by β-arches. The side-chains of amino acids are directed either upward or downward to the plane of the sheet. The hydrophobic side-chains lie between the two sheets, whereas the hydrophilic side-chains point outward. The two sheets are held together by a single disulfide bond.

2.4. Single-Chain Antibodies

Many ways of preparing Fv by enzymatic proteolysis have been tried with variable success, but no general simple method to prepare the Fv fragment from IgG molecule gives consistent results. Genetic engineering principles were first used to make Fv in 1988. The variable domains of light and heavy chains of McPC603 (anti-phosphorylcholine antibody) were cloned into a plasmid pASK22 and expressed in *Escherichia coli* to secrete functional assembled Fv in the bacterial periplasm *(27)*. The thermodynamic and kinetic stability of the hetero-association of the two variable domains was not known. The stability of Fv fragments at low concentration is a limiting factor; because of their tendency to dissociate at higher dilutions, they may not be suitable for experimentation and biomedical applications. In order to stabilize the Fv fragments, and to isolate the minimum binding pocket in its native form, different strategies have been adopted. Glockshuber and colleagues in 1990 *(12)* made a comparative study of three alternative approaches to stabilize V_H and V_L of McPC 603 by crosslinking with glutaraldehyde in the presence of phosphorylcholine, intermolecular disulfide linking *(28)*, and by a peptide-linker sequence. All these approaches produced Fv products that were more stable than the natural Fv fragment in recombinant form (**Fig. 3**).

The single-chain Fv (sFv) is a recombinant polypeptide, expressed from genetically engineered genes, in which the variable amino acid sequences of both the light and heavy chains of a conventional antibody are linked together by a peptide linker *(10,11)*. The carboxy terminus of one variable sequence is linked to the amino terminus of the other variable sequence. The order of variable regions can be either way around, but the V region order may effect the affinity and the level of secretion of the single-chain antibody. Anand and colleagues observed that in the case of the Se155-4 sFv, specific for a trisaccharide epitope of *Salmonella* serotype B *O*-polysaccharide, the V_H-linker-V_L order produces a molecule that has a 10-fold higher affinity for its antigen than the V_L-linker-V_H order, whereas the V_L-linker-V_H molecule yields about 20 times more sFv than V_H-linker-V_L *(29)*. This kind of change in orientation may be caused by steric effects or the changes in the charged molecules on the linker, leading to the perturbation of the binding pockets *(30)*.

Many different names have been assigned to these constructs, i.e., biosynthetic antigen binding sites (BABS), single-chain antigen-binding proteins (SCAB), single-chain antibodies (SCA), or single-chain Fv (scFv or sFv).

2.5. Advantages of sFv

Most of the antibody effector functions, like complement fixation and uptake by the reticulo-endothelial system, are mediated via the Fc region. Heavy-chain constant regions are responsible for effector functions of the antibody *(31)*. Monoclonal antibodies have been used for tumor imaging but the binding of the antibody to nontumor tissues via the Fc region gives high background *(32)*. Because sFv lacks the Fc region, they have no uptake via Fc receptor (FcR); thus, the sFv molecules may be more suitable for targeting and imaging.

The production of recombinant antibodies reduces the risk of contamination with murine-adventitious viruses and murine-oncogenic DNA, which may be carried over when conventional mAbs are produced. The increased ease of purification reduces the cost of producing clinical grade recombinant antibodies.

Single-chain Fv can be genetically manipulated, allowing the effector functions to be altered more easily than is the case with mAb or proteolytic forms of mAb. A number of effector functions can be engineered with sFv gene. Fusion proteins have been made using sFv and enzymes for antibody-directed enzyme prodrug therapy (ADEPT) *(33)*.

2.5.1. Rapid Biodistribution

Pharmacokinetic studies have shown that the sFvs have a much more rapid plasma clearance and whole-body clearance than native antibodies. Comparative pharmacokinetic studies have demonstrated that both the α and β phases of plasma clearance of sFv are faster than those of Fab fragments *(34)*. The pharmacokinetic studies in mice with different forms of CC49 mAb (CC49 is an mAb against B72.3, which reacts with pancarcinoma antigen TAG-72) revealed that the $t_{1/2}\alpha$ of ^{131}I-labeled sFv, Fab, F(ab')$_2$ and intact IgG forms of CC49, was 3.7, 9.1, 26, and 39 min respectively. The $t_{1/2}\beta$ of the same sFv, Fab, F(ab')$_2$, and IgG was 1.5, 1.46, 12, and 113 h, respectively. Because intact antibodies remain in circulation with a half-life of several days, radionuclides or toxic drugs conjugated to the mAb, which are not bound to target tissue, will also remain in circulation for several days, resulting in potential bone marrow toxicity *(35)*. The sFv may reduce the risk of being toxic when bound to toxic drugs or radionuclides because of their faster clearance. Almost 80% of CC49 sFv disappeared from the plasma pool within 15 min in mice and 95% of the sFv was removed from the plasma by 0.5 h in rhesus monkey *(36)*. In the case of rhesus monkeys the $t_{1/2}\alpha$ and $t_{1/2}\beta$ of the CC49 sFv was 3.9 min and 4 h, respectively. Whole-body clearance of sFv is faster than intact antibody. Almost 50% of the sFv was cleared from the body in <5 h and by 24 h most of the sFv was cleared *(36)*. In a clinical trial of an anti carcinoembryonic antigen (CEA) sFv, the median α and β half-lives of the sFv in patients were 0.42 and 5.32 h, respectively, as compared to 28.9 h $t_{1/2}\beta$ of an anti-CEA murine IgG *(37)*.

Because of their smaller size (approx 26–27 kDa), the sFv molecules have a rapid biodistribution, more even distribution in the target tissues, and better tissue penetration as compared to intact antibody or other fragments of antibody molecules. A number of tumor-targeting studies have compared IgG, Fab, F(ab')$_2$, and sFv and shown that the sFv takes approx 30 min to penetrate a tumor mass, whereas an intact antibody takes 2–4 d *(38)*. The immunoglobulin molecules are usually found in higher concentration in the region adjacent to capillaries, whereas distribution of sFv is more even throughout the tumor mass *(39)*.

Antibody–antigen complexes formed during mAb immunotherapy are retained in kidneys and can initiate glomerulitis. Kidney uptake of sFv is less than that of Fab fragments. This may be because of the small size of sFv as compared to the 50 kDa Fab. Molecules of <7 kDa move through the glomerular filter without any hindrance, whereas molecules of more than 60 kDa molecular weight are not filtered *(39)*. The kidney is the main organ of excretion of the sFv in patients. Renal retention of the sFv may be a problem in imaging the tumors that are adjacent to the kidney. When a ^{123}I-labeled anti-CEA sFv was injected in the patients, approx 30% of the injected radiolabeled sFv was excreted in the urine within the first 24 h postinjection *(37)*.

HAMA response is a problem with mAb administration in patients when used for immunodiagnostic and immunotherapeutic purposes, and is seen in almost 50% of patients treated with mAb *(40)*. Repeated exposure to the murine antibody can lead to hypersensitivity reactions resulting from immune complex formation between the HAMA and injected mAb, with such reactions precluding any further therapy with mAb. Murine mAbs against tumor-associated antigens have been used in a number of cancer therapy trials *(41,42)*. Most, though not all, of these early responses are against antigenic determinants in the Fc region of the antibody, not in the F(ab')$_2$ portion of the mouse immunoglobulin *(43)*. The sFv molecules may help in reducing the HAMA response because of reduced size and lack of Fc region. In a small clinical study of an anti-CEA sFv, no evidence of anti-sFv antibodies were seen in the serum of the patients *(37)*.

2.5.2. Imaging

In the case of imaging, nontarget tissue should have a clear demarcation from the targeted tissue by way of difference in contrast. Therefore, the imaging agent that has the least or negligible nonspecific uptake, and sufficient specific binding, is most suitable. Single-chain Fv as compared to intact antibody has negligible or low nonspecific binding, but retains the specific affinity of its parent antibody. Rapid biodistribution and faster clearance of sFv make this molecule a useful imaging agent. Imaging studies of a canine model of active myocardial infarction with technetium-99m-labeled antimyosin sFv have shown that infarct to blood and infarct to normal tissue uptake of sFv facilitate a more rapid infarct visualization than conventional antibodies *(44)*.

A number of sFvs have successfully been used in imaging tumors in mouse models bearing human tumors *(45–49)*. Successful imaging of the tumors is possible only when the tumor-to-blood ratios of the molecules' uptake are high. A number of sFv molecules have been used in mouse models of human tumors to study the uptake of radiolabeled sFvs by the tumors and other organs. One such study has shown that the tumor-to-blood ratios were 13:1 and 24:1 at 24 and 48 h postinjection, respectively, when a ^{125}I-labeled anti-CEA sFv was used in a LS174T human colorectal tumor xenograft model, whereas the ratios for a recombinant chimeric anti-CEA Fab were 6:1 and 11:1 at similar time points in the same model system *(50)*. In a clinical study of eight colorectal carcinoma patients and one breast carcinoma patient, an ^{123}I-labeled anti-CEA sFv gave tumor-to-blood ratios of 5.6:1 after 22 h as compared to a typical anti-CEA antibody ratio of 1.5:1 after 24 h *(33,37)*.

2.6. Fusion Proteins

As discussed in Chapter 1, one of the problems faced with antibody therapy is inadequate cytotoxicity. This is clearly the case with recombinant constructs that lack the Fc region of the molecule. The solution can be to conjugate the antibody to an effector molecule. However, chemical conjugation can damage either the antibody or the effector molecule. In the case of recombinant molecules it is possible to make genetic fusions of the two molecules, resulting in fusion proteins with two properties: the antigen-binding features of the antibody and the effector functions of the partner molecule. The resulting molecule is homogeneous and well defined, in contrast to many chemical conjugates.

2.6.1. Immunotoxins

Recombinant immunotoxins can be used to kill the target/tumor cell by using a specific sFv and a desired toxin *(51)*, when the gene of desired toxin is linked to the gene of sFv to make a fusion protein. In some studies, single-chain Fv immunotoxins have shown enhanced cytotoxicity as compared to chemically linked immunotoxins *(51,52)*. A tripartite immunotoxin (NH_2-DTM1-E6sFv-PE40-COOH) composed of a mutated form of Diphtheria toxin and Pseudomonas exotoxin and a single-chain antibody against human transferrin receptor has comparable cytotoxic effects to that of a conventional immunotoxin *(53)*. A number of sFv immunotoxins have been used in cytotoxic studies. For example, an anti-CD7 sFv-ricin toxin A chain immunotoxin showed inhibition of protein synthesis in vitro in CD7-positive Jurkat cells *(54)*. Similarly, an anti-CD40 sFv-bryodin 1 immunotoxin showed cytotoxic effects against CD40 expressing B-cell lineage non-Hodgkin's lymphoma cell lines *(55)*.

2.6.2. Other sFv-Based Immunoconjugates

In a similar manner to the immunotoxins, other fusion proteins can be produced with such molecules as protein A. The domain of protein A has been linked to the anti-CD3/TcR sFv *(56)* and this could be used to redirect a cytotoxic cell to lyse the target cell via mAb bound to the target cell. Fusion protein between anti-CD3/TcR sFv and the CD4 molecule has been produced to target cytotoxic lymphocytes to HIV infected cells *(57)*.

Better tissue penetration makes sFvs ideal therapeutic agents, in addition to imaging agents. Thus, radionuclides can be delivered in deeper parts of large tumor masses. Fusion proteins of sFv and enzymes may have advantages over other immunoconjugates in targeted tumor therapy *(33)*. They can also be used to target cytokines. In an animal tumor model study, Hakim and colleagues have shown that anti-idiotypic sFv-GM-CSF fusion protein had a protective effect in 38C13 mouse B-cell lymphoma models but the DNA of the construct did not show any effect, whereas both the sFv-IL-1 β peptide fusion protein and DNA of the construct protected mice from the tumor challenge *(58)*.

2.6.3. Bispecific Constructs

Bispecific constructs can be genetically engineered, when a second arm of a different desired specificity is attached to the sFv. Two different sFv molecules can be linked together to make bispecific sFv. Optimal engineering techniques for the production of bispecific sFvs remain to be determined. These recombinant bispecific sFv molecules should be amenable for modifications at the genetic level.

Another class of recombinant antibody molecules similar to the bispecific constructs is called diabodies. Diabodies are antibody fragments with two antigen-binding sites consisting of two associated chains; each chain consists of a heavy- and a light-chain variable domain linked by a peptide spacer *(59,60)*. A bispecific diabody (anti-idiotypic marker on B-cell lymphoma and antimouse CD3) has been shown to mediate specific killing of lymphoma cells by cytotoxic T cells *(61)*. Diabodies have also been used to recruit effector functions *(62,63)*. The diabodies with one specificity to a target antigen and other to a enzyme have also been designed for enzyme immunoassays *(64)*. Other species of sFv-based molecules, such as triabodies and trivalent trimers, have also been described *(65,66)*.

2.6.4. Redirecting Cellular Cytotoxicity

Antigen-specific sFv in conjunction with a universal bispecific construct has been used to redirect cytotoxic cells to kill target cells. Two different sFv fusion proteins U7.6-*myc* (anti-DNP) and OKT9-H6-*myc* (antihuman transferrin receptor) are recognized by an anti-*myc* peptide antibody. The heteroconjugate formed by crosslinking anti-CD3 and anti-*myc* antibodies was utilized to direct human T cells to kill cells from different tumor cell lines coated with sFv-*myc* fusion proteins *(67)*.

2.6.5. Display of sFv Molecules

Single-chain Fv molecules can be genetically conjugated to filamentous phage and cell-surface receptors. When sFv molecules are expressed on the surface of bacteriophages by linking the gene III coat protein of filamentous phage to sFv they are encoded as one unit and expressed as phage antibodies *(68)*. Single-chain Fv molecules have been expressed on the surface of *E. coli* by constructing a fusion gene of sFv and peptidoglycan-associated lipoprotein *(69)*.

2.7. Construction Considerations

In designing the peptide linker for bridging the V_H and V_L domains of the sFv, charge residues of the amino acids, flexibility, solubility, and length of side-chains have to be taken into consideration. The length of the linker must be sufficient to bridge the gap between the carboxy terminus of one variable domain and the amino terminus of the other variable domain, without perturbing the interdomain contacts and structural integrity of domains. The N-terminus and C-terminus distance in the V_H-V_L orientation is about 35 Å in sFv constructs, such as McPC 603, D1.3, and Hy HEL-5; the distance between two termini in V_L-V_H form is 5–11 Å longer *(70)*. Straining of very small linkers may perturb the interaction between V_H and V_L, thus leading to distortion of the binding site. The average amino-acid unit length is about 3.8 Å, so 10 amino acids should be sufficient to span the distance between two termini of variable domains in V_H-V_L orientation. Excessively long linkers may interfere in antigen binding by associating with the binding pocket. Generally 15 amino-acid linkers have been found to be useful in the construction of sFvs.

To avoid misfolding of the sFv, hydrophobic residues are not usually included in linkers *(11)* because they are insoluble and also tend to fold in unusual forms in the presence of water molecules. The $(Gly_4 Ser)_3$ linker, first described by Huston and colleagues, has been found to be a generally suitable linker. The glycines provide flexibility, whereas serine gives solubility to the linker *(11)*.

Other linkers that have been used by a number of investigators include switch region (sequence from carboxy terminus of variable gene and amino terminus of constant region) plus the GGGGS (single-letter amino acid code) linker *(71)*, the 202′ linker of Bird and coworkers *(10)* (EGKSS) (GSGSE) (SKSTQ), and the 212 linker of Bedzyk and colleagues (GSTSG) (SGKSS) (EGKG) *(72)*. Linker residues have also been derived from some naturally existing flexible proteins. Takkinen and colleagues have made an active sFv using a linker derived from 28 residues of cellulase *(73)*. Single-chain molecules have been engineered for other members of the Ig gene superfamily and the same linker design considerations were found to be applicable to them. Novotny and colleagues used the 23 residues of Pro$(Gly_4$-$Ser)_4$-Gly-Ala linker to construct single-chain T-cell receptor (TcR) *(74)*. Turner and colleagues have successfully mutated 6 out of 15 residues of $(Gly_4 Ser)_3$ linker using a phage display system, which resulted in an improved secretion of their sFv *(75)*.

3. Manipulation of the Fc Region

Interface residues of the C_H3 domain of the antibody molecule have been modified using structural-guided phage display technology to promote the formation of stable heterodimers.

A mutant called "knob" was engineered by replacing threonine at position 366 with tryptophan in the C_H3 domain, and a library of the C_H3 "hole" mutants were generated by randomizing residues at positions 366, 368, and 407 (which are in the vicinity of the "knob" mutation in the other partner). The

C_H3 "knob" mutant constructs were fused to a "flag" peptide and C_H3 "hole" library was fused to the gIII of the M13 phage. Phage-displayed stable heterodimers were recovered by panning against an antiflag peptide antibody *(76)*.

A similar technology has been used to stabilize bispecific diabody to produce functional heterodimer *(77)*. Domain interface remodeling can be used to enhance the assembling of the desired domains to yield functional proteins as described above for the C_{H3} domain.

4. Conclusion

Recent advances in the understanding and analysis of antibody structure, increases in the sequence database, and the ability to easily measure the affinity of the molecules have led to the increased enthusiasm to exploit the potential of the antibody-based molecules. At the same time there has been a continual progress in the protein expression systems and molecular biological techniques *(78)*. These developments have given birth to new generation of molecules to target a variety of antigens in various disease conditions.

Future developments in the field of antibody engineering will equip the scientists and clinicians to fully harness the potential of the antibody molecules for immunodiagnostic and immunotherapeutic purposes.

References

1. Glaser, S., Kristensson, K., Chilton, T., Huse, W. (1995) Engineering the antibody combining site by codon-based mutagenesis in a filamentous phage display system, in *Antibody Engineering*, 2nd ed. (Borrebaeck, C. A. K., ed.), Oxford Unversity Press, Oxford, UK, pp. 117–121.
2. Barbas, C. F., III and Burton, D. R. (1996) Selection and evolution of high affinity human anti-viral antibodies. *Trends Biotechnol.* **14,** 230–234.
3. Duenas, M. and Borrebaeck, C. A. K. (1994) Clonal selection and amplification of phage displayed antibodies by linking antigen recognition and phage replication. *Biotechnology* **12,** 999–1002.
4. Boulianne, G. L., Hozumi, N., and Shulman, M. J. (1984) Production of functional chimaeric mouse/human antibody. *Nature* **312,** 643–646.
5. Morrison, S. L., Johnson, M. J., Herzenberg, L. A., and Oi, V.T. (1984) Chimeric human antibody molecules: mouse antigen binding domains with human constant region domains. *Proc. Natl. Acad. Sci. USA* **81,** 6851–6855.
6. Neuberger, M. S., Williams, G. T., Mitchell, E. B., Jouhal, S. S., Flanagan, J. G., and Rabbits, T. H. (1985) A hapten-specific chimaeric IgE antibody with human physiological effector function. *Nature* **314,** 268–270.
7. Better, M., Chang, C. P., Robinson, R. R., and Horwitz, A. H. (1988) *Escherichia coli* secretion of an active chimeric antibody fragment. *Science* **240,** 1041–1043.

8. Jones, P. T., Dear, P. H., Foote, J., Neuberger, M. S., and Winter, G. (1986) Replacing the complementarity-determining regions in a human antibody with those from a mouse. *Nature* **321,** 522–525.

9. Riechmann, L., Foote, J., and Winter, G. (1988) Expression of an antibody Fv fragment in myeloma cells. *J. Mol. Biol.* **203,** 825–828.

10. Bird, R. E., Hardman, K. D., Jacobson, J. W., Johnson, S., Kaufman, B. M., Lee, S. M., Lee, T., Pope, S. H., Riordan, G. S., and Whitlow, M. (1988) Single-chain antigen-binding proteins. *Science* **242,** 423–426.

11. Huston, J. S., Levinson, D., Mudgett-Hunter, M., Tai, M.-S., Novotny, J., Margolies, M. J., Ridge, R. J., Bruccoleri, R. E., and Haber, E., Crea, R. (1988) Protein engineering of antibody binding sites: recovery of specific activity in an anti-digoxin single-chain Fv analogue produced in Escherichia coli. *Proc. Natl. Acad. Sci. USA* **85,** 5879–5883.

12. Glockshuber, R., Malia, M., Pfitzinger, I., and Plückthun, A. (1990) A comparision of strategies to stabilize immunoglobulin Fv fragments. *Biochemistry* **29,** 1362–1367.

13. Verhoeyen, M., Milstein, C., and Winter, G. (1988) Reshaping human antibodies: grafting an antilysozyme activity. *Science* **239,** 1534–1536.

14. Kettleborough, C. A., Saldanha, J., Heath, V. J., Morrison, C. J., and Bendig, M. M. (1991) Humanisation of a mouse monoclonal antibody by CDR grafting: the importance of framework residues on loop confirmation. *Protein Eng.* **4,** 773–783.

15. Reichmann, L., Clark, M., Waldmann, H., and Winter, G. (1988) Reshaping human antibodies for therapy. *Nature* **322,** 323–327.

16. Gussow, D. and Seaman, G. (1991) Humanisation of monoclonal antibodies. *Methods Enzymol.* **203,** 99–121.

17. Rader, C., Cheresh, D. A., Barbas, C. F., 3rd. (1998) A phage display approach for rapid antibody humanisation: designed combinatorial V gene libraries. *Proc. Natl. Acad. Sci. USA* **95,** 8910–8915.

18. Gorman, S. D. and Clark, M. R. (1990) Humanisation of monoclonal antibodies for therapy. *Semin. Immunol.* **2,** 457–466.

19. Padlan, E. A. (1991) A possible procedure for reducing the immunogenicity of antibody variable domains while preserving their ligand-binding properties. *Mol. Immunol.* **28,** 489–498.

20. Pedersen, J. T., Henry, A. H., Searle, S. J., Guild, B. C., Roguska, M., and Rees, A. R. (1994) Comparison of surface accesible residues in human and murine immunoglobulin Fv domains. Implication for the humanization of murine antibodies. *J. Mol. Biol.* **235,** 959–973.

21. Roguska, M. A,, Pedersen, J. T., Keddy, C. A., Henry, A. H., Searle, S. J., Lambert, J. M., Goldmacher, V. S., Blattler, W. A., Rees, A. R., and Guild, B. C. (1994) Humanization of murine monoclonal antibodies through variable domain resurfacing. *Proc. Natl. Acad. Sci. USA* **91,** 969–973.

22. Porter, R. R. (1959) The hydrolysis of rabbit g-globulin and antibodies with crystalline papain. *Biochem. J.* **73,** 119–126.

23. Inbar, D., Hochman, J., and Givol, D. (1972) Localization of the antibody combining site within the variable portion of heavy and light chains. *Proc. Natl. Acad. Sci. USA* **69,** 2659–2662.

24. Hochman, J., Inbar, D., and Givol, D. (1973) An active antibody fragment Fv composed of the variable portions of heavy and light chains. *Biochemistry* **12,** 1130–1135.

25. Sharon, J. and Givol, D. (1976) Preparation of Fv fragment from mouse myeloma XRPC-25 immunoglobulin possessing anti-dinitriphenyle activity. *Biochemstry* **15,** 1591–1594.

26. Kabat, E. A., Wu, T. T., and Bilofsky, H (1978) Variable region genes for immunoglobulin framework are assembled from small segments of DNA—a hypothesis. *Proc. Natl. Acad. Sci. USA* **75,** 2429–2433.

27. Skerra, A. and Plückthun, A. (1988) Assembly of a functional immunoglobulin Fv fragment in Escherichia coli. *Science* **240,** 1038–1041.

28. Brinkmann, U., Reiter, Y., Jung, S. H., Lee, B., and Pastan, I. (1993) A recombinant immunotoxin containing a disulphide-stabilized Fv fragment. *Proc. Natl. Acad. Sci. USA* **90,** 7538–7548.

29. Anand, N. N., Mandal, S., MacKenzie, C. R., Sadowska, J., Sigurskjold, B., Young, N. M., Bundle, D. R., and Narang, S. A. (1991) Bacterial expression and secretion of various single-chain Fv genes encoding proteins specific for a Salmonella serotype B O-antigen. *J. Biol. Chem.* **266,** 21,874–21,879.

30. Huston, J. S., Mudgett-Hunter, M., Tai, M. S., McCartney, J., Warren, F., Haber, E., and Oppermann, H. (1991) Protein engineering of single-chain Fv analogs and fusion proteins. *Methods Enzymol.* **203,** 46–88.

31. Davies, D. R. and Metzger, H. (1983) Structural basis of antibody function. *Ann. Rev. Immunol.* **1,** 87–117.

32. Harwood, P. J., Boden, J., Pedley, R. B., Rawlins, G., Rogers, G. T., and Bagshawe, K. D. (1985) Comparitive tumour localization of antibody fragments and intact IgG in nude mice bearing a CEA-producing human colon tumour xenograft. *Eur. J. Cancer Clin. Oncol.* **21,** 1515–1522.

33. Begent, R. H. and Chester, K. A. (1997) Single-chain Fv antibodies for targeting cancer therapy. *Biochem. Soc. Trans.* **25,** 715–717.

34. Colcher, D., Bird, R., Roselli, M., Hardman, K. D., Johnson, S., Pope, S., Dodd, S. W., Pantoliano, M. W., Milenic, D. E., and Scholm, J. (1990) *In vivo* tumor targeting of a recombinant single-chain antigen-binding protein. *J. Natl. Cancer Inst.* **82,** 1191–1197.

35. Larson, S. M., Raubitschek, A., Reynolds, J. C., Neumann, R. D., Hellstrom, K. E., Hellstrom, I., Colcher, D., Schlom, J., Glatstein, E., and Carrasquillo, J. A. (1989) Comparison of bone marrow dosimetry and toxic effect of high dose ^{131}I-labeled monoclonal antibodies administered to man. *Int. J. Rad. Appl. Instrum. B* **16,** 153–158.

36. Milenic, D. E., Yokota, T., Filpula, D. R., Finkelman, M. A. J., Dodd, S. W., Wood, J. F., Whitlow, M., Snoy, P., and Schlom, J. (1991) Construction, binding properties, metabolism, and tumor targeting of a single-chain Fv derived from the pancarcinoma monoclonal antibody CC49. *Cancer Res.* **51,** 6363–6371.

37. Begent, R. H. J., Verhaar, M. J., Chester, K. A., Casey, J. L., Green, A. J., Napier, M. P., Hope-Stone, L. D., Cushen, N., Keep, P. A., Johnson, C. J., Hawkins, R. E., Hilson, A. J. W., and Robson, L. (1996) Clinical evidence of efficient tumor targeting based on single-chain Fv antibody selected from a combinatorial library. *Nat. Med.* **2,** 979–984.
38. Yokota, T., Milenic, D. E., Whitlow, M., and Schlom, J. (1992) Rapid tumor penctration of a single-chainFv and comparision with other immunoglobulin forms. *Cancer Res.* **52,** 3402–3408.
39. Yokota, T., Milenic, D. E., Whitlow, M., Wood, J. F., Hubert, S. L., and Schlom, J. (1993) Microautoradiographic analysis of the normal organ distribution of radioiodinated single-chain Fv and other immunoglobulin forms. *Cancer Res.* **53,** 3776–3783.
40. Seccamani, E., Tattanelli, M., Mariani, M., Spranzi, E., Scassellati, G. A., and Siccardi, A. G. (1989) A simple qualitative determination of human antibodies to murine immunoglobulins (HAMA) in serum samples. *Nucl. Med. Biol.* **16,** 167–170.
41. Stewart, J., Hird, V., Snook, D., Sullivan, M., Hooker, G., and Courtenay-Luck, N. (1990) Intraperitoneal yttrium-90 labeled monoclonal antibody in ovarian cancer. *J. Clin. Oncol.* **5,** 1890–1899.
42. Hird, V., Maraveyas, A., Snook, D., Dhokia, B., Soutter, W. P., Meares, C., Stewart, J. S. W., Mason, P., Lambert, H. E., and Epenetos, A. A. (1993) Adjuvant therapy of ovarian cancer with radioactive monoclonal antibody. *Br. J. Cancer* **68,** 403–406.
43. Courtenay-Luck, N., Epenetos, A., Moore, R., Larche, M., Pectasides, D., Dhokia, B., and Ritter, M. (1986) Development of primary and secondary immune responses to mouse monoclonal antibodies used in the diagnosis and therapy of malignant neoplasms. *Cancer Res.* **46,** 6489–6493.
44. Nedelman, M. A., Shealy, D. J., Boulin, R., Brunt, E., Seasholtz, J. I., Allen, E., McCartney, J. E., Warren, F. D., Oppermann, H., Pang, R. H. L., Berger, H. J., and Weisman, H. F. (1993). Rapid infarct imaging with a technetium-99m-labeled antimyosin recombinant single-chain Fv: evaluation in a canine model of acute myocardial infarction. *J. Nucl. Med.* **34,** 234–241.
45. Chester, K. A., Begent, R. H., Robson, L., Keep, P., Pedley, R. B., Boden, J. A., Boxer, G., Green, A., Winter, G., Cochet, O., and Hawkins, R. E. (1994) Phage libraries for generation of clinically useful antibodies. *Lancet* **343,** 455–456.
46. George, A. J. T., Jamar, F., Tai, M.-S., Heelan, B. T., Adams, G. P., McCartney, J. E., Houston, L. L., Weiner, L. M., Oppermann, H., and Peters, A. M. (1995) Radiometal labeling of recombinant proteins by a genetically engineered minimal chelation site: technetium-99m coordination by single-chain Fv antibody fusion proteins through a C-terminal cysteinyl peptide. *Proc. Natl. Acad. Sci. USA* **92,** 8358–8363.
47. Tai, M.-S., McCartney, J. E., Adams, G. P., Jin, D., Hudziak, R. M., Oppermann, H., Laminet, A. A., Bookman, M. A., Wolf, E. J., Liu, S., Stafford III, W. F.,

Frand, I., Houston, L. L., Weiner, L. M., and Huston, J. S. (1995) Targeting c-erbB-2 expressing tumors using single-chain Fv monomers and dimers. *Cancer Res.* **55**, 5983s–5989s.

48. Adams, G. P., McCartney, J. E., Wolf, E. J., Eisenberg, J., Tai, M. S., Huston, J. S., Stafford, W., Bookman, M. A., Houston, L. L., and Weiner, L. M. (1995) Optimization of *in vivo* tumor targeting in SCID mice with divalent forms of 741F8 anti-c-erbB-2 single-chain Fv: effects of dose escalation and repeated i.v. administration. *Cancer Immunol. Immunother.* **40**, 299–306.

49. Hu, S., Shively, L., Raubitschek, A., Sherman, M., Williams, L. E., Wong, J. Y., Shively, J. E., and Wu, A. M. (1996) Minibody: A novel engineered anti-carcinoembryonic antigen antibody fragment (single-chain Fv-CH3) which exhibits rapid, high-level targeting of xenografts. *Cancer Res.* **56**, 3055–3061.

50. Verhaar, M. J., Chester, K. A., Keep, P. A., Robson, L., Pedley, R. B., Boden, J. A., Hawkins, R. E., and Begent, R. H. (1995) A single chain Fv derived from a filamentous phage library has distinct tumor targeting advantages over one derived from a hybridoma. *Int. J. Cancer* **61**, 497–501.

51. Chaudhary, V. K., Gallo, M. G., FitzGerald, D. J., and Pastan, I. (1990) A recombinant single-chain immunotoxin composed of anti-tac variable regions and truncated Diptheria toxin. *Proc. Natl. Acad. Sci. USA* **87**, 9491–9494.

52. Chaudhary, V. K., Queen, C., Junghans, R. P., Waldmann, T. A., FitzGerald, D. J., and Pastan, I. (1989) A recombinant immunotoxin consisting of two antibody variable domains fused to Pseudomonas exotoxin. *Nature* **339**, 394–397.

53. Nicholls, P. J., Johnson, V. G., Andrew, S. M., Hoogenboom, H. R., Raus, J. C., and Youle, R. J. (1993) Characterization of single-chain antibody (scFv)-toxin fusion proteins produced *in vitro* in rabbit reticulocyte lysate. *J. Biol. Chem.* **268**, 5302–5308.

54. Pauza, M. E., Doumbia, S. O., and Pennell, C. A. (1997) Construction and characterization of human CD7-specific single-chain Fv immunotoxins. *J. Immunol.* **158**, 3259–3269.

55. Francisco, J. A., Gawlak, S. L., Miller, M., Bathe, J., Russell, D., Chace, D., Mixan, B., Zhao, L., Fell, H. P., and Siegall, C. B. (1997) Expression and characterization of bryodin 1 and a bryodin 1-based single-chain immunotoxin from tobacco cell culture. *Bioconjug. Chem.* **8**, 708–713.

56. Tai, M-S., Mudgett-Hunter, M., Levinson, D., Wu, G-M., Haber, E., Oppermann, H., and Huston, J. S. (1990) A bifunctional fusion protein containing Fc-binding fragment B of Staphylococcal protein A amino terminal to antidigoxin single-chain Fv. *Biochemistry* **29**, 8024–8030.

57. Traunecker, A., Lanzavecchia, A., and Karjalainen, K. (1991) Bispecific single-chain molecules (Janusins) target cytotoxic lymphocytes on HIV infected cells. *EMBO J.* **10**, 3635–3659.

58. Hakim, I., Levy, S., and Levy, R. (1996) A nine-amino acid peptide from IL-1beta augments antitumor immune responses induced by protein and DNA vaccines. *J. Immunol.* **157**, 5503–5511.

59. Holliger, P., Prospero, T., and Winter, G. (1993) "Diabodies": small bivalent and bispecific antibody fragments. *Proc. Natl. Acad. Sci. USA* **90**, 6444–6448.

60. Perisic, O., Webb, P. A., Holliger, P., Winter, G., and Williams, R. L. (1994) Crystal structure of a diabody, a bivalent antibody fragment. *Structure* **2,** 1217–1226.
61. Holliger, P., Brissinck, J., Williams, R. L., Thielemans, K., and Winter, G. (1996) Specific killing of lymphoma cells by cytotoxic T-cells mediated by a bispecific diabody. *Protein Eng.* **9,** 299–305.
62. Holliger, P., Wing, M., Pound, J. D., Bohlen, H., and Winter, G. (1997) Retargeting serum immunoglobulin with bispecific diabodies. *Nat. Biotechnol.* **15,** 632–636.
63. Kontermann, R. E., Wing, M. G., and Winter, G. (1997) Complement recruitment using bispecific diabodies. *Nat. Biotechnol.* **15,** 629–631.
64. Kontermann, R. E., Martineau, P., Cummings, C. E., Karpas, A., Allen, D., Derbyshire, E., and Winter, G. (1997) Enzyme immunoassays using bispecific diabodies. *Immunotechnology* **3,** 137–144.
65. Iliades, P., Kortt, A. A., and Hudson, P. J. (1997) Triabodies: single chain Fv fragments without a linker form trivalent trimers. *FEBS Lett.* **409,** 437–441.
66. Pei, X. Y., Holliger, P., Murzin, A. G., and Williams, R. L. (1997) The 2.0-A resolution crystal structure of a trimeric antibody fragment with noncognate VH-VL domain pairs shows a rearrangement of VH CDR3. *Proc. Natl. Acad. Sci. USA* **94,** 9637–9642.
67. George, A. J. T., Titus, J., Jost, C., Kurucz, I., Perez, P., Andrew, S., Nicholls, P., Huston, J., and Segal, D. (1994) Redirection of T cell-mediated cytotoxicity by a recombinant single-chain Fv molecule. *J. Immunol.* **152,** 1802–1811.
68. McCafferty, J., Griffiths, A. D., Winter, G., and Chiswell, D. J. (1990) Phage antibodies: filamentous phage displaying antibody variable domains. *Nature* **348,** 552–554.
69. Fuchs, P., Breitling, F., Dubel, S., Seehaus, T., and Little, M. (1991) Targeting recombinant antibodies to the surface of Escherichia coli: fusion to a peptidoglycan associated lipoprotein. *Biotechnol. NY* **9,** 1369–1372.
70. Huston, J. S., McCartney, J., Tai, M.-S., Mottola-Hartshorn, C., Jin, D., Warren, F., Keck, P., and Oppermann, H. (1993) Medical applications of single-chain antibodies. *Int. Rev. Immunol.* **10,** 195.
71. McCartney, J. E., Lederman, L., Drier, F. A., Cabral-Denison, N. A., Wu, G. M., Batorsky, R. S., Huston, J. S., and Oppermann, H. (1991) Biosynthetic antibody binding sites: development of a single-chain Fv model based on antidinitrophenol IgA myeloma MOPC 315. *J. Protein Chem.* **10,** 669–683.
72. Bedzyk, W. D., Weidner, K. M., Denzin, L. K., Johnson, L. S., Hardman, K. D., Pantoliano, M. W., Asel, E. D., and Voss, E., Jr. (1990) Immunological and structural characterization of a high affinity anti-fluorescein single-chain antibody. *J. Biol. Chem.* **265,** 18,615–18,620.
73. Takkinen, K., Laukkanen, M. L., Sizmann, D., Alfthan, K., Immonen, T., Vanne, L., Kaartinen, M., Knowles, J. K., and Teeri, T. T. (1991) An active single-chain antibody containing a cellulase linker domain is secreted by Escherichia coli. *Protein Eng.* **4,** 837–841.
74. Novotny, J., Ganju, R. K., Smiley, S. T., Hussey, R. E., Luther, M. A., Recny, M. A., Siliciano, R. F., and Reinherz, E. L. (1991) A soluble, single-chain T-cell

receptor fragment endowed with antigen-combining properties. *Proc. Natl. Acad. Sci. USA* **88,** 8646–8650.

75. Turner, D. J., Ritter, M. A., and George, A. J. T. (1997) Importance of the linker in expression of single-chain Fv antibody fragments: optimisation of peptide sequence using phage display technology. *J. Immunol. Methods* **205,** 43–54.

76. Atwell, S., Ridgway, J. B., Wells, J. A., and Carter, P. (1997) Stable heterodimers from remodeling the domain interface of a homodimer using a phage display library. *J. Mol. Biol.* **270,** 26–35.

77. Zhu, Z., Presta, L. G., Zapata, G., and Carter, P. (1997) Remodeling domain interfaces to enhance hetrodimer formation. *Protein Sci.* **6,** 781–788.

78. Verma, R., Boleti, E., and George, A. J. T. (1998) Antibody engineering: comparison of bacterial, yeast, insect and mammalian expression systems. *J. Immunol. Methods* **216,** 165–181.

4

Phage Display Technology

Michael Johns

1. Introduction

The development of monoclonal antibody (mAb) technology (1) has had a significant impact on many fields of research, in particular immunology. However, the method has limitations. The use of recombinant DNA technology and demonstration by Smith 1985 (2) that peptides can be expressed on the surface of filamentous bacteriophages have permitted the development of a powerful new methodology for the generation and isolation of novel antibody-based reagents for both research and clinical application.

Filamentous bacteriophage (e.g., M13) have a single-stranded DNA genome encapsulated by multiple copies of the major coat protein pVIII (**Fig. 1**). The number of copies of pVIII is variable, thus allowing additional DNA to be incorporated and packaged within the virion without any adverse effects (3). The gene III product, expressed at one end of the bacteriophage, is particularly important in the life cycle of the bacteriophage; it is responsible for infecting male F′-positive bacteria (e.g., *Escherichia coli* strain TG1), transfer of DNA to the bacteria, and initiation of replication (4). In the context of phage display technology it is also the most common (but not only) site for the expression of recombinant proteins, such as sFv (**Fig. 1**). It is possible to express sFv on all copies of the gene III product (5); however, this is the exception rather than the rule.

A variety of peptides and proteins have been expressed on the surface of filamentous phage, including fragments of *Eco*RI endonuclease, IL-3, human growth hormone, alkaline phosphatase, and antibody fragments (2,6–8). As a prerequisite to expressing antibody fragments on the surface of bacteriophage, the heavy and light variable region genes for immunoglobulin must be cloned.

From: *Methods in Molecular Medicine, Vol. 40: Diagnostic and Therapeutic Antibodies*
Edited by: A. J. T. George and C. E. Urch © Humana Press Inc., Totowa, NJ

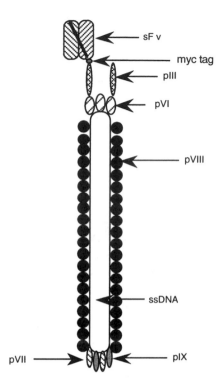

Fig. 1. Diagrammatic representation of a filamentous phage expressing sFv on the gene III product. 2700 copies of the major coat protein (pVIII) encapsulate a single-stranded DNA genome. Five copies of the gene III product cap one end of the phage and are the principal site for expression of recombinant proteins. pVI, pVII, and pIX constitute the other minor coat proteins. Filamentous bacteriophages are approx 1 μ*M* in length and 6–7 nm in diameter.

Typically this is done by polymerase chain reaction (PCR) (*see* Chapter 36) and can be used to clone either specific antibody fragments or families of antibody genes. Cloning families of antibody genes has led to the development of libraries of antibody fragments expressed on the surface of bacteriophage. This chapter is concerned with phage display in the context of antibody engineering and the application of antibody fragments (sFv and Fab) selected from diverse libraries.

2. Phage Display Libraries

A phage lambda system was used originally to screen diverse combinatorial libraries of Fab fragments developed from immunized mice (*9*). However, this method is limited and involves immobilizing the library and screening with soluble labeled antigen. The demonstration that it was possible to express the complete V region genes (cloned as sFv) on the surface of filamentous fd bacteriophage *(10)* initiated the development of large combinatorial libraries (randomly combined V_H and V_L genes, usually in sFv format) expressed on the surface of bacteriophage. During these early studies, it was shown that specific sFv on the surface of phage could be isolated from a mixture of irrelevant phage, expressing no sFv, with enrichments for specific binding of 1000-fold/ round of selection *(10)*. The development of diverse random combinatorial libraries from immunized animals began with the development of a library from mice immunized with phOx. This library was used successfully to select sFv against phOx by affinity chromatography *(11)*. Combinatorial libraries of Fab fragments derived from immunized mice *(12)*, rabbits *(13)*, and vaccinated humans *(14)* have also been developed and successfully screened for useful antibody reagents by panning *(15)*. When generating libraries from immunized individuals, the source of B cells has been shown to be an important issue; more specifically, in certain situations, lymph nodes provide a more appropriate source than peripheral blood *(16)*.

Generating libraries from immunized animals has limitations. Principally, the library has been skewed toward a particular antigen by immunization and consequently a new library must be generated for each antigen you wish to raise an antibody against. The development of naive libraries *(17,18)* (i.e., libraries generated from donors that have not been specifically immunized) offers a number of advantages. First, the same library can be used to select antibodies against a variety of antigens, and furthermore, they allow the possibility of raising human antibodies against specific antigens but negating the problem of immunization.

One of the major considerations when constructing this type of library is how to maximize the number of different specificities contained by the library. This is important for two reasons: it increases the chance of isolating an antibody against the desired antigen and it increases the chance of isolating an antibody fragment of greater affinity. A number of strategies have been developed in order to clone larger and more diverse libraries (of both sFv and Fab fragments) in a quest to increase the chances of successful selection of high-affinity recombinant antibodies. Most notable is the use of PCR *(19)* with randomly generated oligonucleotides to generate random CDR3 regions *(20,21)*. This approach has been used successfully both to help generate random combinatorial libraries from cloned human V_H genes *(21)* and also to generate libraries of existing Fab fragments altered only in the CDR3 region *(22)*. These libraries have been termed semisynthetic.

Nissim et al. *(21)*, have developed a semisynthetic phage library of $>10^8$ different specificities. The library has been made in vitro from 50 cloned human V_H gene segments that have random nucleotide sequences encoding CDR3 lengths of 4–12 residues. Each of the 50 germline V_H segments were amplified using V_H family-based primers. After the addition of restriction sites the PCR products were cloned into pHEN1 (containing λ3 light chain). By introducing an amber stop codon between the gene III and the antibody genes, either whole phage expressing sFv on their surface or sFv alone can be produced depending on the use of suppressor (TG1) or nonsuppressor (HB2151) strains of bacteria. They have used the library to select a variety of sFv against 18 different antigens after four or five rounds of panning. The selected phage-sFv and sFv were used in western blotting and also for epitope mapping and staining of cells. deKruif et al. *(23)* have also constructed a semisynthetic sFv library using cloned human germline V_H genes and synthetic CDR3. However, in contrast to Nissim et al. *(21)*, they have used a 6–15 amino acid CDR3 containing short stretches of fully randomized amino acid residues flanked by regions of limited variability (selected on the frequency of amino acids in the CDR3 of natural antibodies). In doing so the authors reason that this will increase occurrence of phage displaying functionally useful fragments. They also attempted to increase variability by using seven different light chains from both λ and κ subclasses rather than λ3 alone, as used by Nissim et al. *(21)*.

Griffiths et al *(24)* have produced a Fab library of 6.5×10^{10} specificities using a combinatorial infection process, which involves transforming bacteria with a library of heavy chains on a plasmid and then infecting the culture with a library of light chains on a phage and also a Cre recombinase on a separate phage. The Cre recombinase then uses lox P sites within the library vectors to randomly combine H and L chains (from the plasmid and phage vectors) on the same phage replicon within each bacterium. This theoretically can lead to a library as large as the number of infected bacteria. Considering the size of the repertoire of heavy and light chains cloned, if each heavy and light chain were to recombine, a final library of 10^{13} different specificities could theoretically be generated. With the increased size of this library, the authors report antibody fragments of affinities >80-fold higher than those isolated from smaller libraries.

When constructing a phage display library, it should be remembered that different antibodies have different toxic effects on the cells producing them *(25)*. This leads to certain clones being at a great disadvantage and potentially underrepresented or even lost from the library. Recently, attempts have been made to combat the growth disadvantage and vector instability that cells expressing functional sFv-gene III fusions suffer *(26)*. To this end, the phage display systems originally developed have been modified, with consideration being given to all aspects from the PCR primers used in the initial stages to the vector in which the genes are cloned. Some vectors have been adapted specifically for the expression of antibody fragments in the periplasm of Gram-negative bacteria *(26)*. Furthermore, vector systems have now been developed that allow the production of complete antibodies following selection of a Fab expressed on the surface of a phage from a library *(27)*.

The use of phage display technology, however, can still yield antibody fragments of too low an affinity to be useful—either clinically or in research. This problem can be alleviated using chain shuffling *(28)* followed by reselection, i.e., replace either the V_H or V_L with repertoires of V genes and repeat the selection. This was originally demonstrated using an antibody against a hapten *(11)*. However, sFv with a comparable affinity to a mAb, raised by hybridoma technology, have been selected against a protein antigen by this method *(29)*. Error-prone PCR, or chemical mutagenesis of DNA followed by PCR, have been used successfully to randomize antibody genes in attempts to increase affinity. Site-directed random mutagenesis of all three CDRs has also been employed to alter the association and dissociation kinetics of existing sFv by effecting their ability to aggregate *(30)*.

3. Selection from Phage Display Libraries

A great diversity of methods of varying complexity have been developed to isolate specific phage antibodies from diverse libraries, including the use of biotinylated material in solution followed by capture with streptavidin *(29)* and the use of antigen columns. However, the simplest way to select antibody fragments from diverse phage display libraries is by panning. This is a simple, fast, effective method and is described in detail in Chapter 37. Briefly, the antigen of interest is immobilized on a solid surface and after appropriate incubation with the phage antibodies, the unbound phages are washed away and the specifically bound phages are eluted and used to infect bacteria. The phages are then amplified in bacteria and repurified before panning is carried out again. After each round of panning, random phages are selected and tested for their ability to bind specifically to the antigen by enzyme-linked immunosorbent assay (ELISA). Typically, three to six rounds of panning are carried out for each antigen before specifically binding phage antibodies are isolated *(18,21)*.

This basic protocol has been adapted in a number of ways to direct selection toward a particular antigen. For example, competitive elution of bound phage using mAbs has been used to develop human sFvs against predefined epitopes that previously were only recognized by animal-derived mAbs *(31)*. The basic method has also been modified to allow isolation of antibodies to specific epitopes on only one member of a group of closely related molecules. To this end, related soluble protein (not encoding the epitope of interest) can be added to the phage during selection against an immobilized antigen, thereby keeping phages that react to the irrelevant antigen in solution and hopefully increasing the chance of isolating specific phage antibodies against the epitope of interest.

Selection has also been achieved against antigens in solution. This can be achieved by biotinylation of the antigen of interest followed by incubation with the phage antibodies and subsequent capture of the antigen-bound phage antibodies using streptavidin-coated magnetic beads. Reducing the amount of antigen present in each round of selection provides a simple means of selecting for the highest affinity binders *(29)*. A modification of this method has been used to select a panel of Fab fragments against cell surface molecules captured from cell lysates by pre-existing antibodies *(32)*. Comparison of the affinity of sFvs selected by panning on immobilized antigen vs selection in solution showed better affinities for those sFvs selected in solution. Furthermore, selection of sFv against immobilized antigen preferentially selected for dimerizing sFv (with mutation in the V_H-V_L interface), which had lower affinity than the monomeric sFv isolated against biotinylated antigen in solution *(29)*.

The use of immobilized antigen in all the above ways has an obvious limitation: You must know and have purified the antigen of interest before selection can be performed. Phage display technology has been extended to allow selection of phage against uncharacterized or unavailable antigen in its native configuration by screening against cells known to express the antigen of interest *(33–35)*. The initial studies were performed on human red blood cells and the selected sFvs were able to substitute for mAbs in agglutination tests *(33)*. This method has been extended such that selection of phage against antigens on subpopulations of cells defined by pre-existing mAbs is possible *(36)*. After incubation of the cells with the phage, nonbound phages were removed by washing and a subpopulation of leukocytes defined using labeled anti-CD3 and anti-CD20 mAbs. The population defined by CD3 and CD20 was then isolated using FACS and the bound phage eluted and amplified before the next round of selection. This method reasons that phage interacting with common antigens will be absorbed by the nonselected population, thus increasing the chance of successful selection of an sFv against a specific antigen after fewer rounds of selection. This method has been modified to allow selection of phage antibodies against populations of cells without the use of FACS *(35)*.

With the development of larger and more diverse libraries, better and more powerful selection procedures have to be developed. Duenas and Borrebaeck *(37)* have developed a system in which antigen recognition and phage replication have been linked. This system requires noninfectious phages that are complimented (and therefore "made infectious") when the Fab on the surface of the phage recognizes its antigen fused to the M13 bacteriophage gene III product. Furthermore, this SAP system has been used to show the selection of Fabs on the basis of kinetics *(38)*; high-affinity clones are selected at lower concentrations of the antigen-gene III fusion protein and low-affinity clones at higher doses of the antigen. Varying contact times were also used to bias selection toward different dissociation rates for the antibodies in question. The use of dissociation rate constants has recently been used to differentiate between two different pre-existing Fab phages. Antigen was immobilized on a biosensor chip and the phage flowed over the surface. Specifically bound phages were eluted and analyzed. This method has been expanded to select sFv from phage libraries after chain shuffling of a previously selected antibody as well as from immunized libraries *(39)*. The use of BIAcore measurements has been employed in combination with ELISA for detection of high-affinity clones. Schier et al. *(29)* have used a BIAcore-based method to further select phage antibodies, already shown to be positive by ELISA, on the basis of affinity. The advantage of this method is that it can distinguish not only between the affinity of the clones but also the relative proportions of monomeric, dimeric, and multivalent sFv present in a crude periplasmic extract of the sFv in question, thus allowing screening without purification of the sFv.

The development of large phage display libraries and sophisticated selection procedures outlined above have been combined to produce many useful reagents. Antibodies have been isolated against novel determinants, including those previously found to be poorly immunogenic or highly conserved *(40)* across species and therefore hard to raise antibodies against. Furthermore, phage display technology has allowed basic characterization by epitope mapping of important molecules, such as gp120 (HIV), that have proven difficult to analyze in detail by nuclear magnetic resonance (NMR) or X-ray crystallography.

References

1. Kohler, G. and Milstein, C. (1975) Continuous culture of fused cells secreting antibody of predefined specificity. *Nature* **256**, 495–497.
2. Smith, G. P. (1985) Filamentous fusion phage: novel expression vectors that express cloned antigens on the virion surface. *Science* **228**, 1315–1317.
3. Sambrook, J., Fritsch, E. F,. and Maniatis, T. (1989) *Molecular Cloning: A Laboratory Manual*. Cold Spring Harbor Laboratory Press, Cold Spring Harbor, NY.
4. Dulbecco, R. and Ginsberg, H. S. (1988) *Virology*, 2nd ed., Lippincott, London, UK.
5. MacKenzie, R. and To, R. (1998) The role of valency in the selection of anti-carbohydrate single chain Fvs from phage display libraries. *J. Immunol. Methods* **220**, 39–49.

6. Bass, S., Greene, R., and Well, J. A. (1990) Hormone phage: an enrichment method for variant proteins with altered binding properties. *Proteins Struct. Funct. Genet.* **8,** 309–314.

7. McCafferty, J., Jackson, R. H., and Chiswell, D. (1991) Phage-enzyme: expression and affinity chromatography of functional alkaline phosphatase on the surface of bacteriophage. *Protein Eng.* **4,** 955–961.

8. Gram, H., Strittmatter, U., Lorenz, M., Gluck, D., and Zenke, G. (1993) Phage display as a rapid gene expression system: production of bioactive cytokine-phage and generation of neutralising monoclonal antibodies. *J. Immunol. Methods* **161,** 169–176.

9. Huse, W. D., Sastry, L., Iverson, S. A., Kang, A. S., Alting, M. M., Burton, D. R., Benkovic, S. J., and Lerner, R. A. (1989) Generation of a large combinatorial library of the immunoglobulin repertoire in phage lambda. *Science* **246,** 1275–1281.

10. McCafferty, J., Griffiths, A. D., Winter, G., and Chiswell, D. J. (1990) Phage antibodies: filamentous phage displaying antibody variable domains. *Nature,* **348,** 552–554.

11. Clackson, T., Hoogenboom, H. R., Griffiths, A. D., and Winter, G. (1991) Making antibody fragments using phage display libraries. *Nature* **352,** 624–628.

12. Barbas, C. F. 3rd, Kang, A. S., Lerner, R. A., and Benkovic, S. J. (1991) Assembly of combinatorial antibody libraries on phage surfaces: the gene III site. *Proc. Natl. Acad. Sci. USA* **88,** 7978–7982.

13. Lang, I. M., Barbas, C. F. 3rd, and Schleef, R. R. (1996) Recombinant rabbit Fab with binding activity to type-1 plasminogen activator inhibitor derived from a phage-display library against human alpha-granules. *Gene* **172,** 295–298.

14. Zebedee, S. L., Barbas, C. F. 3rd, Hom, Y. L., Caothien, R. H., Graff, R., DeGraw, J., Pyati, J., LaPolla, R., Burton, D. R., Lerner, R. A., et al. (1992) Human combinatorial antibody libraries to hepatitis B surface antigen. *Proc. Natl. Acad. Sci. USA* **89,** 3175–3179.

15. Parmley, S. F. and Smith, G. P. (1988) Antibody-selectable filamentous fd phage vectors: affinity purification of target genes. *Gene* **73,** 305–318.

16. Yip, Y. L., Hawkins, N. J., Clarke, M. A., and Ward, R. L. (1997) Evaluation of different lymphoid tissue sources for the construction of human immunoglobulin gene libraries. *Immunotechnology* **3,** 195–203.

17. Marks, J. D., Hoogenboom, H. R., Bonnert, T. P., McCafferty, J., Griffiths, A. D., and Winter, G. (1991) Bypassing immunisation: human antibodies from V-gene libraries displayed on phage. *J. Mol. Biol.* **222,** 581–597.

18. Davies, E. L., Smith, J. S., Birkett, C. R., Manser, J. M., Anderson-Dear, D. V., and Young, J. R. (1995) Selection of specific phage-display antibodies using libraries derived from chicken immunoglobulin genes. *J. Immunol. Methods* **186,** 125–135.

19. Orlandi, R., Gussow, D. H., Jones, P. T., and Winter, G. (1989) Cloning immunoglobulin variable domains for expression by the polymerase chain reaction. *Proc. Natl. Acad. Sci. USA* **86,** 3833–3837.

20. Hoogenboom, H. R. and Winter, G. (1992) By-passing immunisation. Human antibodies from synthetic repertoires of germline VH gene segments rearranged in vitro. *J. Mol. Biol.* **227,** 381–388.
21. Nissim, A., Hoogenboom, H. R., Tomlinson, I. M., Flynn, G., Midgley, C., Lane, D., and Winter, G. (1994) Antibody fragments from a 'single pot' phage display library as immunochemical reagents. *EMBO J.* **13,** 692–698.
22. Barbas, C. F. 3rd, Bain, J. D., Hoekstra, D. M., Lerner, R. A. (1992) Semisynthetic combinatorial antibody libraries: a chemical solution to the diversity problem. *Proc. Natl. Acad. Sci. USA* **89,** 4457–4461.
23. deKruif, J., Boel, E., and Logtenberg, T. (1995) Selection and application of human single chain Fv antibody fragments from a semi-synthetic phage antibody display library with designed CDR3 regions. *J. Mol. Biol.* **248,** 97–105.
24. Griffiths, A. D., Williams, S. C., Hartley, O., Tomlinson, I. M., Waterhouse, P., Crosby, W. L., Kontermann, R. E., Jones, P. T., Low, N. M., Allison, T. J., et al. (1994) Isolation of high affinity human antibodies directly from large synthetic repertoires. *EMBO J.* **13,** 3245–3260.
25. Knappik, A. and Pluckthun, A. (1995) Engineered turns of a recombinant antibody improve its in vivo folding. *Protein Eng* **8,** 81–89.
26. Krebber, A., Bornhauser, S., Burmester, J., Honegger, A., Willuda, J., Bosshard, H. R., and Pluckthun, A. (1997) Reliable cloning of functional antibody variable domains from hybridomas and spleen cell repertoires employing a reengineered phage display system. *J. Immunol. Methods* **201,** 35–55.
27. Persic, L., Roberts, A., Wilton, J., Cattaneo, A., Bradbury, A., and Hoogenboom, H. R. (1997) An integrated vector system for the eukaryotic expression of antibodies or their fragments after selection from phage display libraries. *Gene* **187,** 9–18.
28. Kang, A. S., Jones, T. M., and Burton, D. R. (1991) Antibody redesign by chain shuffling from random combinatorial immunoglobulin libraries. *Proc. Natl. Acad. Sci. USA* **88,** 11,120–11,123.
29. Schier, R., Bye, J., Apell, G., McCall, A., Adams, G. P., Malmqvist, M., Weiner, L. M., and Marks, J. D. (1996) Isolation of high-affinity monomeric human anti c-erbB-2 single chain Fv using affinity-driven selection. *J. Mol. Biol.* **255,** 28–43.
30. Deng, S. J., MacKenzie, C. R., Hirama, T., Brousseau, R., Lowary, T. L., Young, N. M., Bundle, D. R., and Narang, S. A. (1995) Basis for selection of improved carbohydrate-binding single-chain antibodies from synthetic gene libraries *Proc. Natl. Acad. Sci. USA* **92,** 4992–4996.
31. Meulemans, E. V., Nieland, L. J., Debie, W. H., Ramaekers, F. C., and van-Eys, G. J. (1996) Phage displayed antibodies specific for a cytoskeletal antigen. Selection by competitive elution with a monoclonal antibody. *Hum. Antibodies Hybridomas* **6,** 113–118.
32. Sawyer, C., Embleton, J., and Dean, C. (1997) Methodology for selection of human antibodies to membrane proteins from a phage-display library. *J. Immunol. Methods* **204,** 193–203.

33. Marks, J. D., Ouwehand, W. H., Bye, J. M., Finnern, R., Gorick, B. D., Voak, D., Thorpe, S. J., Hughes Jones, N. C., and Winter, G. (1993) Human antibody fragments specific for human blood group antigens from a phage display library. *Biotechnology* **11,** 1145–1149.

34. Dziegiel, M., Nielsen, L. K., Andersen, P. S., Blancher, A., Dickmeiss, E., and Engberg, J. (1995) Phage display used for gene cloning of human recombinant antibody against the erythrocyte surface antigen, rhesus D. *J. Immunol. Methods* **182,** 7–19.

35. Palmer, D. B., George, A. J., and Ritter, M. A. (1997) Selection of antibodies to cell surface determinants on mouse thymic epithelial cells using a phage display library. *Immunology* **91,** 473–478.

36. deKruif, J., Terstappen, L., Boel, E., and Logtenberg, T. (1995) Rapid selection of cell subpopulation-specific human monoclonal antibodies from a synthetic phage antibody library. *Proc. Natl. Acad. Sci. USA* **92,** 3938.

37. Duenas, M. and Borrebaeck, C. A. (1994) Clonal selection and amplification of phage displayed antibodies by linking antigen recognition and phage replication. *Biotechnol. NY* **12,** 999–1002.

38. Duenas, M., Malmborg, A. C., Casalvilla, R., Ohlin, M., Borrebaeck C. A. (1996) Selection of phage displayed antibodies based on kinetic constants. *Mol. Immunol.* **33,** 279–285.

39. Malmborg, A. C., Duenas, M., Ohlin, M., Soderlind, E, and Borrebaeck, C. A. (1996) Selection of binders from phage displayed antibody libraries using the BIAcore biosensor. *J. Immunol. Methods* **198,** 51–57.

40. Palmer, D. B., Crompton, T., Marandi, M. B., George, A. J. T., and Ritter, M. A. (1999) Intrathymic function of the cortical epithelial cell surface antigen gp200-MR6 single-chain antibodies to evolutionarily conserved determinants disrupt mouse thymus development. *Immunology* **96,** 236–245.

II

ANTIBODIES IN MEDICINE

5

Prospects for the Application of Antibodies in Medicine

Herman Waldmann

1. Introduction

The evolution of therapeutic agents in medicine has been based around a standard set of principles. These include:

1. A defined need.
2. Specificity for the disease process to be controlled.
3. Ease and cost of discovery and production.
4. Stability and consistency of the product and its performance.
5. Capacity to amplify the desired therapeutic with limited toxicity.
6. Scope for patent protection and therefore profit opportunities.
7. User-friendly application.
8. Compatibility with regulatory requirements.

It is, therefore, not surprising that antibodies have significant appeal as therapeutics. Their remarkable specificity, well defined biochemical and biophysical properties, stability in adverse environments, natural capacity to seduce complement and cellular amplification events, and the abundant technology to ensure their high level expression in cell lines are all attractive features that have brought antibody diagnostics and therapeutics into prominence in the last 30 years, indeed ever since Köhler and Milstein made their momentous discovery.

Acknowledging the many very fine chapters in this volume, I do not intend to duplicate information that the reader has or will be exposed to. Instead, I highlight emerging areas that may soon have sufficient impact to reverse the seemingly negative attitude of the biotechnology and pharmaceutical industries toward antibody therapy. I focus my attention on two issues.

From: *Methods in Molecular Medicine, Vol. 40: Diagnostic and Therapeutic Antibodies*
Edited by: A. J. T. George and C. E. Urch © Humana Press Inc., Totowa, NJ

Table 1
Sources of Human Therapeutic Antibodies

Chimeric antibodies
Humanized antibodies
Somatic hybrids from mice transgenic for human Ig genes
Phage libraries from human lymphocytes
Epstein-Barr virus immortalization
Somatic hybrids with human lymphocytes
Single-cell PCR

First, I discuss the immunogenicity problem, which has constrained thinking about antibodies as agents to be used on only a limited number of occasions in the individual patient. Second, I consider the opportunities for treatment of certain diseases, where antibodies may be used as short term therapy to gain long-term effects.

2. The Immunogenicity Problem
2.1. Introduction

It has been recognized for some time, and it is not surprising that rodent antibodies are immunogenic in human patients. The consequence of this is the neutralization of the therapeutic agent and difficulty in readministration because of the unpredictable pharmacokinetics and risks of hypersensitivity reactions. For this reason it has been generally accepted that antibodies should be selected or engineered to be as "human" as possible. **Table 1** lists some ways in which "human" antibodies may be derived.

Some very amusing discussions have taken place claiming that certain forms of antibody are more human than others. This has led to major misconceptions that have been valuable for stock prices but not for science. The issue is really one of trying to understand why the immune system of a patient should or should not respond to a therapeutic antibody. Two factors should be considered:

1. Humans will be naturally tolerant to conserved sequences in most abundant proteins, and therefore will be tolerant of human immunoglobulin-constant regions. However, by the structural nature of antibodies one should expect no tolerance to allotypic variants nor to variable region sequences based on different CDRs between antibodies.
2. For immunogenicity, there is a requirement that T-helper cells recognize "foreign" peptides that are bound to the MHC Class II of an antigen-presenting cell. This can be avoided if one prevents such processing, or if the peptides that are bound are those to which we are already tolerant.

On the basis of the above points there is no special reason why "human" antibodies will not be immunogenic on repeated administration. Certainly, the fewer the number of foreign epitopes the less will be the immunogenicity, but it is not the case that "human" antibodies will always be nonimmunogenic, and anti-idiotypic antibodies have indeed been observed in patients re-treated with certain humanized monoclonal antibodies (mAbs).

The long-term future for antibody therapeutics must depend on elimination of the immunogenicity problem. This, I argue, can be resolved through an understanding and exploitation of the principles of immunological tolerance.

2.2. Cell Binding or Antibody Aggregation Is Required for Immunogenicity

One of the classic discoveries in immunological tolerance came nearly 40 years ago with the finding of Chiller and Weigle *(1)* that monomeric (deaggregated) human immunoglobulin could not immunize mice, but rather would tolerize both the T- and B-cell populations. In contrast, heat-aggregated immunoglobulin or human immunoglobulin in adjuvant would always immunize. The issue of antibody immmunogenicity for therapeutic antibodies was reconsidered by us in 1986 *(2,3)*, when we observed that rat antibodies directed to mouse white blood cells were always immunogenic, whereas non-cell–binding antibodies were not, but actually behaved as tolerogens. In some way the binding of antibody to white blood cells simulated aggregation and provides some intrinsic adjuvanticity. Although a detailed explanation of why cell-bound antibodies come to immunize is not yet available, these findings do give optimism that the anti-Ig response to therapeutic antibodies can be prevented. How might that be?

It is now known that xenogeneic anti-Ig responses are, as predicted, CD4 T-(helper) cell-dependent *(4)*. The implication of this finding was that CD4 T cells were recognizing processed peptides of the therapeutic antibody, bound to MHC Class II. We argued that if it were possible to tolerize T-helper cells to these MHC Class II-bound peptides then B cells would be deprived of their help, and so no anti-Ig response could be mounted.

Where a rodent antibody is processed for APC presentation in the human, we would expect there to be many epitopes (some from the H and some from the L chain) that might be seen as foreign on host MHC. Any humanized antibody would also generate many processed peptides, but the host immune system would be naturally tolerant of all those peptides derived from antibody-constant regions, leaving just a few (involving CDR residues) as potential immunogens. This and comparable arguments for B cells are why humanized antibodies are less immunogenic overall.

Given this background, how then might we permanently avoid anti-Ig responses? One avenue that we have been investigating *(5)* has been that of embracing two forms of a therapeutic antibody as ingredients of every therapeutic course. The first of these would be a minimal mutant of the cell-bound form, mutated in one or two residues to be non-cell binding. This mutant would be used in the first stage of the therapeutic procedure to establish immunological tolerance. Once tolerance has been induced, the second stage therapeutic course of the wild-type (cell-binding form) would begin, in the knowledge that tolerance would preclude any anti-Ig response. This strategy has succeeded in rodent models in our laboratory *(5)*, and we see no reason why it should not work in the clinic.

A potential disadvantage of this strategy, that two antibody products would have to be produced for every one therapeutic agent, is outweighed by the opportunity to offer useful antibodies on multiple occasions to the same patient. In tolerizing T cells to monomer (or deaggregated) Ig , one is tolerizing to all the foreign epitopes. Intuitively, it seems that it would be more difficult to tolerize to all foreign processed peptides of a xenogeneic antibody than the few peptides of a human(ized) variant, and so we advocate a combination of humanization and tolerance induction as a failsafe.

More sophisticated antibody engineering will, in time, also offer another way to reduce immunogenicity. This will aim to avoid the creation of immunogenic peptides that could bind to the groove of MHC Class II. Current knowledge of processing mechanisms and MHC Class II motifs does not yet enable this type of engineering, but it is inevitable that this should eventually be possible.

3. Short-Term Therapy and Long-Term Effects

3.1. Immunosuppression

One of the major goals in the practice of immunosuppression has been to use a short course of immunosuppression to achieve long-term effects in autoimmune diseases and in transplantation. Most current immunosuppressive agents are small drugs, which act intracellularly, all carrying the baggage of undesirable side effects and in most circumstances needing long-term, if not indefinite, administration.

Cells of the immune system sense their environments with surface-bound receptors and use these for numerous functions necessary to immunity—namely, antigen recognition, interaction with antigen presenting cells and cytokines, migration through lymphoid tissues to blood and back, and ultimately homing to tissues, responsiveness to chemokines, and the interaction of effector cells with their targets.

All of these surface receptor functions could be considered as potential targets for which drugs could be developed. For the adhesive interactions many of the interactions between receptors and their ligands are low affinity, and involve molecular interactions with many surface contact points. It has not been an easy matter to find small drugs with desirable pharmacokinetics, that can specifically block these interactions. For that reason antibodies have filled the vacuum. Many pharmaceutical and biotechnology companies have been uncomfortable with the notion of antibodies as drugs, arguing that eventually a small drug strategy would supervene. One reasonable concern has been that of immunogenicity—the assumption that all antibodies would eventually elicit neutralizing antiglobulin responses if given for long enough. In part that anxiety was allayed with the development of numerous ways of rendering antibodies very human-like, as discussed above. Other factors have included the need for parenteral administration, cost of production, and the depressing cost of patent licence fees that affect most aspects of antibody engineering.

To my mind, though, pharmaceutical companies have not yet grasped the notion that the best way to control the immune system is to exploit its own resources that have evolved over millions of years. The immune system has had to evolve mechanisms to produce the correct type of response to a defined stimulus, and to be able to turn off that response once its job is done. It has also developed strategies to ensure no damaging responses to self. All these controls require that lymphocytes sense their microenvironment through their surface receptors. What better way to control lymphocyte function than to block these surface receptors. What better agents to use than antibodies themselves. These molecules have evolved as hardy proteins resisting a wide range of adverse conditions, have extended half-lives, and are endowed with at least two binding sites per molecule. As drugs they are easily expressed, easily purified, and monitored.

The realization that antibodies to adhesion receptors or their ligands could be used to induce tolerance came with studies in rodents directed to enabling the acceptance of transplanted tissues *(6,7)*. Short therapeutic courses of CD4 and CD8 antibody combinations (which depleted T cells) had a longer immunosuppressive effect than could be accounted for by lymphocyte depletion or antibody presence. A subsequent graft of donor tissue many months after the primary graft had been administered demonstrated that tolerance had indeed been achieved.

Subsequent work demonstrated that antibodies that blocked function rather than depleted lymphocytes were equally good *(7)*, if not better, at achieving tolerance. A detailed investigation of mechanisms has demonstrated that long-term tolerance is maintained in these models, by a selected set of regulatory

CD4 T cells that ensure long-term "infectious tolerance" *(8,9)*. As long as the antigen remains in the system it sustains (or continues to vaccinate) these regulatory cells so they remain dominant, thus preventing aggression toward that antigen while allowing normal immune responses that protect the animal against infection.

A feature of infectious tolerance that may have clinical potential is the finding that tolerance to one antigen (say A) will enable tolerance to spread to further antigens (B, C, etc.) if they are linked to A on the same cell *(9)*. We have termed this linked suppression, and shown it to be dependent on regulatory CD4 T cells.

On reflection we have come to consider these therapeutic antibodies as a selective blindfold, holding back aggression while permitting regulation to develop. Transplantation tolerance has since been obtained with antibodies to CD3, CD40L, CD18, and with the fusion protein CTLA4-Ig *(10–16)*. We assume that similar mechanisms operate to maintain tolerance in these examples, although these still need to be resolved. Whatever the mechanisms turn out to be, the conclusion is that the potential for induction of therapeutic tolerance is intrinsic to the host, and that a wide range of different antibodies can be used to harness this.

The notion that small drugs may also be able to do this remains to be explored. However, the redundancy of signaling systems within cells may prove a constraint. For example, if cyclosporine were to inhibit the expansion of regulatory cells in the way it does immunocompetent cells, then although it is a powerful immunosuppressant, it might never be adequate to permit the emergence of a robust "infectious tolerance."

3.2. Is Tolerance Likely to Be Clinical Reality with Antibody Immunosuppression?

The transplant community has accepted that tolerance must be the ultimate goal in transplantation. Numerous experiments in rodents and more recently in primates attest to that. There is, however, a major problem in trying to achieve transplantation tolerance in the clinic. This is a direct result of the previous improvements in small-drug immunosuppression. Graft survival rates are so good generally at a year after transplantation that it is hard to justify any new protocol, and the process to conduct trials to show improvements can be very expensive and extensive. An interesting compromise has been that described as "Prope Tolerance" *(17)* whereby a short course of monoclonal antibody (mAb) therapy with CAMPATH-1H was given to deplete lymphocytes and the patient then maintained on monotherapy with half-dose cyclosporine. The preliminary results of this approach look encouraging enough to contemplate this sort of antibody + drug combination becoming the next stage of immuno-

Table 2
Approaching Tolerance with Antibodies

Transplantation	Autoimmune disease
Prope tolerance	Abolish inflammation, e.g., antitumor necrosis factor in RA
Complex cell therapies involving hemopoietic stem cells	Short-term therapy with nondepleting antibodies (e.g., diabetes, lupus, hyperthyroidism)
Use of linked suppression to achieve immune regulation	Short-term therapy with depleting antibodies, e.g., vasculitis, multiple sclerosis
Gene therapy to donor kidney to reduce immunogenicity	Short-term antibody depletion combined with marrow transplantation to replace defective hemopoietic genotype

suppressive practice. Even if the goal of complete tolerance is not realized for ethical reasons, the halfway house strategy outlined above may be sensible to ensure that the patient is always receiving some, albeit low, doses of immunosuppression, guarding against any factor that might precipitate a rejection event.

Current practice in the management of autoimmune diseases makes it equally difficult to identify if tolerance or reprogramming of the immune system can be elicited. It is perhaps in the difficult area of the vasculitides that the notion of short-term therapy for long-term effects can be said to have been demonstrated *(18)*. A short course of CAMPATH-1H antibody seems to enable patients to come up with other immunosuppressive agents with prolonged remissions. Relapses could be retreated with similar benefit.

Because T-cell recovery is relatively slow in adults following lymphocyte ablation, autoimmune diseases with a relatively good prognosis may not merit such powerful agents. In this set (e.g., juvenile diabetes, SLE, hyperthyroidism) the introduction of nonlytic antibodies selected for low toxicity (e.g., nonactivating CD3, CD18, CD40L, CD4) may likely be considered appropriate, and we can expect physicians to cautiously assess these agents as opportunities arise. The tolerogenic effects of equivalent antibodies in rodents are well documented, and the hazards seem small. **Table 2** summarizes some of the antibody-based approaches to achieving tolerance in the mature immune system.

4. Antibodies in Cancer Therapy

The challenge in cancer therapy is to be able to kill or inactivate a sufficient enough number of cancer cells to prevent relapse. The likelihood that a single agent, such as an antibody, would be sufficient to achieve a long-lasting remis-

Table 3
Emerging Issues in Cancer Therapy with Antibodies

Operational specificity vs precise specificity
Amplifying desired effector mechanisms
Evoking tumor dormancy
Helping tumor cells die (assisted suicide)
Improved chelation chemistry
Synergistic and adjuvant therapy
Targeting the blood supply
Avoiding antibody immunogenicity

sion is generally considered small. For that reason the ultimate value of an antibody may only be realized in combination with the other therapeutic modalities: surgery, chemotherapy, irradiation, and therapeutic vaccination. This introduction only highlights issues showing which concepts are beginning to change, largely a result of thinking beyond the traditional magic-bullet ideas.

4.1. Some Examples of Lateral Thinking in Cancer Therapy (see Table 3)

4.1.1. Specificity

The field has long been preoccupied with the notion that the most desirable antibody would be one that is truly tumor-specific, i.e., directed to an antigen found just on tumor cells and not on normal tissue. In reality the number of such tumor-specific antigens is small, and what really matters is operational specificity, reflected in whether one can get an adequate tumor kill with acceptable toxicity even if the antibody is reactive with normal tissues. This is best illustrated in the blood and immune systems, which can comfortably tolerate loss of differentiated cells as a price for treatment of leukemia, because multipotential stem cells can respond to replenish the depleted cell types. Less obviously, but equally relevant, one can see how antibodies might kill accessible (e.g., in the bone marrow) micrometastases from epithelial cancers without damaging normal epithelium, because the latter may be protected behind basement membranes and less amenable to antibody aggression.

4.1.2. Density and Quality of Antigen

The amount of antigen on the cell surface is one factor that may determine whether an antibody would harness sufficient natural effector mechanisms adequate to kill. However, antigen density alone is not sufficient, as it has become clear (empirically) that some surface antigens make good targets for lysis (e.g., CD52) and others poor targets, (e.g., CD45), even though the latter can be very abundant on the cell surface *(19)*.

For antibodies that block function or for those that deliver signals, then antigen density may be less significant. A growing optimism is emerging around the notion that cancer cells may be "signaled" by certain antibodies that would encourage them to become dormant, undergo apoptosis *(20)*, or become more sensitive to other therapeutic modalities. In many instances cells will evade destruction if they generate antigen-loss variants or if the effector mechanisms are just not powerful enough. The latter has been the subject of controversy ever since mAb therapy began. The issue has very much been one of whether natural effector mechanisms are adequate, whether they can be amplified, or whether indeed they need to be supplemented by targeted drugs, toxins, or radioisotopes. Whatever the amplification strategy, attention needs to be paid to bystander destruction of cells in the vicinity, and this is where choice of radioisotope, prodrug, or synergistic agent will be crucial.

4.2. Targeting the Blood Supply of Cancers

One of the major problems of antibody therapy in cancer is that of penetration of the antibody into the tumor. Large antibodies do not diffuse as well as small nutrients into the tumor mass. An emerging field is one that takes account of the fact that cancers grow together with their own blood vasculature to supply nutrients. If one could block the process of neo-angiogenesis or target the endothelium of cancer cells to artificially occlude vessels through a thrombotic reaction reaction, this could supplement other therapies directed to the cancer itself.

References

1. Chiller, J. M., Habicht, G. S., and Weigle, W. O. (1970) Cellular sites of immunologic unresponsivenss. *Proc. Natl. Acad. Sci. USA* **65**, 551–556.
2. Benjamin, R. J. and Waldmann, H. (1986) Induction of tolerance by monoclonal antibody therapy. *Nature* **320**, 449–451.
3. Benjamin, R. J., Cobbold, S. P., Clark, M. R., and Waldmann, H. (1986) Tolerance of rat monoclonal antibodies: implications for serotherapy. *J. Exp. Med.* **163**, 1539–1552.
4. Isaacs, J. D. and Waldmann, H. (1994) Helplessness as a strategy for avoiding antiglobulin responses to therapeutic monoclonal antibodies. *Therapeutic Immunol.* **1**, 303–312.
5. Gilliland, L. K., Walsh, L. A., Frewin, M. R., Wise, M., Tone, M., Hale, G., Kioussis, D., and Waldmann, H. (1999) Elimination of the immunogenicity of therapeutic antibodies. *J. Immunol.* **162**, 3663–3671.
6. Cobbold, S. P., Martin, G., Qin, S., and Waldmann, H. (1986) Monoclonal antibodies to promote marrow engraftment and tissue graft tolerance. *Nature* **323**, 164–166.

7. Qin, S., Wise, M., Cobbold, S., Leong, L., Kong, Y.-C., Parnes, J. R., and Waldmann, H. (1990) Induction of tolerance in peripheral T cells with monoclonal antibodies. *Eur. J. Immunol.* **20,** 2737–2745.

8. Qin, S., Cobbold, S. P., Pope, H., Elliott, J., Kioussis, D., and Waldmann, H. (1993) Infectious transplantation tolerance. *Science* **12(259),** 974–977.

9. Davies, J. D., Leong, L. Y. W., Mellor, A., Cobbold, S. P., and Waldmann, H. (1996) T-cell suppression in transplantation tolerance through linked recognition. *J. Immunol.* **156,** 3602–3607.

10. Isobe, M., Suzuki, J., Yamazaki, S., and Sekiguchi, M. (1996) Acceptance of primary skin graft after treatment with anti-intercellular adhesion molecule-1 and anti-leukocyte function-associated antigen-1 monoclonal antibodies in mice. *Transplantation* **62(3),** 411–413.

11. Chavin, K. D., Qin, L., Lin, J., Yagita, H., Bromberg, J. S. (1993) Combined anti-CD2 and anti-CD3 receptor monoclonal antibodies induce donor-specific tolerance in a cardiac transplant model. *J. Immunol.* **151,** 7249–7259.

12. Krieger, N. R., Most, D., Bromberg, J. S., Holm, B., Huie, P., Sibley, R. K., Dafoe, D. C., Alfrey, E. J. (1996) Coexistence of Th1- and Th2-type cytokine profiles in anti-CD2 monoclonal antibody-induced tolerance. *Transplantation* **62,** 1285–1292.

13. Chatenoud, L., Thervett, E., Primo, J., and Bach, J. F. (1994) Anti-CD3 antibody induces long-term remission of overt autoimmunity in non-obese diabetic mice. *Proc. Natl. Acad. Sci. USA* **91,** 123–127.

14. Lenschow, D. J., Zeng, Y., Thistlethwaite, J. R., Montag, A., Brady, W., Gibson, M. G., Linsley, P. S., and Bluestone, J. A. (1992) Long-term survival of xenogeneic pancreatic islet grafts induced by CTLA4lg. *Science* **57,** 789.

15. Pearson, T. C., Alexander, D. Z., Winn, K. J., Linsley, P. S., Lowry, R. P., and Larsen, C. P (1994) Transplantation tolerance induced by CTLA4-Ig. *Transplantation* **57(12),** 1701–1706.

16. Steurer, W., Nickerson, P. W., Steele, A. W., Steiger, J., Zheng, X. X., and Strom, T. B. (1998) Ex vivo coating of islet cell allografts with murine CTLA4/Fc promotes graft tolerance. *J. Immunol.* **155(3),** 1165.

17. Calne, R., Friend, P., Moffatt, S., Bradley, A., Hale, G., Firth, J., Bradley, J., Smith, K., and Waldmann, H. (1998) Prope tolerance, perioperative Campath 1H, and low-dose cyclosporin monotherapy in renal allograft patients. *Lancet* **351,** 1701,1702.

18. Lockwood, C. M., Thiru, S., Steard, S., Hale, G., Isaacs, J., Wraight, P., Elliott, J., and Waldmann, H. (1996) Treatment of refractory Wegener's granulomatosis with humanized monoclonal antibodies. *Q. J. Med.* **89,** 903–912.

19. Bindon, C. I., Hale, G., and Waldmann, H. (1988) Importance of antigen specificity for complement-mediated lysis by monoclonal antibodies. *Eur. J. Immunol.* **18,** 1507–1514.

20. Coney, L. R., Daniel, P. T., Sanborn, D., Dhein, J., Debatin, K. M., Krammer, P. H., and Zurawski, V. R. (1994) Apoptotic cell death induced by a mouse-human anti-APO-1 chimeric antibody leads to tumor regression. *Int. J. Cancer* **58,** 562–567.

6

Antibodies for Neoplastic Disease

Solid Tumors

Ian T. W. Matthews

1. Introduction

The ease with which polyclonal, monoclonal, and engineered antibody fragments can be prepared allows access to a series of reagents with high selectivity and affinity. These reagents therefore have long held promise as a means of influencing the growth and spread of malignant disease. Over a number of decades therapeutic antibodies have been developed either as single entities or conjugated to a variety of potential disease-ameliorating agents.

Single entity antibodies can have their effects either through antigen- or nonantigen-binding site interactions leading to, for instance, complement fixation or T cell activation. Conjugates of antibodies have been prepared both by chemistry and by molecular biology, leading to a range of reagents conjugated to protein toxins, organic toxins, chelating agents, radioisotopes, enzymes, and photosensitizers. This chapter will be restricted to some modern clinical experiences with a variety of antibodies with and without toxic passengers in the most difficult area of cancer therapy, the solid tumor.

2. Immunotoxins

The word "toxin" can be applied to a number of low- and high-mol wt agents either directly antitumor-progressive, or as in the case of photodynamic therapy and prodrugs, indirectly antitumor progressive. The clinical use of immunotoxins has found success in the therapy of lymphoma (*1*) and leukemia (*2*) but has been spectacularly unsuccessful in the treatment of solid tumors. The apparent ease with which xenograft-bearing mice could be cured spurred on a number of clinical trials, the conclusions of which were far from positive.

From: *Methods in Molecular Medicine, Vol. 40: Diagnostic and Therapeutic Antibodies*
Edited by: A. J. T. George and C. E. Urch © Humana Press Inc., Totowa, NJ

Recently, for instance, a monoclonal antibody (mAb) (791T) that recognizes a 72 kDa glycoprotein on colorectal and ovarian carcinomas and an osteogenic sarcoma was conjugated to ricin A chain (XMMCO-791/RTA) and administered as a Phase I trial to 12 patients with metastatic colorectal carcinoma. The conclusion (3) of this trial was that a number of severe toxic side effects were seen but no antitumor effect was apparent. In a further study (4), eight patients with leptomeningeal neoplasia (although not a classical solid tumor) were treated by intraventricular administration of an antitransferrin antibody (454A12) linked to recombinant ricin A chain. Admin-istered doses of <120 μg showed little toxicity and although tumor burden was reduced it was not cleared in any of the patients.

Despite the intense effort in the biotechnology of this area there are few modern published clinical studies of immunotoxins in the treatment of solid tumors. Within this biotechnology area lie some elegant molecular biology and conjugation chemistry, which has lead to the construction of precise conjugates with optimum antibody activity and optimum toxin effect on release from their conjugates. In this last point lies one of the reasons for the poor clinical showing of these reagents. In general the protein-based toxins need to be within the cell to have their full toxic effects realized and will therefore cause little bystander cell death. In general the low-mol-wt organic toxins should have a greater effect if released extracellularly (cf. enzyme-activated prodrugs), allowing a greater chance of bystander cell death.

This bystander cell death is of considerable importance since the heterogeneous nature of human tumors means that not all the tumor cells will express enough, or indeed any, of the antibody recognition epitope. A group at the Bowman Gray School of Medicine in Winston-Salem, NC, is developing an innovation in this area by genetically engineering human lymphokine-activated killer lymphocytes (LAK cells) to produce their own immunotoxin (5).

This toxin is comprised of a single-chain antibody directed against a cancer-specific antigen (HER-2) linked to the cytotoxic domain of Pseudomonas exo-toxin-A. It is hoped that tumor-infiltrating lymphocytes can be made to release their immunotoxin at the tumor site and also call in other lymphocytes to increase the therapeutic potential. Other, perhaps more conventional, work in this area is aimed at the targeting of some of the newer and extremely toxic natural products, such as calicheamicin (6) and maytansinoid (7). Accumulated knowledge in this area has identified the main areas of difficulty in the successful treatment of solid tumors with immunotoxins. These difficulties include the immunological response to large toxin conjugates, the generally poor absolute localization amount, which is sublethal to the tumor, the intratumoral pressure inhibiting toxic substance diffusion, the lack of antigen homogeneity within human tumors, and finally, side effects resulting from nontarget tissue uptake. It was hoped that many of the above difficulties could be overcome by the use of targeted therapeutic radioactive nuclides.

3. Radioimmunotherapy

The targeting of therapeutic radioisotopes has its attractions, not least because of the real possibility of bystander tumor cell death, leading to the successful management of some solid tumors, particularly those of a smaller size and expressing high densities of antigen.

Depending on the therapeutic setting a number of radionuclides with different properties can be selected for linking to mAbs. A few of these would include b emitters ^{90}Y, ^{131}I, ^{186}Re, ^{188}Re, ^{177}Lu, ^{153}Sm, and γ emitters, such as ^{211}At or ^{212}Bi. Once again, in lymphoma the use of radioimmunotherapy is close to being used as a standard treatment *(8)*. In solid tumors, however, clinical success has been limited *(9)* although there have been some notable exceptions. Animal experiments suggest that radioimmunotherapy is superior to chemotherapy, particularly in an adjuvant setting *(10)*. A number of clinical studies have been conducted in a range of solid tumors. Although these studies have been conducted under different disease stage circumstances, positive conclusions can be drawn regarding the effectiveness of this type of therapy. A number of studies have been conducted in ovarian cancer with either minimal disease or advanced disease. In a study conducted on 52 patients with epithelial ovarian cancer, an antibody against human milk fat globulin (HMFG1) was linked to ^{90}Yt and administered intraperitoneally to patients who had previously been treated by surgery and chemotherapy. Twenty-one of these patients were considered to be disease free and therefore this treatment was classified as adjuvant therapy. The conclusion of this study was that after follow-up of 3–62 mo patients with advanced ovarian cancer who achieved complete remission following conventional therapy would probably benefit from this treatment *(11)*.

Another group studied the effect of ^{131}I-labeled antibody (MoV18) on 13 patients with ovarian cancer and a dose of 3700 MBq injected intraperitoneally produced five complete remissions, five stable disease, and three progressive disease *(12)*. Of nine recent studies selected at random from the literature (1987–1994), only two reported no response to this therapy, which suggests intraperitoneal injection of high levels of radiolabeled mAb can have a positive effect on the treatment of patients with minimal and advanced disease.

Colorectal carcinoma has also been studied clinically for its ability to yield to radioimmunotherapy. A study with an ^{131}Y isotope labeled mAb to carcinoembryonic antigen (CEA) was administered intraperitoneally to 41 patients with gastrointestinal tumors. The final total tumor dose given was greater than normal at 8900 cGy; this, however, produced 10 complete remissions and six partial remissions (13). Perhaps a more typical study involved an [131]Y monoclonal (A33) that was given to 23 patients at an injected activity of 1110–3478 MBq, giving a maximum tolerated dose of 75mCi/m^2 to the bowel. This treatment achieved four mixed responses but little toxicity (14). Of 10 recent trials only two reported any complete remissions, although most did report some partial or mixed response. It is probable that in an adjuvant setting these radiolabeled reagents have a positive effect but for gross disease more studies need to be carried out to determine which antibody/radiolabel and what treatment schedule has the most beneficial effect. The apparent lack of major toxic side effects may also be of considerable importance affecting the quality of life in patients with advanced disease. Colorectal carcinoma is not considered to be radiosensitive. Therefore, any beneficial effects with this type of treatment could be considered positive for continuing these studies.

Gliomas are tumors that should lend themselves to this type of therapy mainly because of the potential for intratumor administration. In one major study 24 patients who had already been treated by surgery, radiotherapy, and chemotherapy were treated with two mouse monoclonal anti-tenascin antibodies (BC-2 and BC-4) labeled with [131]I. The antibodies were administered in an escalating dose ranging from 15–57 mCi, which in some cases was repeated up to four times. The mean radiation dose to thetumor was 36.5 cGy/MBq of injected [131]I. This treatment resulted in three complete remissions (15 mo), three partial remissions (11 mo), and five tumor stabilizations (9 mo) (15). In another study using a mixture of antibodies to epidermal growth factor receptor and placental alkaline phosphatase a total tumor dose of up to 12.5 Gy was given, which produced 6 out of 10 clinical improvements and two radiographic regressions (16). Despite being radioinsensitive, radioimmunotherapy of gliomas should produce life-lengthening treatment, perhaps particularly with two- or three-step treatment schedules (17) and also as a part of combination therapy.

A number of other malignancies that have been treated with this type of reagent include melanoma, breast, lung, liver, neuroblastoma, and prostate. Of these, the most promising is the use of radioimmunotherapy in liver tumors. Of five recent clinical studies in a variety of liver tumors, complete remissions were noted in three of these studies (18–20) and partial remissions in the remainder (21,22).

A consequence of any form of therapy involving radioactivity is the potential for rapid regrowth of malignant cells that have not been subject to a lethal dose of radioactivity. This more than anything can be a major impedance to a successful therapeutic outcome. Perhaps this could be overcome by the use of growth inhibiting compounds administered at the appropriate time. With or without any additional therapy this type of radioactivity-based antibody-guided therapy is becoming an important addition to the clinical anticancer armorarium. As an alternative, antibody based focusing of the body's own multifactorial defenses against malignancies remains a tantalizing prospect.

4. Bispecific Antibodies

It has been hoped that the ability to simultaneously bind two different antigens or one antigen and one hapten could produce reagents that would be simple to label with a variety of disease-modifying agents. These haptens or antigens have included toxins, cytotoxics, radioactive compounds, prodrugs, or even cell-surface proteins that can focus the body's own cellular defenses against cancer by crosslinking cell surface receptors of two different cell types. Bispecific antibodies could be considered the magic bullet of magic bullets. These reagents can potentially be made even more useful by the construction of bispecific single-chain antibody fragments that are smaller (~50 kDa) and therefore penetrate further, and may be without the kidney- and liver-retaining effector functions *(23)*.

Many of the modern clinical studies have concentrated on the use of bispecific antibodies as immune modulating agents in attempts to focus the attentions of T-lymphocytes generating a local immune response against any malignancy. For this approach to be successful these reagents must be able to activate immune effector pathways, such as complement fixation and antibody-dependent cell-mediated cytotoxicity (ADCC) aimed primarily at the tumor. Patient trials to date show that peripheral blood mononuclear cells can be activated ex vivo acquiring tumor targeting and tumor growth inhibiting characteristics. In one such study *(24)* 28 ovarian cancer patients with limited intraperitoneal disease and after first-line therapy were treated with in a Phase II trial with two intraperitoneal 5 d cycles of activated peripheral blood mononuclear cells activated and retargeted by a bispecific antibody (OCTR). This antibody was directed to CD3 on T cells and the folate receptor on ovarian cancer cells. Despite, as it is documented, unfavorable tumor characteristics, 7 of the 28 showed complete or partial intraperitoneal responses with strict surgical evaluation. In most cases, however, the disease relapsed outside the peritoneal cavity and in one case, despite complete intraperitoneal response, there was progressive disease in the retroperitoneal lymph nodes. It was concluded that locoregional immunotherapy of ovarian cancer with this bispecific antibody can result in tumor regression.

Improvements in systemic tumor response are, however, needed before this approach with this particular antibody is to be useful as an adjunctive treatment following chemotherapy in patients with minimal disease. To treat large numbers of patients it would, however, be beneficial to have this activation and refocusing take place in vivo. Bispecific antibody, MDX-210, is a chemically prepared construct comprising a Fab fragment raised against the Her-2/neu proto-oncogene product and crosslinked to an anti-CD64 Fab. The Her-2/neu proto-oncogene product, human epidermal growth factor receptor 2 (p185HER2), is overexpressed in 20–30% of ovarian and breast cancers and CD64 is the high-affinity Fc IgG receptor. This antibody allows effective targeting of cytotoxic monocyte-derived macrophages and interferon-treated neutrophils in vitro. This antibody was used in a Phase Ia/Ib clinical trial in patients with advanced breast or ovarian cancer. The antibody was administered as either a single dose or multiple doses ranging from 0.35–10.0 mg/m^2.

Even at high doses the antibody was well tolerated, hypotension being the most serious side effect. Out of 10 patients on the single-dose regimen that could be evaluated, one patient with metastatic breast cancer had a partial response and one with metastatic ovarian cancer had a mixed response. Of eight patients on the multidose regimen that could be evaluated, one patient with metastatic breast cancer had stable disease for 5 mo. The conclusion of this study (25) was that MDX-210 would be effective for treating patients with tumors that overexpress HER-2/neu and particularly when the disease is minimal. It is early in the clinical use of these reagents and more understanding will be required to determine which of the immune effector pathways is the most important for tumor killing, or perhaps getting the right blend of a number of them. These reagents will undoubtedly take their place in the cancer clinic, but it remains to be seen whether their main target will be the solid or disseminated tumor, and whether antibodies can be designed to allow administration of a large amount to maximize their specific effects without a concomitant increase in side effects.

5. Neat Antibody

The use of unconjugated antibody to facilitate tumor cell death through an adjuvant effect is attractive. If such an antibody could be administered in a large amount without undue side effects in a minimal but still life-threatening disease, then this type of therapy could be beneficial. An antibody chosen for such a study (26) was against the epithelial antigen 17-1A and the disease was resected Dukes' stage C colorectal carcinoma. The patient population (189), who were free of observable residual tumor, was divided into two groups; an observation regimen or postoperative treatment with 500 mg 17-1A antibody followed by monthly infusions of 100 mg. After a median follow-up of 5 yr the antibody-treated group had a reduced death rate of 30% and a decreased recurrence rate of 27%. The side effects were reported as minor; the most serious were four steroid responsive anaphylactic reactions.

The conclusion was that adjuvant therapy with this antibody to 17-1A extends life and prolongs remission in patients with colorectal cancer of Dukes' stage C, although the exact mechanism or mechanisms of tumor cell death are still unclear.

6. Idiotypic Network Immunization

Antibodies have a molecular weight and composition that makes them good antigens; thus, antibodies can be made against antibodies. Antibodies are categorized as having three major antigenic determinants: isotypic, allotypic, and idiotypic. The isotypic determinants distinguish the C regions of the H-chain (and subclasses) and the L-chain types. Each isotype is encoded by a distinct gene that is characteristic for a particular mammalian species and is present in all members of that species. Allotypic determinants reflect genetic polymorphism of immunoglobulins within one species. The idiotypic determinants exist as a result of unique structures generated by the hypervariable subregions (complementarity-determining regions; CDR) on H and L chains. Idiotypic antigenic determinants (idiotopes) are classified, according to the antibodies raised against them, as α-idiotopes (outside the antigen binding region), β-idiotopes (close to the antigenic binding region), and γ-idiotopes (against the binding region). Anti-idiotypic antibodies (antibodies to idiotopes) can be formed naturally or induced artificially by external introduction of antibody and are defined serologically by the reaction of anti-idiotypic antibodies (Ab2) with antibodies bearing the idiotopes (Ab1).

The presence of self-generated anti-idiotypic antibodies is explained in the idiotypic network theory *(27)*, which suggests that the formation of anti-antibodies has an immune regulatory function, and that the initial antigen can be reflected in a so-called mirror image anti-idiotypic antibody (Ab2).

The mirror image anti-idiotypic antibody has been used as a surrogate antigen to stimulate the immune response in a number of clinical trials. In one study *(28)* that comprised two clinical trials a mouse mAb (MF11-30) that carried the internal image of the human high-mol-wt-melanoma-associated antigen (HMW-MAA) was administered without adjuvant, subcutaneously to patients with stage IV malignant melanoma on d 0, 7, and 28. Additionally, if anti-anti-idiotypic antibodies were not seen then further anti-idiotypic antibody was given.

The first trial saw 16 patients given an initial dose of 0.5 mg/injection rising to 4 mg/injection. In the second trial the antibody was administered at a dose of 2 mg/injection since this dose had previously been shown to induce an anti-anti-idiotypic response. Over the duration of the treatment (34 wk) little toxicity was seen in either trial and from the second trial one patient achieved a complete remission with disappearance of multiple abdominal lymph nodes for a duration of 95 wk. Minor responses were seen in three other patients.

The conclusion of this study was that MF11-30 mouse anti-idiotypic antibody bearing an internal reflection of the HMW-MAA might be useful for specific immunotherapy of melanoma patients. A further immunotherapy trial *(29)* by the same group used a different anti-idiotypic antibody (MK2-23) but against the same melanoma antigen. Here the anti-idiotypic antibody was administered with adjuvant and as a carrier conjugate to increase the immunogenicity. This treatment induced humoral anti-HMW-MAA immunity in about 60% of the immunized patients, which was associated with a statistically significant increase in duration of survival.

In another study *(30)* the generation of an anti-idiotypic antibody network has been suggested as the mechanism by which the administered antibody has been effective. Ab3 antibodies were observed in 47% of patients with metastatic colorectal carcinoma after administration of mouse mAb 17-1A (Ab1). Patients who developed Ab3 responses survived significantly longer than patients who did not; 80 wk as opposed to 38 wk. Once again it is suggested that the production of an antiidiotypic response can have a positive outcome on the progression of this difficult-to-manage disease.

In a further study *(31)* ovarian cancer patients received an anti-CA125 mouse mAb (Ab1, B43.13) and the immune status was investigated by measuring the anti-idiotypic (Ab2), anti-anti-idiotypic (Ab3), anti-isotypic, interferon-γ, and CA125 levels. Of 50 patients treated, 26 had elevated Ab2 levels and out of these 26 patients 11 had high Ab3 levels. Eight of 22 patients had elevated interferon-γ levels. The tentative conclusion to this study was that there was a association between survival of these patients and anti-idiotypic induction.

The generation of an anti-idiotypic cascade for the purposes of cancer immunotherapy is a highly complex process and the in vivo characteristics in relation to therapeutic effect are little understood. Any of the antibodies that have tumor-binding characteristics produced in an anti-idiotypic cascade could have the right effector functions to trigger a cytotoxic effect or act in a cytotoxic manner either individually or in concert. The human anti-idiotypic antibody 105AD7 derived from an antibody to the tumor antigen gp72 has been shown to induce antitumor cellular responses in animal studies and to prolong survival in patients with metastatic colorectal carcinoma. Results of a number of ex vivo studies *(32)* with treated and nontreated patients showed that at 1–2 wk postimmunization, significant killing of autologous tumor cells occurred that was not due to natural killer cell activity. Two to three weeks post-immunization, however, enhanced natural killer cell activity was seen. These findings suggest that human antibody 105AD7 immunization of patients with metastatic colorectal carcinoma enhances cytotoxicity by a specific and a nonspecific nature.

The immunization of patients with either primary (Ab1) or secondary (Ab2) antibodies for cancer therapy may be of great importance, as with radio-immunotherapy, selecting the disease, and the stage that is most susceptible to this approach will be vital. Increasing scientific understanding of each of the many effector functions that could increase an antibody's cytotoxic effect may also allow further design of disease-specific cytotoxic antibodies.

7. Conclusion

Major advances in the treatment of solid tumors may come from a number of different areas. These could include targeting of a genetically altered form of the body's own defenses, as highlighted earlier with the antibody immunotoxin secreting T-lymphocytes, or by replacing deleted or mutated genes by gene therapy. Harnessing the destructive power of target selective/replicating viruses may also be fruitful. The use of compounds that have their effects on restricting the blood supply allows a longer retention of a potential disease-altering agent. Additionally, affecting the blood-supply-forming capabilities of solid tumors with antiangiogenic compounds could have considerable consequences for solid tumor therapy. The use of cancer cells as vaccines is achieving a recent revival by showing early promise in metastatic melanoma.

If any of the above antibody-based therapies are to have any real effect on human survival it is important to marry the therapy to the disease and not to ask too much of these reagents. Radioimmunotherapy and unconjugated antibody therapy will have a role to play in the clinic; the degree of success of this role will be disease-specific, regimen-specific, antibody-specific, and isotope-specific. Determining whether these reagents will have a bigger impact if administered with other forms of treatment, old and experimental, may also be fruitful. The window of opportunity for these reagents may be closing and new windows opening for some of the newer chemical, biochemical, and biological modalities. Are there lessons to be learned from the past use of antibody-based reagents, which have been with us for many years?

References

1. Liu, S. Y. and Press, O. W. (1997) The potential for immunoconjugates in lymphoma therapy. *Haematol. Oncol. Clin. North Am.* **11**, 987–1006.
2. Frankel, A. E., Laver, J. H., Willingham, M. C., Burns, L. J., Kersey, J. H., and Vallera, D. A. (1997) Therapy of patients with T-cell lymphomas and leukemias using an anti-CD7 monoclonal antibody-ricin A chain immunotoxin. *Leuk. Lymphoma* **26**, 287–298.
3. LoRusso, P. M., Lomen, P. L., Redman, B. G., Poplin, E., Bander, J. J., and Valdivieso, M. (1995) Phase I study of monoclonal antibody-ricin A chain

immunoconjugate Xomazyme-791 in patients with metastatic colon cancer. *Am. J. Clin. Oncol.* **18,** 307–312.

4. Laske, D. W., Muraszko, K. M., Oldfield, E. H., DeVroom, H. L., Sung, C., Dedrick, R. L. Simon, T. R., Clandrea, J., Copeland, C., Katz, D., Greenfield, L., Groves, E. S., Houston, L. L., and Youle, R. J. (1997) Intraventricular immunotoxin therapy for leptomeningeal neoplasia. *Neurosurgery* **41,** 1039–1049.

5. Chen, S. Y., Yang, A. G., Chen, J. D., Kute, T., King, C. R., Collier, J., Cong, Y., Yao, C., and Huang, X. F. (1997) Potent antitumour activity of a new class of tumour-specific killer cells. *Nature* **385,** 78–80.

6. Yarranton, G. (1998) Antibody-calicheamicin conjugates for the treatment of cancer. Antibody Engineering. New Technology, Application and Commercialisation. IBC event code IB 146. March 2–3, The Royal Society, London, UK.

7. Liu, C., Tadayoni, B. M., Bourret, L. A., Mattocks, K. M., Derr, S. M., Widdison, W. C., Kedersha, N. L., Ariniello, P. D., Goldmacher, V. S., Lambert, J. M., Blattler, W. A., and Chari, R. V. (1996) Eradication of large colon tumor xenografts by targeted delivery of maytansinoids. *Proc. Natl. Acad. Sci. USA* **93(16),** 8618–8623.

8. Press, O. W., Eary, J. F., Appelbaum, F. R., Martin, P. J., Badger, C. C., Nelp, W. B., Glenn, S., Butchko, G., Fisher, D., Porter, B., Matthews, D. C., Fisher, L. D., and Bernstein, I. D. (1993) Radiolabelled-antibody therapy of B-cell lymphoma with autologous bone marrow support. *N. Engl. J. Med.* **329,** 1219–1224.

9. Goldenberg, D. M., ed. (1995) *Cancer Therapy with Radiolabelled Antibodies.* CRC, Boca Raton, FL.

10. Blumenthal, R. D., Sharkey, R. M., Natale, A. M., Kashi, R., Wong, G., and Goldenberg, D. M. (1994) Comparison of equitoxic radioimmunotherapy and chemotherapy in the treatment of human colonic cancer xenografts. *Cancer Res.* **54,** 142–151.

11. Hird, V., Maraveyas, A., Snook, D., Dhokia, B. Soutter, W. P., Meares, C., Stewart, J. S., Mason, P., Lambert, H. E., and Epenetos, A. A. (1993) Adjuvant therapy of ovarian cancer with radioactive monoclonal antibody. *Br. J. Cancer* **68(2),** 403–406.

12. Canevari, S., Miotti, S., Bottere, F., Valota, O., and Colnaghi, M. I. (1993) Ovarian carcinoma therapy with monoclonal antibodies. *Hybridoma* **12,** 501–507.

13. Riva, P., Tison, V., Arista, A., et al. (1993) Radioimmunotherapy of gastrointestinal cancer and glioblastomas. *Int. J. Biol. Markers* **8,** 192–197.

14. Welt, S., Divgi, C. R., Kemeny, N., et al. (1994) Phase I/II study of iodine 131-labelled monoclonal antibody A33 in patients with advanced colon cancer. *J. Clin. Oncol.* **12,** 1561–1571.

15. Riva, P., Arista, A., Tison, V., et al. (1994) Intralesional radioimmunotherapy of malignant glioma. An effective treatment in recurrent tumours. *Cancer* **73,** 1076–1082.

16. Kalofonos, H. P., Pawlikowska, T. R., Hemingway, A., et al. (1989) Antibody guided diagnosis and therapy of brain gliomas using radiolabelled monoclonal

antibodies against epidermal growth factor receptor and placental alkaline phosphatase. *J. Nucl. Med.* **30,** 1636–1645.

17. Grana, C., Chinol, M., Magnani, P., Corti, A., Sidoli, A., Siccardi, A. G., and Paganelli, G. (1996) In vivo tumour targeting based on the avidin-biotin system. *Tumour Targeting* **2,** 230–239.

18. Stillwagon, G. B., Order, S. E., Klein, J. L., et al. (1987) Multi-modality treatment of primary nonresectable intrahepatic cholangiocarcinoma with I-131 anti-CEA: a Radiation Therapy Oncology Group Study. *Int. J. Radiat. Oncol. Biol. Phys.* **13,** 687–695.

19. Order, S. E., Stillwagon, G. B., Klein, J. L., et al. (1985) Iodine-131-antiferritin, a new treatment modality in hepatoma: a Radiation Therapy Oncology Group Study. *J. Clin. Oncol.* **3,** 1573–1582.

20. Order, S. E., Vriesendorp, H. M., Klein, J. L., and Leichner, P. K. (1988) A phase I study of 90yttrium antiferritin: dose escalation and tumour dose. *Antibody Immunoconj. Radiopharm.* **1,** 163–168.

21. Zeng, Z. C., Tang, Z. Y., Xie, H., et al. (1993) Radioimmunotherapy for unresectable hepatocellular carcinoma using 131-Hepama-1 mAb: preliminary results. *J. Cancer Res. Clin. Oncol.* **119,** 257–259.

22. Siegel, J. A., Pawlyk, D. A., Lee, R. E., et al. (1990) Tumor, red marrow and organ dosimetry for 131I-labelled anti-carcinoembryonic antigen monoclonal antibody. *Cancer Res.* **50,** 1039s–1042s.

23. Thirion, S., Motmans, K., Heyligen, H., Janssens, J., Raus, J., and Vandevyver, C. (1997) Mono- and bispecific single-chain antibody fragments for cancer therapy. *Euro. J. Can. Prev.* **5,** 507–511.

24. Canevari, S., Stoter, G., Arienti, F., Bolis, G., Colnaghi, M. I., Di Re, E. M., and Eggermont, A. A. (1995) Regression of advanced ovarian carcinoma by intraperitoneal treatment with autologous T lymphocytes retargeted by a bispecific antibody. *J. Natl. Cancer Inst.* **87,** 1463–1469.

25. Valone, F. H., Kaufman, P. A., Guyre, P. M., Lewis, L. D., Memoli, V. Deo, Y., Graziano, R., Fisher, J. L., Meyer, L., Mrozek-Orlowski, M., et al. (1995) Phase Ia/Ib trial of bispecific antibody MDX-210 in patients with advanced breast or ovarian cancer that over-expresses the proto-oncogene HER-2/neu. *J. Clin. Oncol.* **13,** 2281–2292.

26. Riethmuller, G., Schneider-Gadicke, E., Schlimok, G., Schmiegel, W., Raab, R., Hoffken, K., Gruber, R., Pichlmaier, H., Hirche, H., Pichlmyr, R., et al. (1994) Randomised trial of monoclonal antibody for adjuvant therapy of resected Dukes' C colorectal carcinoma. German Cancer Aid 17-1A Study Group. *Lancet* **343,** 1177–1183.

27. Jerne, N. K. (1974) Towards a network theory of the immune system. *Ann. Immunol. C* **25,** 373–389.

28. Mittleman, A., Chen, Z. J., Kageshita, T., Yang, H., Yamada, M., Baskind, P., Goldberg, N., Ahmed, T., and Arlin, Z. (1990) Active specific immunotherapy in patients with melanoma. A clinical trial with mouse antiidiotypic monoclonal antibodies elicited with syngeneic anti-high-molecular-weight-melanoma-associated antigen monoclonal antibodies. *J. Clin. Invest.* **86,** 2136–2144.

29. Mittelman, A., Wang, X., Matsumoto, K., and Ferrone, S. (1995) Antiidiotypic response and clinical course of the disease in patients with malignant melanoma immunized with mouse antiidiotypic monoclonal antibody MK2-23. *Hybridoma* **14,** 175–181.

30. Frodin, J. E., Faxas, M. E., Hagstrom, B., Lefvert, A. K., Masucci, G., Nilsson, B., Steinitz, M., Unger, P., and Mellstedt, H. (1991) Induction of anti-idiotypic (ab2) and anti-anti-idiotypic (ab3) antibodies in patients treated with the mouse monoclonal antibody 17-1A (ab1). Relation to the clinical outcome-an important antitumoral effector function? *Hybridoma* **4,** 421–431.

31. Madiyalakan, R., Sykes, T. R., Dharampaul, S., Sykes, C. J., Baum, R. P., Hor, G., and Noujaim, A. A. (1995) Antiidiotypic induction therapy: evidence for the induction of immune response through the idiotype network in patients with ovarian cancer after administration of anti-CA125 murine monoclonal antibody B43.13. *Hybridoma* **14,** 199–203.

32. Durrant, L. G., Buckley, T. J., Denton, G. W., Hardcastle, J. D., Sewell, H. F., and Robins, R. A. (1994) Enhanced cell-mediated tumor killing in patients immunized with human monoclonal antiidiotypic antibody 105AD7. *Cancer Res.* **54,** 4837–4840.

7

The Application of Monoclonal Antibodies in the Treatment of Lymphoma

Martin J. Glennie, Jamie Honeychurch, Ruth R. French, and Alison L. Tutt

1. Introduction

Monoclonal antibodies (mAbs) appear to offer many benefits for the treatment of cancer and in particular lymphoma (*1*). They are natural products that can be made with precise specificity and in almost unlimited amounts. In addition, mAbs can be selected or engineered to efficiently recruit the body's effector systems, such as complement and natural killer cells, against the unwanted cells in much the same way as they might destroy an invading pathogen. Unfortunately, progress in the clinic has been slow, and the cytotoxic activity achieved with mAb in vitro has failed to be transferred into patients. Despite this rather disappointing outcome, recent results in treating non-Hodgkin's lymphoma (NHL) and chronic lymphocytic leukemia (CLL) with anti-CD20 and anti-CD52 (CAMPATH 1) mAb suggest, at least for certain neoplasms, that the situation may be changing (*2,3*). Stevenson and colleagues (personal communication) have recently achieved more than 70% complete responses in posttransplant lymphoma treated with a chimeric anti-CD20 mAb, and Maloney and co-workers (*2*) recently reported a 50% response rate in relapsed, low-grade, NHL, with a 10–11 mo duration. Encouragingly, patients in these studies did not raise antibody responses to the treatment anti-CD20 mAb and, unlike the situation following therapy in many lymphomas with anti-idiotype (Id) mAb, the emergence of antigen-negative tumors has not been seen (*4*). To underline its clinical success, anti-CD20 mAb (Rituximab) has now become the first anticancer mAb to become licensed by the FDA for lymphoma treatment. One of the most encouraging aspects of Rituximab treatment is that, in addition to its therapeutic activity, which appears to match that of more con-

From: *Methods in Molecular Medicine, Vol. 40: Diagnostic and Therapeutic Antibodies*
Edited by: A. J. T. George and C. E. Urch © Humana Press Inc., Totowa, NJ

ventional chemotherapy in a similar setting, it has very few adverse effects and can be given to patients who are in poor condition with advanced disease. Early experience suggests that it will be this lack of adverse effects that will be its most attractive feature.

Perhaps the most disappointing aspect of the work to date with anti-CD20 mAb has been the low frequency of complete remissions (CR) (approx 8%). Failure to eradicate all tumor shows that the treatment conditions have yet to be optimized or, as has been pointed out by many workers, mAbs are not ideal reagents for dealing with bulky disease and may be more appropriate in the setting of minimal disease. In this regard it will be interesting to see how this reagent performs as "first-line" therapy in NHL before the patient's immune system has become damaged by disease and therapy. Encouraging results are already appearing from a study in which anti-CD20 mAb is being used in combination with chemotherapy. Although the results are still preliminary and based on a small number of patients, Czuczman and colleagues *(5)* have found a higher than expected number of molecular CR (bcl-2 negative by PCR) can be obtained using this approach. It remains to be seen if these CR transform into improved clinical results. The importance of combination therapy is supported by recent in vitro studies showing that treatment with anti-CD20 mAb can sensitize neoplastic B cells to various chemotherapeutic agents *(6)*.

2. A Role for Transmembrane Signaling in mAb Therapy?

The question being asked by many workers in the immunotherapy field is why anti-CD20 mAb appears clinically effective when many other mAbs have failed. The most straightforward explanation is that anti-CD20 mAb has been studied more intensively than other antilymphoma mAb and consequently has had much greater opportunity to succeed. Although there is probably some truth in this observation, it is also clear that the CD20 molecule has many properties that make it an ideal mAb target *(7,8)*. CD20 is a B-cell specific membrane molecule that is expressed at relatively high levels on most B-cell malignancies. Structural studies show that it is a member of a small family of molecules that appear to traverse the plasma membrane four times. This configuration requires that both the amino- and carboxyl-terminal domains are cytoplasmic with only one small extracellular peptide loop (41 amino acids) to provide the epitope for mAb binding. Although the function of CD20 is not known, extensive evidence shows it is involved with cell signaling and may be important in Ca^{2+} regulation *(8)*. CD20 is known to be very resistant to antigenic modulation and, even during the first in vivo studies using mouse mAb *(7)*, it was found that unlike most other targets CD20 remained on the cell surface following crosslinking by mAb treatment. This lack of internalisation is clearly very important because it allows mAb maximum opportunity to recruit effectors. Finally, it should not be overlooked that Rituximab anti-CD20 mAb is a genetically engineered chimeric reagent with mouse-variable regions and human-constant regions giving it the effector functions of human IgG1 *(2)*. Together, these factors ensure very effective recruitment of both complement and cellular effectors as measured in vitro, which may be sufficient to explain the reported successes of anti-CD20 mAb in patients. However, it should be remembered that, despite some 20 yr of study, we still have a very poor understanding of how mAbs remove tumor cells in vivo, other factors may also be important. As an alternative explanation for therapeutic activity, a number of workers are now looking at the ability of mAb to generate direct cytotoxic effects in the tumor cells by delivering transmembrane signals. Perhaps certain mAbs, by crosslinking plasma membrane proteins, can reorganize them in such a way that the target cells respond to the inappropriate signaling by modulating their growth or even undergoing programmed cell death (apoptosis).

Although there is little evidence as yet to support or exclude this mechanism of action for anti-CD20 mAb, data suggest that it plays an important part in the success of anti-Id mAb in the treatment of NHL *(9)*. Vuist and colleagues *(9)* have reported that in a trial of 34 NHL patients treated with tailor-made mouse anti-Id mAb, 68% of whom responded to treatment, a striking correlation was seen between the ability of the individual anti-Id mAb to trigger transmembrane signals in a patient's lymphoma cells and the clinical response observed. Only mAbs that were able to activate tyrosine phosphorylation produced therapeutic responses when the patient was treated. The exact reason why anti-Id mAb should behave in this way is not clear. However, it is likely that, in crosslinking the surface Ig on neoplastic B cells, the anti-Id mimics a response often seen following exposure of normal B cells to excess antigen or self antigen, which leads to anergy and clonal deletion. In addition to these observations in patients, it has been known for many years that anti-IgM mAb, when crosslinking the surface B-cell receptor (BCR) on various B cells, normal and neoplastic, results in growth arrest and apoptosis *(10)*. Generally, it is evident that immature B cells are more sensitive to anti-IgM induced growth arrest. This probably relates to the ease with which early B cells can be tolerized by self antigens. However, even the growth of mature cells can be perturbed provided sufficient crosslinking of the BCR is provided *(11)*. Interestingly, in our experience anti-Id mAb are not particularly effective as crosslinking reagents, probably because they bind monogamously or univalently rather than bigamously like most anti-Fcμ mAb *(10)*. Such differences in binding patterns could explain some of the variation seen in patient responses reported by Vuist and colleagues *(9)*.

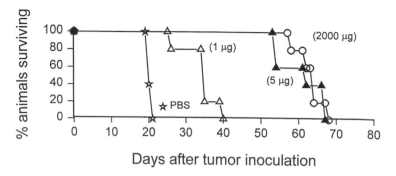

Fig. 1. Immunotherapy of mouse lymphoma (A31) with rat anti-Id mAb. Groups of matched mice (5/group) were given 10^5 fresh tumor cells on day 0 by intravenous (i.v.) injection. The mice were then treated with 1, 5, or 2000 µg of IgG anti-Id mAb per mouse as indicated on day 3 (i.v.) and their survival monitored. As explained in the text, anti-Id mAb was highly effective at prolonging animal survival, but all mice eventually succumbed to tumor due to the emergence of variant tumors that are probably defective in BCR signaling *(12)*.

3. Animal Studies Point to a Signaling Mechanism for mAb Treatment

The role of transmembrane signaling with anti-Id mAb is also supported by studies in animals. We find that, in certain models, very small amounts of mAbs are required to give profound therapeutic responses (*see* **Fig. 1**). Such levels (1 µg/mouse) of mAb are far below the predicted amounts needed to coat the tumor cells in vivo for killing by natural effectors such as complement or NK cells. It seems much more likely that such amounts would be sufficient to trigger transmembrane signals following limited crosslinking of the BCR. A second line of support comes from the work of Vitetta and co-workers *(12)*, who have shown that a high percentage of BCL_1 tumor cells emerging in mice that have been immunized with idiotypic IgM (from BCL_1 tumor), are genetic variants that no longer signal effectively via their BCR. For example, the variant cells had alterations in their expression of the signaling proteins Syk, HS1, and/or Lyn. In this regard, it is interesting to note that in **Fig. 1**, even following 2 mg of anti-Id mAb/mouse, none of the animals survived beyond day 70. We now know that the majority of emerging tumours are variants that are phenotypically normal with regard to surface Id expression but resistant to the anti-Id mAb. Interestingly, these variant cells show a level of sensitivity in cytotoxicity assays (complement and cellular killing) that is unchanged compared with that of the parental tumor. However, when these cells are reused in immunotherapy with anti-Id mAb, their growth is unperturbed, showing that they can avoid the immunological pressure exerted by the mAb. Together, these results suggest that sensitivity to immunotherapy is dependent not on the ability to recruit natural effectors to be lethal but on signaling pathways in the cell.

Studies from this laboratory have now extended this animal work with syngeneic B-cell lymphomas and a panel of potential therapeutic mAb that includes anti-Id, CD19, CD21, CD22, CD38, CD40, CD72, CD74, CD86, and MHC class II. Unfortunately anti-CD20 mAb is not yet available for the mouse. The results show that there is no obvious correlation between the cytotoxic activity of mAb in vitro with their therapeutic performance in vivo. Despite a number of mAb being active in complement and cellular cytotoxicity assays, particularly those binding at high levels, such as anti-MHC class II, only two reagents, anti-Id (see **Fig. 1**) and anti-CD40 mAb, were consistently therapeutic in a range of mouse models *(13)*. In addition, we have recently found some limited therapeutic activity with anti-CD19 and anti-CD21 mAb in certain lymphoma lines, such as BCL_1, but not in all models. All other mAbs were without significant therapeutic activity and failed to show any protection in tumor-bearing mice even when given early in the course of the disease.

Explaining this apparent lack of activity with most mAbs is difficult, but suggests that despite in vitro activity, natural effectors do not operate efficiently in vivo with mAb-coated tumor cells and is somewhat reminiscent of the situation in the clinic where most reagents have failed to benefit patients. The mechanisms operating with anti-Id and anti-CD40 are unknown. However, as discussed earlier, it appears reasonable to expect that, as in the human NHL, the anti-Id mAb operates, at least partially, via transmembrane signaling mechanisms that can control tumor growth and may lead to apoptosis. The therapeutic activity of the anti-CD40 mAb is more difficult to explain. In vitro studies show that it binds at comparatively low levels to most tumor cells and is consequently quite poor at recruiting effectors. We speculate that anti-CD40 mAb immunotherapy may also involve signaling to the tumor cells but could also include a stimulating effect on the mouse immune system.

CD40 is a major co-stimulatory molecule on B cells and antigen-presenting cells. It is normally engaged by CD40 ligand on helper T cells during immune responses and appears to be necessary for driving B-cell proliferation and rescuing them from the tolerogenic signals delivered via the BCR. However, work from Funakoshi and colleagues *(14)* has recently shown that the situation is slightly different in many B-cell malignancies in which anti-CD40 mAb, if crosslinked appropriately, can result in profound growth arrest of cultured cells. When used in SCID/xenograft models, these researchers found the same anti-CD40 mAb was effective in protecting mice from tumor development. At least part of this in vivo activity appears to depend on the direct signaling activity of the anti-CD40 mAb because it is partially effective even in the absence of FcR-expressing effector cells. Our animal work has extended these observations and shown that anti-CD40 mAb is highly therapeutic even in syngeneic lymphoma models. Interestingly, in vitro we found no evidence of growth arrest, but rather the anti-CD40 mAb tended to stimulate growth. This result does not agree with those of Funakoshi and co-workers (*14*), who reported only growth arrest in various lymphoma lines. Similarly, growth arrest has been reported by Baker and colleagues (*15*) when anti-CD40 mAb was added to certain Burkitt's cell lines. Despite these inconsistencies, it is clear that anti-CD40 mAb can be therapeutically very active and that part of its mechanism of action may result from inhibitory signaling. It is important to note that in normal B cells, signaling via CD40, leads to profound phenotypic changes, including upregulation of adhesion molecules, costimulatory receptors, and the apoptosis-inducing Fas molecule, and that in certain circumstances such surface changes can result in B-cell depletion. Goodnow and co-workers (*16*) have shown that during immune responses the Fas pathway may be an important mechanism for preventing inappropriate activation of bystander B cells. They were able to demonstrate that if B cells were engaged via CD40 (using CD40 ligand-expressing T helper cells) but had not bound multivalent antigen via their BCR, then Fas expression was upregulated and the cells were deleted via a Fas/Fas ligand interaction. It is possible that similar phenotypic changes occur following anti-CD40 mAb treatment of neoplastic B cells and that such changes allow the removal of tumor in a similar manner. In recent work with various mouse B-cell lymphomas, we have found that anti-CD40 mAb operates with very interesting kinetics in which tumor cells continue to proliferate normally for 3–4 d after mAb treatment and only then do their numbers start to decline compared with untreated controls (*13*). This picture is very different to the situation following anti-Id mAb treatment where cells undergo rapid growth arrest. Investigations are underway to establish the mechanism by which anti-CD40 mAb operates in vivo. Although the relatively slow kinetics of anti-CD40 mAb-treatment would be consistent with upregulation and activation of surface Fas (*16*), preliminary data show only small changes in Fas expression following anti-CD40 mAb treatment. As an alternative explanation we are also considering whether the anti-CD40 mAb, rather than, or in addition to, delivering a direct cytotoxic effect on the tumor, may also deliver its action via stimulation of the normal immune system. Our recent unpublished data shows that anti-CD40 mAb therapy is highly dependent on intact T-cell function and consequently that we see comparatively little therapeutic activity with anti-CD40 mAb following T-cell depletion.

4. Therapeutic mAb Require Fc Regions

Although much of our data are consistent with at least part of the therapeutic activity of mAb being via transmembrane signaling it is clear that with anti-Id

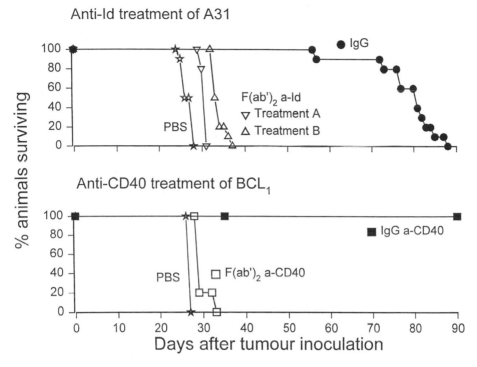

Fig. 2. F(ab')$_2$ mAb is ineffective in delivering tumor immunotherapy. Groups of 10 matched mice were given 10^5 fresh lymphoma cells (A31 in CBA mice; BCL$_1$ in BALB/c mice) on day 0 by i.v. injection. The A31-carrying mice were treated with PBS (day 1); IgG anti-Id (5 μg on day 1); F(ab')$_2$ anti-Id (Treatment A= 5 μg/day on days 1, 2, 5, and 7); or F(ab')$_2$ anti-Id (treatment B = 20 μg/d on days 1, 2, 3, 4, and 5), as indicated. The BCL$_1$-carrying mice were treated with: PBS (days 9, 10, 11, and 12); IgG anti-CD40 (0.5 mg on days 9, 10, 11, and 12); or F(ab')$_2$ anti-CD40 (1 mg on days 9, 10, 11, and 12) as indicated. For mAb reagents, removing the Fc from the IgG has abolished almost all therapeutic activity showing that FcR interactions are very important.

and anti-CD40 mAb treatment, the Fc region of the reagents still plays an important part in the therapeutic process. **Figure 2** shows two mouse models in which anti-Id or anti-CD40 mAb have been used to protect (A31 treated with anti-Id mAb) or cure (BCL$_1$ treated with anti-CD40 mAb) lymphoma-bearing mice. These results are impressive and unlike those achieved with any other mAb specificity to date in these models, but they can only be obtained when intact IgG is used. When these mAb were converted to F(ab')$_2$ fragments by limited digestion with pepsin, the therapeutic activity was almost completely lost. Both mAb are rat IgG2a isotypes. In view of the difference in half-life of rat IgG2a (30 h) and F(ab')$_2$ fragments (9 h), we have attempted, especially with the F(ab')$_2$ anti-Id mAb, to compensate for this difference by increasing the amount of F(ab')$_2$ derivative given. Therefore it appears unlikely that the loss of therapeutic activity arises from differences in metabolic survival and is more likely due to the signaling properties of these two derivatives.

As F(ab')$_2$ and IgG are both bivalent, then we would expect them to have similar cell-signaling activity. In vitro studies support this assumption showing that both are equally effective in inhibiting B-cell growth (10). However, it is also true that on normal B cells F(ab')$_2$ fragments of anti-μ polyclonal antisera are sometimes stimulatory, whereas IgG molecules from the same sera are not (17). This difference in activity has been attributed to the ability of IgG Ab to crosslink FcRII (CD32) and thereby recruit phosphatase activity into the BCR complex, which results in cessation of signaling events. This inhibitory activity of the CD32 is attributable to its ability to interact with phosphatase molecules via its cytoplasmic immunoreceptor tyrosine inhibition motif (ITIM). However, we do not think CD32 expressed on B-cell lymphoma constitutes an important signaling pathway in terms of explaining why some mAb work in therapy, in particular because a number of cell lines, such as the Burkitt's line Ramos, which lack FcR, are still highly sensitive to anti-BCR mAb-mediated growth arrest (10).

Finally, **Fig. 3** hypothesizes on the importance of Fc:FcR, not as deliverers of direct negative signals to the tumor cells as discussed, but in terms of their ability to increase the crosslinking activity of mAb. It is clear from a number of in vitro culture systems that FcR-expressing cells can influence the crosslinking activity of mAb. By providing a multivalent array of FcR, even low-affinity receptors such as CD32, will increase the crosslinking of Ab-coated target cells markedly. Fc:FcR interactions of this type have been shown to increase the signaling activity of mAb in the CD40 culture system where, as discussed, normal B cells are maintained on a feeder layer of CD32-expressing L-cells and anti-CD40, plus IL-4 (18), and have been shown to increase the level of modulation and internalization of Ab-complexes from the surface of Ab-coated target cells (19). Similarly, signaling via the TCR with anti-CD3 mAb is also greatly enhanced by FcR-expressing effector cells. Shan and colleagues (20) have now shown that FcR-expressing effector cells, as a result of increased crosslinking activity, can also promote the level of apoptosis induced by anti-CD20 mAb bound to B-cell targets.

As a result of such evidence, we now feel that it is quite likely that the difference in therapeutic activity of IgG and F(ab')$_2$ in vivo could result from differences in signaling activity as a result of molecular crosslinking. The nature of the FcR-expressing cells responsible in this system is not known.

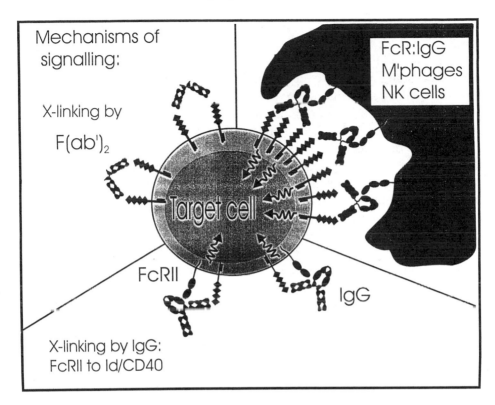

Fig. 3. The mechanism of mAb-medicated therapy in vivo. Despite 20 yr of intensive investigation we are still surprisingly ignorant of how mAbs control lymphoma growth in vivo. The latest results suggest that therapeutically effective mAbs may be those that exert a direct cytotoxic effect on tumor cells. This property is probably dependent on the ability of the mAb to crosslink key signaling molecules. Here, we show situations in which the crosslinking and signaling activity of mAb can be influence by its valency, its ability to interact with FcRII on the lymphoma cells, which will modulate signaling activity; and interaction with FcR bearing effector cells (*see* text for details).

Theoretically they would not need to be cytotoxic in the normal sense and could be any FcR-expressing cells capable of hypercrosslinking cell-bound mAb, such as NK cells, monocytes, platelets, or, in some cases, even the B-cell lymphoma itself.

5. The Future

The developments in Ab engineering that have occurred over the last 10–15 yr have primarily been aimed at improving the effector-recruiting activity of Ab, e.g., by inserting human-constant regions. In view of our current findings, it may be felt that such improvements were not critical to the success of therapeutic mAb such as anti-CD20. However, such structural changes can improve the signaling activity of the mAb. Engineering has improved interaction with human FcR, reduced immunogenicity, and, probably most important of all, it has extended the metabolic survival of the therapeutic mAb. Rodent mAb normally has a half-life in humans of no more that 24 h, but following chimerization or humanization this may be extended to more than 10 d, and in the case of the recent anti-CD20 mAb trial serum Ab could be detected for several months after treatment *(2)*. This sustained immunological pressure on the lymphoma cells is probably very important in terms of delivering growth-controlling signals. In particular, it will allow tumor cells that are cycling slowly to receive sustained transmembrane signaling from the Ab as they pass through each stage of the cell cycle. The requirement for sustained signaling by the mAb in this way may explain some of the very slow responses that are seen in clinical trials *(2)*.

For the future, it is important that we develop derivatives with not only the appropriate signaling activity, but also with increased crosslinking activity. Already Woolf and co-workers *(21)* and Ghetie and colleagues *(22)* have shown that certain mAbs perform better when delivered as dimers. For example, an anti-CD19 mAb gave improved protection from tumors in mice when used as a dimer rather than as a monomer, and this activity was attributed to its increased crosslinking activity. Perhaps small, multivalent, mAb derivatives or fusion proteins point the way forward. This approach has already been attempted with multivalent peptides that crosslink the surface BCR of lymphoma cells *(23)*. As an alternative, we have data to suggest that mAb derivatives constructed as bispecific Ab (BsAb) may also operate by performing a similar signaling role in the target cells, but achieve this by crosslinking two cell surfaces together *(24)*. These BsAb probably operate via the same mechanism as IgG in terms of delivering negative signaling to the tumor, but because they bind to effector cells, such as CD3 on T cells, with increased affinity and no blocking compared with that of the Fc:FcR interaction, they appear to deliver a more potent therapeutic effect. The impressive data from Demanet and colleagues *(25)* with [anti-CD3 × anti-Id] BsAb in two mouse lymphoma models underlines the potency of these reagents showing that they can far outperform IgG anti-Id mAb. In this work, just 5 µg of BsAb given at day 9 of tumor development was able to cure most animals, an achievement not seen with any IgG-based therapy. If, as speculated, these BsAb are delivering antilymphoma activity as a result of crosslinking activity on the target, then one way forward will be to design derivatives that perform this role more effectively. For example, it may be possible to achieve tumor-cell crosslinking, and consequent therapy, with BsAb designed to recruit noneffector cells, such as red blood cells, platelets, or B cells, on to the tumor cell surface. An advantage of this approach would be the selection of surface molecules on the adopted "effector" cells that did not modulate and therefore would maintain the Ab derivative at the cell surface for long periods. Furthermore, even if these derivatives were designed to recruit more conventional effectors, such as T cells and myeloid cells, then this could be achieved through molecules that did not activate the effector cells and would thereby avoid one of the major complications of existing BsAb, that of toxicity. BsAb, such as [anti-CD3 × antitumor], have resulted in significant toxicity which has restricted systemic use in clinical trials *(26)*.

Understanding the mechanisms by which Ab and Ab derivatives operate in vivo would appear to be an absolute requirement if we are to extend their use in patients. It is quite clear that, for most derivatives, simply recruiting natural effectors is not adequate to destroy unwanted cells in vivo. A fuller understanding will not only improve application in the hematological malignancies, but may eventually extend their use to solid tumors.

References

1. Dillman, R. O. (1994) Antibodies as cytotoxic therapy. *J. Clin. Oncol.* **12,** 1497–1515.
2. Maloney, D. G., Grillo-Lopez, A. J., White, C. A., et al. (1997) IDEC-C2B8 (Rituximab) anti-CD20 monoclonal antibody therapy in patients with relapsed low-grade non-Hodgkin's lymphoma. *Blood* **90,** 2188–2195.
3. Osterborg, A., Dyer, M. J. S., Bunjes, D., et al. (1997) Phase II multicentre study of human CD52 antibody in previously treated chronic lymphocytic leukemia. *J. Clin. Oncol.* **15,** 1567–1574.
4. Meeker, T. C., Lowder, J., Cleary, M. L., Stewart, S., Warnke, R., Sklar, J., and Levy, R. (1985) Emergence of idiotype variants during treatment of B-cell lymphoma with anti-idiotype antibodies. *New Engl. J. Med.* **312,** 1658–1665.
5. Czuczman, M. S., Grillo-Lopez, A. J., Jonas, C., Gordon, L., Saleh, M., White, C. A., Varns, C., and Rogers, J. (1995) IDEC-C2B8 and CHOP chemoimmunotherapy of low-grade lymphoma. *Blood* **86(suppl 1),** 55a.
6. Demiden, A., Lam, T., Alas, S., Hariharan, K., et al. (1997) Chimeric anti-CD20 (IDEC-C2B8) monoclonal antibody sensitizes a B cell lymphoma cell line to cell killing by cytotoxic drugs. *Cancer Biother. Radiopharm.* **12,** 177–186.
7. Press, O. W., Appelbaum, F., Ledbetter, J. A., et al. (1987) Monoclonal antibody-1F5 (anti-CD20) serotherapy of human B-cell lymphoma. *Blood* **69,** 584–591.
8. Tedder T. F. and Engel, P. (1994) CD20: a regulator of cell-cycle progression of B lymphocytes. *Immunol. Today* **15,** 450–454.

9. Vuist, W. M., J., Levy, R., and Maloney, D. G. (1994) Lymphoma regression induced by monoclonal anti-idiotype antibodies correlates with their ability to induce Ig signal transduction and is not prevented by tumor expression of high levels of bcl-2 protein. *Blood* **83,** 899–906.

10. Cragg, M. S., Zhang, L., French, R. R., and Glennie, M. J. (1999) Analysis of the interaction of monoclonal antibodies with surface IgM on neoplastic B cells. *Br. J. Cancer* **79,** 850–857.

11. Parry, S. L., Hasbold, J., Holman, M., and Klaus, G. G. B. (1994) Hypercross-linking surface IgM or IgD receptors on mature B-cells induces apoptosis that is reversed by costimulation with IL-4 and anti-CD40. *J. Immunol.* **152,** 2821–2829.

12. Vitetta, E. S., Tucker, T. F., Racila, E., et al. (1997) Tumor dormancy and cell signaling. V. Regrowth of the BCL_1 tumor after dormancy is established. *Blood* **89,** 4425–4436.

13. Tutt, A. L., French, R. R., Illidge, T. M., et al. (1998) Monoclonal antibody therapy of B-cell lymphoma: signaling activity on tumor cells appears more important than recruitment of effectors. *J. Immunol.* **161,** 3176–3185.

14. Funakoshi, S., Longo, D. L., and Murphy, W. J. (1996) Differential in vitro and in vivo antitumor effects mediated by anti-CD40 and anti-CD20 monoclonal antibodies against human B-cell lymphomas. *J. Immunother.* **19,** 93–101.

15. Baker, M. P., Eliopoulos, A. G., Young, L. S., et al. (1998) Prolonged phenotypic, functional, and molecular change in group I Burkitt lymphoma cells on short-term exposure to CD40 ligand. *Blood* **92,** 2830–2843.

16. Rathmell, J. C., Townsend, S. E., Xu, J. C. C., et al. (1996) Expansion or elimination of B cells in vivo: dual roles for CD40 and Fas (CD95)-ligands modulated by the B cell antigen receptor. *Cell* **87,** 319–329.

17. Tridandapani, S., Kelley, T., Cooney, D., et al. (1997) Negative signaling in B cells: SHIP Grbs Shc. *Immunol. Today* **18,** 424–427.

18. Banchereau, J., Bazan, F., Blanchard, D., et al. (1994) The CD40 antigen and its ligand. *Annu. Rev. Immunol.* **12,** 881–922.

19. Schroff, R. W., Klein, R. A., Farrell, M. M., and Stevenson, H. C. (1984) Enhancing effects of monocytes on modulation of a lymphocyte membrane antigen. *J. Immunol.* **133,** 2270–2277.

20. Shan, D., Ledbetter, J. A., and Press, O. W. (1998) Apoptosis of malignant human B cells by ligation of CD20 with monoclonal antibody. *Blood* **91,** 1644–1652.

21. Wolff, E. A., Schreiber, G. J., Cosand, W. L., and Raff, H. V. (1993) Monoclonal antibody homodimers: enhanced antitumor activity in nude mice. *Cancer Res.* **53,** 2560–2565.

22. Ghetie, M.-A., Podar, E. M., Ilgen, A., et al. (1997) Homodimerization of tumor-reactive monoclonal antibodies markedly increases their ability to induce growth arrest or apoptosis of tumor cells. *Proc. Natl. Acad. Sci. USA* **94,** 7509–7514.

23. Renschler, M. R., Wada, H. G., Fok, K. S., and Levy, R. (1995) B-lymphoma cells are activated by peptide ligands of the antigen-binding receptor or by anti-idiotype antibody to induce extracellular acidification. *Cancer Res.* **55,** 5642–5647.

24. Honeychurch, J., Cruise, A., Tutt, A. L., and Glennie, M. J. (1997) Bispecific Ab therapy of B-cell lymphoma: target cell specificity of antibody derivatives appears critical in determining therapeutic outcome. *Cancer Immunol. Immunother.* **45,** 171–173.

25. Demanet, C., Brissinck, J., Leo, O., et al. (1994) Role of T-cell subsets in the bispecific antibody (anti-idiotype x anti-CD3) treatment of the BCL₁ lymphoma. *Cancer Res.* **54,** 2973–2978.

26. Kroesen, B. J., Helfrich, W., Molema, G., and deLeij, L. (1998) Bispecific antibodies for treatment of cancer in experimental animal models and man. *Adv. Drug Del. Rev.* **31,** 105–129.

8

Antibodies for Inflammatory Disease

Effector Cells

Richard Smith

1. Introduction

Their inherent specificity makes antibodies attractive immunotherapeutic agents. Definition of appropriate therapeutic strategies requires parallel identification of potential target molecules and the immunotherapeutic mechanisms to be recruited by antibodies targeting these molecules. Regardless of the target antigen, antibodies may modify immune responses by:

1. Killing target cells (cytotoxic or depleting antibodies);
2. Blocking molecular interactions;
3. Modulating target molecules from the surface of cells; or
4. Modifying cell function as a consequence of signal transduction by ligated molecules.

In addition to their inherent specificity, the ability to modify antibody-constant regions in order to selectively recruit these mechanisms of action greatly increases the appeal of antibodies as therapeutic agents. Importantly, these strategies may be recruited to passively suppress or to actively modulate immune responses. Finally, the ability to modify antibody-constant regions in order to minimize antiglobulin responses facilitates the use of these molecules as therapeutic agents. The development of antibodies capable of modifying inflammatory autoimmune disease processes illustrates many of these principles.

The ideal scenario for development of a therapeutic monoclonal antibody (mAb) would be to focus on a disease or diseases in which the pathogenic mechanisms are known, develop an effective therapeutic strategy in an animal

From: *Methods in Molecular Medicine, Vol. 40: Diagnostic and Therapeutic Antibodies*
Edited by: A. J. T. George and C. E. Urch © Humana Press Inc., Totowa, NJ

model in which the same mechanisms are acting, and then develop a molecule for use in humans that recruited the same mechanisms. Immunopathogenic mechanisms are poorly defined in many inflammatory autoimmune diseases, making selection of appropriate animal models difficult. However, data from human disease supports the suggestion that organ-specific autoimmune diseases are T-cell dependent and development of antibodies against the cellular components of the inflammatory autoimmune disease process therefore focuses largely (although not exclusively, *vide infra*) on T lymphocytes.

2. Immune Responses in Inflammatory Diseases

Inflammatory immune responses contribute to the pathogenesis of many human autoimmune diseases, including multiple sclerosis, rheumatoid arthritis, and type 1 diabetes mellitus. They may also contribute to clinical transplant rejection. Selection of target molecules for therapeutic antibodies requires reference to the mechanisms operating in these pathological immune responses. Two cellular components are central to the inflammatory immune response: antigen-specific helper T (Th) lymphocytes acting to focus and coordinate the response, and nonantigen-specific effector cells (predominantly macrophages), which mediate tissue damage (**Fig. 1**). Therapeutic antibodies may target either of these cell types, the cytokines that co-ordinate their activity (e.g., interferon-γ) or macrophage effector function (e.g., anti-TNF-α). Antibodies targeting cytokines have been discussed in Chapter 9). Here we will focus on antibodies recognizing the cellular components of the inflammatory response.

In common with other T cells, Th cells recognize antigen through binding of their cell surface TcR to MHC/peptide complexes (**Fig. 2**). Helper T cells are characterized by expression of the CD4 molecule and recognition of peptide antigen complexed with major histocompatibility complex (MHC) class II molecules. The CD3 molecule is noncovalently associated with the TcR and is an essential component of the antigen recognition apparatus mediating signal transduction following binding of the TcR to antigen MHC complexes. Activation of naive T cells requires a costimulatory signal in addition to this antigen-specific signal. This is delivered by binding of antigen presenting cell (APC) ligands (either CD80 or CD86) to T cell CD28 (reviewed in **refs.** *1,2*). A second T cell ligand with a negative regulatory role (CTLA-4) also binds these APC molecules (reviewed in **ref.** *3*). Finally, CD40–CD40L interactions appear essential to effective delivery of T-cell costimulation (*4,5*). Antibodies targeting these pathways alone or in combination have been shown to be effective in prevention and treatment of inflammatory autoimmune disease in experimental models.

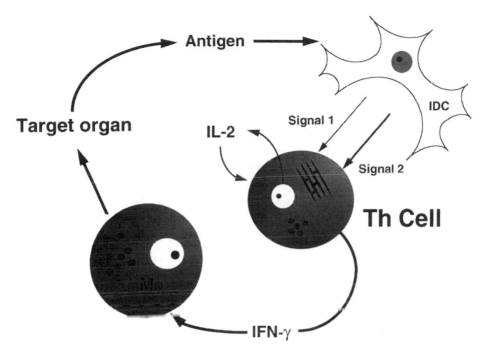

Fig. 1. Cellular interactions in inflammatory autoimmune disease. The effector cells in inflammatory autoimmune disease are predominantly macrophages. The activity of these cells is coordinated by antigen-specific helper T (Th) cells. Activation of Th cells requires antigen presentation by "professional" antigen presenting such cells as interdigitating dendritic cells (IDC). Interferon-γ released by Th cells is essential for macrophage activation.

3. How May Specificity Be Achieved?

The Holy Grail of immunotherapy is antigen-specific tolerance induction. Two strategies may be employed to achieve this: targeting of molecules unique to the deleterious response or use of immunotherapeutic antibodies at a time when the predominant response is that which is being targeted. The only moieties that are unique to a particular deleterious inflammatory immune response are the components of the trimolecular complex of TcR/peptide/MHC molecule. Experimentally, antibodies targeting the TcR-variable regions have been used effectively (6). However, in clinical disease limited heterogeneity of TcR usage appears to be the norm (7), making it difficult to define specificities allowing development of this strategy for clinical use. Theoretically, antibodies against a specific MHC/peptide complex would also be immunosuppressive and specific for the deleterious immune response (8). Few such antibodies

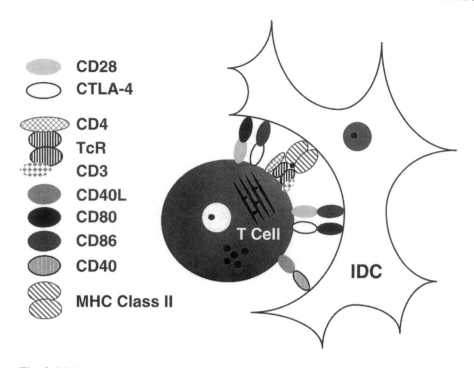

Fig. 2. Molecular interactions in T-cell priming. T-cell activation requires the coordinated interaction of a number of ligand pairs on the APC and T cell. Signal 1 is provided by antigen-specific interactions between the T cell receptor (TcR) on the T cell and peptide/MHC class II complex on the APC. The CD4 and CD3 molecules play an essential role in this interaction. Signal 2 is provided by the T-cell costimulatory ligand CD28 binding to either CD80 or CD86 on the APC. CD80 and CD86 may bind also to T-cell CTLA-4 delivering an inhibitory signal to the T cell. CD40 binding to CD40-L mediates upregulation of APC costimulatory ligands and may itself deliver a costimulatory signal.

have been described and none been extensively developed. Furthermore, as with antibodies targeting TcR-variable regions, such strategies are unlikely to be applicable to outbred populations.

Many of the molecules identifying Th cells and macrophages are unique to these cells. Immunosuppressive antibodies recognizing these cell-specific molecules thus achieve greater specificity than is possible with pharmacological agents. If therapy is then administered at a time when the dominant immune response is the one that must be controlled, the predominant effect will be on this immune response. If such a strategy is coupled to targeting of molecules upregulated on T-cell activation, further specificity is achieved. Such a strategy has been exploited to greatest effect in transplantation, with antibodies recognizing the α chain of the IL-2 receptor (CD25) *(9,10)*. Experimental inflammatory autoimmune disease may be treated also using anti-CD25 antibodies *(11)*. Small numbers of patients with rheumatoid arthritis have been treated with an anti-IL-2R antibody with limited symptomatic improvement *(12)*. Antibodies recognizing CD7, a second molecule upregulated on activation of T cells, have also been used in small numbers of patients. Unfortunately, only limited followup has been reported for these patients *(13,14)*.

It is important to recognize that when clinical disease is manifest, T-cell activation and much tissue damage will already have occurred. In such instances passively immunosuppressive agents, including antibodies, will have little opportunity to influence the outcome of immune activation and it is perhaps not surprising that immunosuppressive agents are of little use in clinical diseases, such as multiple sclerosis. Therapeutic agents able to induce tolerance may similarly have little effect on the disease episode during which they are first administered, but subsequent episodes of disease may be inhibited because of re-education of the immune system. In a relapsing remitting model of central nervous system (CNS) inflammatory autoimmune disease in mice (chronic relapsing experimental autoimmune encephalomyelitis), administration of a noncytotoxic anti-MHC class II antibody at the time of a disease episode had no effect on either the disease severity or length of the attack during which the antibody was administered. However, the severity and number of subsequent disease episodes were significantly reduced (**Table 1**). Importantly, in this model immune responses to other foreign antigens were not subsequently affected.

4. Pharmacokinetic Requirements of Therapeutic Antibodies

The pharmacokinetic requirements of a therapeutic antibody are determined by which of the above mechanisms is to be recruited. Access to lymphoid tissues is essential and may be better for immunoglobulin fragments than for intact immunoglobulin. Importantly, plasma half-life is a surrogate for the most important measurement: cell surface half-life. A short plasma half-life may be driven by effective binding to a target molecule *(15)*. Thus, if a "single hit" is all that is required or if binding is high affinity and the target molecule shows stable expression, repeated administration may be unnecessary despite a short plasma half-life. Furthermore, a prolonged cell surface half-life may not be necessary and indeed may be detrimental if the aim is to modify rather than prevent T-cell activation. Thus, with blockade of costimulation delayed administration may be optimum *(16)*, with prolonged administration exacerbating disease in some models *(17)*.

Table 1
Chronic Relapsing Experimental Autoimmune Encephalomyelitis:
Effect of Noncytotoxic Anti-MHC Class II Antibody Treatment[a]

Treatment	First round		First relapse		Second relapse	
	Incidence	Mean max grade	Incidence	Mean max grade	Incidence	Mean max grade
OX6[b]	0/7	0	0/7	0	0/7	0
OX6[c]	6/7	2.1	5/7	1.9	3/7	1.1
MOPC21	7/8	1.6	7/8	2.0	6/8	1.9

[a]CREAE was induced by administration of 1 mg subcutaneously in the flank on two occasions 7 d apart.

[b]For prevention of disease 1 mg OX6 (anti-MHC class II) was administered the day before and the day after each administration of antigen.

[c]For treatment of disease 10 doses of 250 μg OX6 were administered daily from the first signs of relapse. Animals were only treated for the first relapse. Control animals received MOPC21 both the day before and the day after each administration of antigen and daily for 10 d from the first signs of relapse. Disease was scored daily for 120 d from initial administration of antigen using an accepted scheme *(23)*.

5. Antigenic Targets

5.1. MHC Class II

Although unlikely to be used in clinical practice, the history of the use of anti-MHC class II antibodies illustrates many of these principles. The generation of antibodies recognizing MHC class II was central to elucidation of the role of the class II molecule as a restriction element for presentation of antigen to CD4[+] Th cells. Initial work used these antibodies in vitro to block binding of the TcR to MHC class II/peptide complexes, demonstrating the efficacy of antibodies as simple antagonists. When used in vivo the situation is more complex. First, the ability to act as a competitive antagonist remains. However, in vivo these antibodies have a number of other actions (reviewed in **ref. *18***). They modulate MHC class II from the surface of target cells and comodulate other molecules from the cell surface, e.g., other MHC class II molecules *(19,20)*, CD19/TAPA-1 (R. M. S., unpublished observations). Second, cytotoxic anti-MHC class II antibodies deplete antigen-presenting cells, resulting in profound immunosuppression. As with other therapeutic mAbs, the ability of anti-MHC class II antibodies to elicit signal transduction through the MHC class II molecule is less often considered as a therapeutic mechanism. Signal transduction by the MHC class II molecules is central to normal function of antigen-presenting cells and B-cell activation *(21,22)*. With naive B cells such signal transduction contributes to target cell depletion by driving apoptosis. In

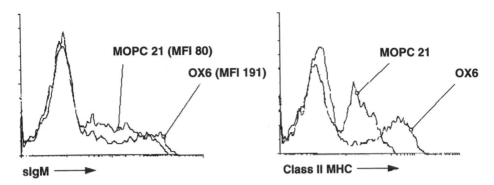

Fig. 3. Phenotypic changes in B cells following noncytotoxic anti-MHC class II antibody treatment. Biozzi AB/H mice were given 1 mg OX6 or isotype-matched control antibody intraperitoneally on each of three consecutive days. Five days after the first dose splenic B-cell MHC class II and surface IgM expression was examined by flow cytometry.

contrast, antigen-experienced B cells are driven to proliferate and differentiate by ligation of MHC class II. It is thus of interest that following anti-MHC class II antibody treatment B cells show upregulated levels of MHC class II and surface IgM (**Fig. 3**). Effects of this signal transduction on effector cell function, antigen presentation, and in turn on the developing autoimmune response, remain poorly defined. Finally, simple blockade of target molecules may interfere with the coordinated interactions required in order to initiate the immune response resulting in immunomodulation.

In different models anti-MHC class II antibodies recruit all of the above actions. For therapeutic use this is important, because cytotoxicity would be undesirable, but is not a prerequisite for therapeutic activity. In animal models three 1-mg doses of a noncytotoxic anti-MHC class II antibody do not prevent T-cell priming but are able to prevent development of clinical EAE *(23)*. Thus, selection of an appropriate antibody allows desirable effects to be retained and deleterious effects to be avoided. Concerns about side effects have precluded clinical development of anti-MHC class II antibodies. However, these mechanisms available to anti-MHC class II antibodies (blockade of cellular interactions, modulation of surface molecules, depletion of cells, modification of cell function) are the same mechanisms that may be recruited by antibodies of a wide range of specificities. Importantly, in different settings these basic mechanisms may have different effects on the immune response; i.e., may be immunosuppressive or modulatory. Thus, target cell depletion may be passively immunosuppressive but may also be a prerequisite for tolerance induction; modulation of MHC molecules may passively inhibit antigen presentation but by alteration of the density of ligands for TcR engagement may also affect the phenotype of the T cell *(24)*, resulting in immunomodulation rather than immunosuppression.

5.2. CD4

In keeping with the central role of CD4 in Th cell activation, antibodies targeting CD4 are effective immunotherapeutic agents. Initial studies demonstrated tolerance induction to both foreign antigen and transplantation antigens with antibodies that depleted Th cells. Subsequent studies have shown that in some models tolerance induction may be optimum with noncytotoxic antibodies *(25)*. Thus, these antibodies have the potential to fulfill the ultimate demand of immunotherapy; short-term treatment with long-term effect as a consequence of tolerance induction to the target antigen. Specificity is achieved by virtue of the timing of antibody administration. The use of both depleting and nondepleting anti-CD4 antibodies has been extended to clinical disease (rheumatoid arthritis, psoriasis, systemic lupus erythematosus, and multiple sclerosis), but with only temporary benefit. The most impressive results have been seen in systemic vasculitis when a nondepleting rat antihuman CD4 antibody was combined with the humanized CAMPATH 1H (C1H) antibody *(26,27)*. The relative contribution of these two antibodies is unclear, but these results would be in keeping with the suggestion that some degree of depletion is required in order to facilitate the immunotherapeutic actions of noncytotoxic anti-CD4 antibodies. A humanized version of this rat anti-CD4 antibody has been used either alone or in conjunction with C1H in refractory psoriasis and rheumatoid arthritis *(28)*. The anti-CD4 antibody effectively coated peripheral blood CD4+ T cells, resulting in transient disappearance of CD4+ T cells from peripheral blood and more sustained modulation of CD4 from their surface. CD4 expression returned within 2 wk of stopping treatment and was back to baseline at 1 mo. In most patients CD4 counts were within the normal range at 1 mo following treatment. The therapeutic effect was, however, transient in most patients. In general the results of clinical use of anti-CD4 antibodies have been disappointing in comparison with the impressive experimental results. Reference to our original scheme suggests a number of possible reasons. Although definitive proof is lacking it seems likely that T cells are central to the disease process and their lack of efficacy is therefore unlikely to be caused by selection of an inappropriate target. However, anti-CD4 antibodies have been shown to modify immune responses through a range of mechanisms, including steric hindrance of TcR/CD4 binding to MHC/peptide *(29)*, inhibition of p56^{lck} association with CD3 *(30)*, modulation of CD4 from the T cell surface *(31)*, and transduction of a negative signal to T cells *(32)*. Furthermore, both depleting and nondepleting antibodies may be effective, and tolerance induction has been shown to be the result of either immune deviation or induction of anergy in different models. Finally, it is not clear if all antibodies are equally effective, and the characteristics of those that are effective are incompletely defined. Thus, it is possible that the lack of clinical efficacy is attributable to inappropriate antibody selection with a failure to recruit appropriate mechanisms. Furthermore, Isaacs has calculated that 600 g of antibody would need to be given to a 70-kg adult if an equivalent dosage regimen to that shown to be effective in experimental models were to be given to patients. In keeping with this, dose escalation is associated with an improved response and more recent studies are using higher doses of anti-CD4 antibody with greater clinical effect (reviewed in **ref. 33**).

5.3. CD3

The CD3 molecule is both a marker for T cells (Tc and Th) and central to T-cell activation. Anti-CD3 antibodies modify immune responses by transient T-cell depletion and modulation of the CD3/TcR complex from the surface of T cells. A murine antibody against the ε chain of the CD3 molecule (OKT3) has been used extensively to prevent and treat human transplant rejection (*see* Chapter 10). In the NOD mouse model of T-cell-dependent autoimmune diabetes mellitus, administration of a short course of anti-CD3 antibody within 7 d of the onset of overt diabetes achieved antigen-specific immunomodulation with prevention of disease *(34)*. Thus, anti-CD3 antibodies are very effective immunosuppressive agents and may facilitate tolerance induction. However, in clinical use intact anti-CD3 antibodies are associated with significant morbidity resulting from a cytokine-mediated first dose response. This response is dependent on antibody binding to FcR. $F(ab')_2$ fragments and an aglycosyl variant of this antibody have been developed, neither of which bind FcR *(35,36)*. These molecules are both effective immunomodulatory agents and avoid many of the side effects seen with the parent antibody.

5.4. CAMPATH Antibodies

The CAMPATH 1 series of antibodies recognize the CD52 antigen expressed on all leukocytes. They were developed for use in hematological malignancy and bone marrow transplantation where cytotoxicity was required. Target cell depletion may be achieved in three ways. First, conjugation of antibodies of appropriate specificity with toxic moieties will generate an antibody capable of highly efficient killing. Alternatively, unconjugated antibodies may be cytotoxic through either complement fixation or recruitment of FcR-positive effector cells. Development of the CAMPATH series of antibodies has defined in great detail the requirements for optimum in vivo killing, recruitment of cell-mediated killing being essential. Humanized antibodies have also been generated to minimize antiglobulin responses. Development of these antibodies thus illustrates the potential for manipulation of antibody-molecule-constant regions in order to optimize their effector function and biocompatibility. These antibodies have not been widely used in autoimmune disease. However, in problematic cases cytotoxic antibodies may be advantageous because they avoid the nonimmunological side effects of the alternative pharmacological agents (e.g., cyclophosphamide). Small numbers of patients with autoimmune disease have been treated effectively with CAMPATH 1H either alone or in conjunction with other antibodies (e.g., anti-CD4) as discussed above.

5.5. Blockade of Costimulation

The definition of the ligand pairs mediating T-cell costimulation has led to the investigation of the immunotherapeutic potential of antibodies binding these molecules. Antibodies targeting the T-cell ligands CD28 and CTLA-4 have not been extensively developed for in vivo use. However, the history of the development of our understanding of these molecules emphasizes the dangers in ignoring the potential for signal transduction following binding of intact antibody to target cells. Initial studies defining the role of CD28 as a costimulatory receptor used both intact antibody and monovalent Fab' fragments, demonstrating that bivalent antibodies were able to substitute for accessory cells in delivery of costimulatory signals and that monovalent Fab' fragments blocked delivery of this signal, inhibiting T-cell activation (37). Despite this demonstration of signal transduction by anti-CD28 antibodies, initial studies using intact anti-CTLA-4 antibodies assumed them to act only as competitive antagonists. The demonstration of inhibition of T-cell activation by anti-CTLA4 antibody was thus taken to demonstrate that CTLA-4 was analogous to CD28 in its action. Subsequently it has been demonstrated that anti-CTLA-4 antibodies act not as competitive antagonists but deliver a negative signal to the T cell (38,39). In keeping with this, in vivo blockade of CTLA-4 may exacerbate experimental autoimmune disease (40).

In experimental studies of inflammatory autoimmune disease the APC ligands for these T-cell costimulatory receptors have more often been targeted. Three strategies have been used: targeting of CD80 and CD86 simultaneously using either CTLA-4 expressed as an Ig fusion protein or a combination of anti-CD80 and anti-CD86 antibodies, the selective use of anti-CD80 or anti-CD86 antibodies, and the combination of reagents targeting APC costimulatory ligands with anti-CD40 antibodies. CTLA-4-Ig may be considered as a bivalent immunoglobulin that retains Fc binding ability. CTLA-4-Ig has been shown to be effective in a wide range of animal models of inflammatory autoimmune disease (reviewed in **ref. 2**), its effect being potentiated by combination with anti-CD40 antibody *(41)*. CTLA4-Ig has been suggested to preferentially block Th1 type responses *(42,43)*, although the mechanism of this effect remains unclear. The effects of anti-CD80 and anti-CD86 antibodies used alone are conflicting. In acute experimental autoimmune encephalomyelitis (EAE) anti-CD80 antibody prevents, whereas anti-CD86 antibody exacerbates, disease *(17,44)*. In this work anti-CD86 antibody inhibited Th2 cytokine production and enhanced IFN-γ production *(44)*. Anti-CD86, but not anti-CD80 antibody, inhibits in vitro IL-5 production by murine TcR transgenic T cells (D. Wraith, personal communication). However, in the NOD mouse model of diabetes the converse is seen *(45)*, with anti-CD86 preventing and anti-CD80 exacerbating disease. Furthermore, in a relapsing remitting model of EAE treatment with anti-CD80 during remission exacerbated disease *(46)*. These findings are difficult to reconcile but suggest the possibility of distinct roles for the CD80 and CD86 molecules rather than duplication and redundancy. It has been suggested that these differences are caused by differential expression or differential binding to CD28 and CTLA-4. However, the signal detectable in T cells following binding of CD80 or CD86 to CD28 is remarkably similar *(47–49)*. Thus, it is difficult to see how this differential expression of CD80 and CD86 could influence T-cell phenotype as a consequence of their differential binding to T-cell ligands. In contrast, CD80 and CD86 are capable of signal transduction and deliver distinct signals to B cells *(50,51)*. Ligation of human B-cell CD86 supports IgG4 and IgE class-switching; both IL-4-dependent processes and CD86 have been shown to preferentially support IL-4 production *(44,52)*. Thus, it is possible that either CD80 or CD86 can fulfil the minimum requirement of binding to the T-cell ligands delivering a costimulatory signal, but that CD80 and CD86 differ in their influence on T-cell phenotype following priming resulting from differential transduction of signals to APC by the CD80 and CD86 molecules. Such an effect may not be seen using transfectants expressing CD80 and CD86 or fixed APC, which may not respond to or deliver the appropriate signals (e.g., **ref. 47**). Importantly, intact bivalent antibody molecules or Ig fusion proteins may mediate complex cell surface and intercellular interactions (**Fig. 4**). Often overlooked is their ability to approximate FcR to target molecules and to crosslink FcR on adjacent cells delivering a distinct signal to these cells. Optimum use of these molecules will require resolution of these issues. Given that initial work with CD28 and subsequent work with CTLA-4 testify to the dangers of not appreciating the potential for signal transduction, it is disappointing that little work has been performed using monovalent molecules that do not bind FcR to block these interactions.

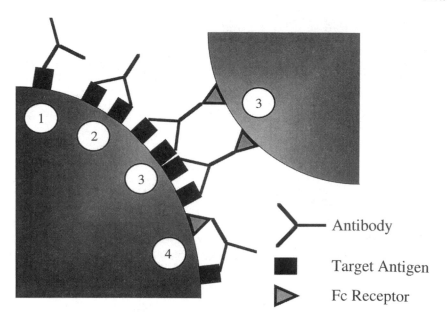

Fig. 4. Cell surface interactions mediated by antibodies or Ig fusion proteins. Intact antibodies may transduce signals to target cells through four distinct mechanisms:

1. For some target antigens binding of antibody, without crosslinking, may be adequate.
2. Alternatively, bivalent antibody may be required in order to crosslink target molecules (e.g. members of immunoglobulin superfamily).
3. Binding of antibody to FcR on one cell and target antigen on an adjacent cell may provide higher valency crosslinking of the target antigen but also approximate FcR on the adjacent cell delivering a signal to this cell also.
4. Intact antibody may crosslink the target antigen and FcR on the same cell.

6. Summary

A large number of therapeutic antibodies targeting the inflammatory autoimmune response have been developed. Their efficacy in clinical use still falls significantly short of the expectation generated by experimental results. This may in part be explained by a failure of therapeutic antibodies to recruit the same mechanisms shown to be effective in animal models. However, the inherent specificity of antibody molecules and the ability to manipulate antibodies to achieve optimum therapeutic actions ensures that they remain attractive therapeutic agents.

Acknowledgments

Work in the author's laboratory is supported by the National Kidney Research Fund, Fujisawa UK Ltd., Grifols UK Ltd., and Celltech Therapeutics.

References

1. Chambers, C. A. and Alison, J. P. (1997) Co-stimulation in T cell responses. *Curr. Opin. Immunol.* **9**, 396–404.
2. Lenschow, D. J., Walunas, T. L., et al. (1996) CD28/B7 system of T cell costimulation. *Ann. Rev. Immunol.* **14**, 233–258.
3. Saito, T. (1998) Negative regulation of T cell activation. *Curr. Opin. Immunol.* **10**, 313–321.
4. Grewal, I. S., Foellmer, H. G., et al. (1996) Requirement for CD40 ligand in costimulation induction, T cell activation and experimental allergic encephalomyelitis. *Science* **273**, 1864–1867.
5. Yang, Y. and Wilson, J. M. (1996) CD40 ligand-dependent T cell activation: requirement of B7-CD28 signaling through CD40. *Science* **273**, 1862–1864.
6. Acha-Orbea, H., Mitchell, D. J., et al. (1988) Limited heterogeneity of T cell receptors from lymphocytes mediating autoimmune encephalomyelitis allows specific immune intervention. *Cell* **54**, 263–273.
7. Acha-Orbea, H. (1993) T-cell receptors in autoimmune disease, in *Monoclonal Antibodies and Peptide Therapy in Autoimmune Diseases,* vol. 59 (Bach, J.-F., ed.), Marcel Dekker, New York, pp. 131–142.
8. Aharoni, R., Teitelbaum, D., et al. (1991) Immunomodulation of experimental allergic encephalomyelitis by antibodies to the antigen-Ia complex. *Nature* **351**, 147–150.
9. Waldmann, T. A. (1993) The IL-2/IL-2 receptor system: a target for rational immune intervention. *Immunol. Today* **14**, 264–269.
10. Van Gelder, T. and Weimar, W. (1997) Potential of anti-interleukin-2 receptor monoclonal antibodies in solid organ transplantation. *Biodrugs* **8**, 46–55.
11. Kuttler, B., Kauert, C., et al. (1997) Anti-CD25/CsA therapy induced a CD4+ T cell-mediated tolerance in BB/OK rats. *Immunobiology* **197**, 243.
12. Kyle, V., Coughlan, R. J., et al. (1989) Beneficial effect of monoclonal antibody to interleukin 2 receptor on activated T cells in rheumatoid arthritis. *Ann. Rheumatic Dis.* **48**, 428–429.
13. Kirkham, B., Pitzalis, C., et al. (1991) Monoclonal antibody therapy in rheumatoid arthritis: the clinical and immunological effects of a CD7 monoclonal antibody. *Br. J. Rheumatol.* **30**, 459–463.
14. Kirkham, B., Thien, F., et al. (1992) Chimeric CD7 monoclonal antibody therapy in rheumatoid arthritis. *J. Rheumatol.* **19**, 1348–1352.
15. Williams, I. R. and Perry, L. L. (1985) A double determinant sandwich immunoassay for quantitation of serum monoclonal anti-I-A antibody. *J. Immunol. Methods* **85**, 279–294.

16. Sayegh, M. H., Akalin, E., et al. (1995) CD28-B7 blockade after alloantigenic challenge in vivo inhibits Th1 cytokines but spares Th2. *J. Exp. Med.* **181,** 1869–1874.
17. Racke, M. K., Scott, D. E., et al. (1995) Distinct roles for B7-1 (CD-80) and B7-2 (CD-86) in the initiation of experimental allergic encephalomyelitis. *J. Clin. Invest.* **96,** 2195–2203.
18. Vladutiu, A. O. (1991) Treatment of autoimmune diseases with antibodies to class II major histocompatibility complex antigens. *Clin. Immunol. Immunopathol.* **61,** 1–17.
19. Fultz, M., Finkelman, F. D., et al. (1984) In vivo administration of anti-I-A antibody induces the internalization of B cell surface I-A and I-E without affecting the expression of surface immunoglobulin. *J. Immunol.* **133,** 91–97.
20. Kruisbeek, A. M., Titus, J. A., et al. (1985) In vivo treatment with monoclonal anti-I-A antibodies: disappearance of splenic antigen-presenting cell function concomitant with modulation of splenic cell surface I-A and I-E antigens. *J. Immunol.* **134,** 3605–3614.
21. Wade, W. F., Davoust, J., et al. (1993) Structural compartmentalization of MHC class II signaling function. *Immunol. Today* **14,** 539–545.
22. Scholl, P. R. and Geha, R. S. (1994) MHC class II signalling in B-cell activation. *Immunol. Today* **15,** 418–422.
23. Smith, R. M., Morgan, A., et al. (1994) Anti-class II MHC antibodies prevent and treat EAE without APC depletion. *Immunology* **83,** 1–8.
24. Constant, S., Pfeiffer, C., et al. (1995) Extent of T cell receptor ligation can determine the functional differentiation of naive CD4+ T cells. *J. Exp. Med.* **182,** 1591–1596.
25. Waldmann, H. and Cobbold, S. (1998) How do monoclonal antibodies induce tolerance? A role for infectious tolerance? *Ann. Rev. Immunol.* **16,** 619–644.
26. Lockwood, C. M., Thiru, S., et al. (1993) Long-term remission of intractable systemic vasculitis with monoclonal antibody therapy. *Lancet* **341,** 1620–1622.
27. Lockwood, C. M., Thiru, S., Stewart, S. (1996) Treatment of refractory Wegener's granulomatosis with humanized monoclonal antibodies. *QJM* **89,** 903–912.
28. Isaacs, J. D., Burrows, N., Wing, M., et al. (1997) Humanized anti-CD4 monoclonal antibody therapy of autoimmune and inflammatory disease. *Clin. Exp. Immunol.* **110,** 158–166.
29. Marrack, P., Endres, R., et al. (1983) The major histocompatibility complex-restricted antigen receptor on T-cells. II. Role of the L3T4 product. *J. Exp. Med.* **158,** 1077–1091.
30. Rudd, C. E., Trevillyan, J. M., et al. (1988) The CD4 receptor is complexed in detergent lysates to a protein-tyrosin kinase (pp58) from human T lymphocytes. *Proc. Natl. Acad. Sci. USA* **85,** 190–194.
31. Bartholomew, M., Brett, S., et al. (1995) Functional analysis of the effects of fully humanized anti-CD4 antibody on resting and activated human T cells. *Immunology* **85,** 41–48.

32. Bank, I. and Chess, L. (1985) Perturbation of the T4 molecules transmits a negative signal in T-cells. *J. Exp. Med.* **162,** 1294–1303.
33. Isaacs, J. D. (1999) Does immunotherapy have a role? *Questions and Uncertainties in Rheumatology* (Bird, H. and Snaith, M., eds.), Blackwell Science, Oxford, UK, pp. 207–228.
34. Chatenoud, L., Thervet, E., et al. (1994) Anti-CD3 antibody induces long-term remission of overt autoimmunity in nonobese diabetic mice. *Proc. Natl. Acad. Sci. USA* **91,** 123–127.
35. Bolt, S., Routledge, E., et al. (1993) The generation of a humanized, non-mitogenic CD3 monoclonal antibody which retains in vitro immunosuppressive properties. *Eur. J. Immunol.* **23,** 403–411.
36. Routledge, E. G., Falconer, M. E., et al. (1995) The effect of aglycosylation on the immunogenicity of a humanized therapeutic CD3 monoclonal antibody. *Transplantation* **60,** 847–853.
37. Harding, F. A., McArthur, J. G., et al. (1992) CD28-mediated signalling co-stimulates murine T cells and prevents induction of anergy in T-cell clones. *Nature* **356,** 607–609.
38. Jenkins, M. K. (1994) The ups and downs of T cell costimulation. *Immunity* **1,** 443–446.
39. Walunas, T. L., Lenschow, D. J., et al. (1994) CTLA-4 can function as a negative regulator of T cell activation. *Immunity* **1,** 405–413.
40. Karandikar, N. J., Vanderlugt, C. L., et al. (1996) CTLA-4: a negative regulator of autoimmune disease. *J. Exp. Med.* **184,** 783–788.
41. Larsen, C. P., Elwood, E. T., et al. (1996) Long-term acceptance of skin and cardiac allografts after blocking CD40 and CD28 pathways. *Nature* **381,** 434–438.
42. Khoury, S. J., Akalin, E., et al. (1995) CD28-B7 costimulatory blockade by CTLA4Ig prevents actively induced experimental autoimmune encephalomyelitis and inhibits Th1 but spares Th2 cytokines in the central nervous system. *J. Immunol.* **155,** 4521–4524.
43. Akalin, E., Chandraker, A., et al. (1996) CD28-B7 T cell costimulatory blockade by CTLA4Ig in the rat renal allograft model. *Transplantation* **62,** 1942–1945.
44. Kuchroo, V. K., Das, M. P., et al. (1995) B7-1 and B7-2 costimulatory molecules activate differentially the Th1/Th2 developmental pathways: application to autoimmune disease therapy. *Cell* **80,** 707–718.
45. Lenschow, D. J., Ho, S. C., et al. (1995) Differential effects of anti-B7-1 and anti-B7-2 monoclonal antibody treatment on the development of diabetes in the nonobese diabetic mouse. *J. Exp. Med.* **181,** 1145–1155.
46. Vanderlugt, C. L., Karandikar, N. J., et al. (1997) Treatment with intact anti-B7-1 mAb during disease remission enhances epitope spreading and exacerbates relapses in R-EAE. *J. Neuroimmunol.* **79,** 113–118.
47. Lanier, L. L., O'Fallon, S., et al. (1995) CD80 (B7) and CD86 (B70) provide similar costimulatory signals for T cell proliferation, cytokine production, and generation of CTL. *J. Immunol.* **154,** 97–105.

48. Ghiotto-Ragueneau, M., Battifora, M., et al. (1996) Comparison of CD28-B7.1 and B7.2 functional interaction in resting human T cells, Phosphatidylinositol 3-kinase association to CD28 and cytokine production. *Eur. J. Immunol.* **26,** 34–41.

49. Nunes, J. A., Battifora, M., et al. (1996) CD28 signal transduction pathways. A comparison of B7-1 and B7-2 regulation of the MAP kinases: ERK2 and Jun kinases. *Mol. Immunol.* **33,** 63–70.

50. Hirokawa, M., Kuroki, J., et al. (1996) Transmembrane signaling through CD80 (B7-1) induces growth arrest and cell spreading of human B lymphocytes accompanied by protein tyrosine phosphorylation. *Immunol. Lett.* **50,** 95–98.

51. Jeannin, P., Delneste, Y., et al. (1997) CD86 (B7-2) on human B cells. *J. Biol. Chem.* **25,** 15,613–15,619.

52. Freeman, G. J., Boussiotis, V. A., et al. (1995) B7-1 and B7-2 do not deliver identical costimulatory signals, since B7-2 but not B7-1 preferentially costimulates the initial production of IL-4. *Immunity* **2,** 523–532.

9

Antibodies for Inflammatory Disease

Cytokines

Peter C. Taylor

1. Introduction

Cytokines are small proteins and major mediators of local intercellular communication required for an integrated response to a variety of stimuli in immune and inflammatory responses. By binding their cognate receptors on target cells, these short-lived molecules play a role in many important biological processes, including cell proliferation, activation, death, and differentiation. During an inflammatory response many cytokines are synthesized by a wide range of cell types, including leukocytes and fibroblasts. Some cytokines are proinflammatory, such as interleukin-1 (IL-1) and tumor necrosis factor α (TNF-α); others, such as interleukin-10 (IL-10) and transforming growth factor β (TGF-β), exert predominantly anti-inflammatory effects. However, it is now understood that many cytokines, for example, interferon-γ (IFN-γ), with chiefly proinflammatory activity, can also in some instances have anti-inflammatory properties. Similarly, cytokines with predominantly anti-inflammatory activity, such as IL-10 and TGF-β, may also exhibit proinflammatory properties and therefore have pathogenic potential. Paracrine or autocrine pathways involving cytokines with either pro- or anti-inflammatory activity can lead to reverberating networks determining whether chronic inflammation results.

1.1. Cytokine Antagonists as Therapeutic Agents and Probes of Pathogenesis

The availability of specific high-affinity antagonists to proinflammatory cytokines affords the opportunity to evaluate any potential therapeutic benefits in a pathological setting, while also investigating the biology of a given

From: *Methods in Molecular Medicine, Vol. 40: Diagnostic and Therapeutic Antibodies*
Edited by: A. J. T. George and C. E. Urch © Humana Press Inc., Totowa, NJ

cytokine by means of specific blockade in vivo. The first demonstration of the efficacy of specific cytokine blockade in the treatment of human chronic inflammatory disease was the use of chimeric anti-TNF-α monoclonal antibodies (mAbs) to treat patients with rheumatoid arthritis (RA) *(1)*. Other biological agents employed with a view to inhibit proinflammatory cytokine activity in RA include soluble cytokine receptors, cytokine receptor antagonists, fusion proteins combining cytokines or soluble cytokine receptors with human Fc constructs, or polyethylene glycol and counterregulatory cytokines, which oppose actions of the targets of cytokines (i.e., IL-10 or IL-4 opposing the effects of TNF-α and IL-1).

Means to inhibit processing or synthesis of IL-1 or TNF are also under consideration.

For the purposes of this chapter, I shall focus on the use of antibodies to cytokines in the treatment of RA, with particular emphasis on agents targeting TNF-α.

2. Rheumatoid Arthritis

Rheumatoid arthritis (RA) is a common human disease, with a prevalence of about 1%. The clinical presentation is heterogeneous, with a wide spectrum of age of onset, degree of joint involvement, and severity. At the onset of symptoms it is difficult to predict which patients will follow a more severe disease course. In past decades the treatment strategy for RA has been based on the premise that the disease prognosis is generally favorable. However, the majority of patients with a more aggressive disease evolution become clinically disabled within 20 yr, and for those with severe disease or extra-articular features the mortality is equivalent to that of patients with three-vessel coronary artery disease or stage IV Hodgkin's lymphoma *(2)*. Thus, the notion that RA is a benign disease has been discredited.

The traditional treatment of RA is represented by a pyramidal approach, starting with nonsteroidal anti-inflammatory drugs and progressing to so-called disease-modifying agents, such as gold, sulfasalazine, and methotrexate (MTX). However, up to 90% of patients with aggressive synovitis have radiological evidence of bone erosion within 2 yr of diagnosis, despite treatment *(3)*. Such observations have led to a recent trend toward much earlier use of disease-modifying antirheumatic drugs in the pharmacological management of disease. However, it can not be stated unequivocally that any treatment halts the destructive process responsible for erosion of cartilage, bone, and soft tissues.

Recent therapeutic advances have accompanied progress in defining the pathogenesis of RA. Although there is abundant evidence that RA is an immune-mediated disease, there are many unresolved questions. For example, is RA primarily an autoimmune disease? Is the initiating agent infectious, a self antigen, or both? To what extent does the course of the disease depend on systemic or joint-specific events?

RA is characterized by chronic inflammation of synovial joints, with synovial proliferation and infiltration by blood-derived cells, in particular, memory T cells, macrophages, and plasma cells, all of which show signs of activation *(4,5)*. The augmented cell mass is sustained by prominent development of new blood vessels. In the chronic phase of disease, capillaries and postcapillary venules are particularly evident in the sublining region, histological sections sometimes demonstrating mononuclear and polymorphonuclear leukocytes in close aposition to vascular endothelium and probably in the process of margination and adhesion prior to migration into the inflamed tissue. Synovium becomes markedly hyperplastic and locally invasive at the interface of cartilage and bone, with progressive destruction of these tissues in the majority of cases. This invasive tissue is referred to as "pannus," comprising mainly lining cells with the appearance of proliferating mesenchymal cells with very little sublining lymphocytic infiltration. The accompanying destruction of bone and cartilage is thought to be principally mediated by cytokine-induced degradative enzymes, especially matrix metalloproteinases. In most cases the principal manifestation of rheumatoid disease is in the synovial joint (**Fig. 1**), but there is also evidence of systemic involvement; for example, the upregulation of acute phase proteins, and in severe cases, involvement of other organs.

2.1. Role of Cytokines in the Pathogenesis of RA

Cytokines derived from macrophages and fibroblasts are abundant in the rheumatoid synovium. These include IL-1, TNF-α, granulocyte-macrophage colony stimulating factor (GM-CSF), interleukin-6 (IL-6), and numerous chemoattractant cytokines known as chemokines. Many of these factors are of importance in regulating inflammatory cell migration and activation. By contrast, given the extent of synovial inflammation and lymphocytic infiltration, factors produced by T cells, for example, IFNγ, interleukin-2 (IL-2), and interleukin-4 (IL-4), are surprisingly sparsely expressed *(6,7)*.

Studies from a number of laboratories have confirmed the expression of this extensive range of proinflammatory cytokines in human synovial tissue samples regardless of differences in donor disease duration, severity, or even drug therapy *(8)*. Such observations imply prolonged cytokine expression in rheumatoid synovium, contrasting with the transient production induced by mitogenic stimulation. This hypothesis was confirmed by the finding of proinflammatory cytokine production in dissociated RA synovial membrane cell cultures over several days in the absence of extrinsic stimulation *(9)*. This observation suggested the presence of signals regulating prolonged cytokine

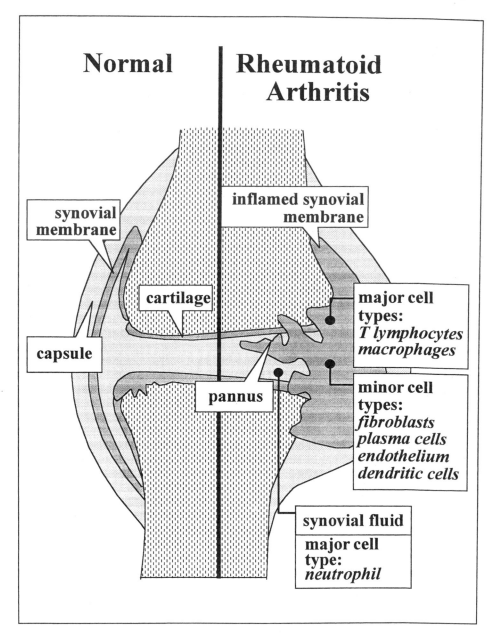

Fig. 1. Synovial joint in health and rheumatoid arthritis indicating cellular components and sites of destruction in diseased joint.

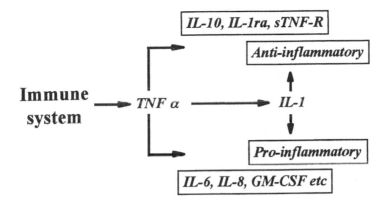

Fig. 2. Cytokine cascade in rheumatoid arthritis.

synthesis within the RA synovial membrane cell cultures. A key observation, in the face of a heterogeneous population of cells producing numerous cytokine and other noncytokine messengers, was that in RA synovial cell cultures, addition of anti-TNF antibodies strikingly reduced the production of other proinflammatory cytokines, including IL-1, GM-CSF, IL-6, and IL-8 *(10)*. Furthermore, using the same RA synovial cell culture system, blockade of IL-1 by means of the IL-1 receptor antagonist results in reduced IL-6 and IL-8 production, but not that of TNF-α *(11)*. These observations support the concept that TNF-α occupies the dominant position at the apex of a proinflammatory cytokine network (**Fig. 2**). As a pleiotropic cytokine with the ability to enhance synovial proliferation and production of prostaglandins, metalloproteinases *(12)*, and cytokines, TNF-α was seen as representing a potential therapeutic target in RA.

In the chronic inflammatory situation in rheumatoid synovium there is also upregulation of multiple anti-inflammatory mediators but at a level insufficient to suppress synovitis. There is abundant expression of IL-10 *(13)* and TGF-β both in latent and active form *(14,15)*. Naturally occurring cytokine inhibitors, such as interleukin-1 receptor antagonists (IL-1ra) and soluble TNF receptors, the specific inhibitors of IL-1 and TNF α respectively *(16)*, are also upregulated in the rheumatoid joint.

3. TNF-α as a Mediator of Disease

As long ago as 1893 it was noted that severe infection may lead to reduction in the bulk of a malignant tumor *(17)*, an observation now attributed to infection-induced release of cytotoxic cytokines, such as TNF-α. TNF-α was purified *(18)* and the gene encoding it cloned *(19–21)* in the mid 1980s. Since then

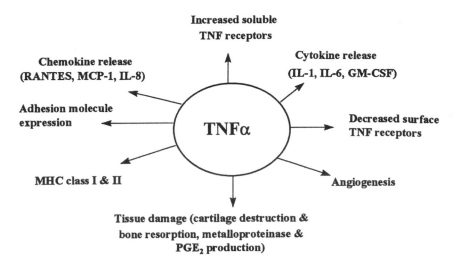

Fig. 3. The biological activities of TNF-α.

many biological properties have been reported in addition to the induction of cachectia and tumor lysis that led to its discovery *(22)* (**Fig. 3**).

TNF-α is synthesized as a protein with a molecular weight of 26 kDa and comprising 233 amino acids. This proprotein is cleaved by TNF-α-converting enzyme (a specific metalloproteinase), yielding a monomeric 17-kDa molecule comprising 157 amino acids. Under physiological conditions, TNF-α exists as a noncovalently bound, cone-shaped homotrimer *(23)*. The biological activity of TNF-α is mediated by crosslinking of membrane-bound receptors, which exist in two isoforms; TNF receptor I (TNFRI, p55) and TNF receptor II (TNFRII, p75) *(24)*. The extracellular domains of both receptors can be shed such that the soluble forms retain the ability to bind TNF-α, thus limiting acute TNF-α-induced effects *(25,26)*.

It is not possible to detect TNF-α in the peripheral blood of healthy humans *(27)* even by means of very sensitive assays (with a 200 attomolar detection limit equivalent to 12×10^5 TNF trimers in 1 mL of plasma) based on the extremely high binding specificity and affinity of p55 TNF receptor for TNF-α. By contrast, TNF-α is detectable in up to nanomolar concentrations in a variety of infectious diseases and inflammatory diseases, including acute septic shock, bacterial meningitis, cerebral malaria, adult respiratory distress syndrome, AIDS, Crohn's disease, and RA *(28)*. High concentrations of plasma TNF-α also occur in therapy-associated syndromes, such as Jarisch-Herxheimer reaction *(29)*, and subsequent to infusion of anti-CD3 mAbs for the treatment of acute graft rejection *(30)*. It might be predicted that TNF-α blockade would be of therapeutic benefit in several of these disease states.

3.1. Strategies to Block TNF-α

The effects of released TNF-α can be antagonized by anti-TNF-α antibodies or soluble TNF-α receptors. A number of other endogenous or synthetic anti-TNF-α agents inhibit synthesis of the molecule. Endogenous agents include cytokines, such as IL-4 *(31)*, IL-10 *(32)*, and TGF-β *(33)*, in addition to noncytokine mediators, such as corticosteroids *(34)*, adenosine *(35,36)*, histamine *(37)*, and nitric oxide *(38,39)*. Drugs may interfere with TNF production at a number of points in the synthetic pathway. Thus, TNF-α transcription is suppressed by pentoxifyline, a phosphodiesterase inhibitor, and TNF-α translation is inhibited by dexamethasone *(34)*. The half-life of TNF-α mRNA is decreased by thalidomide *(40)*.

4. Anticytokine Antibodies as Therapeutic Agents: Clinical Research and Trials

4.1. Chimeric Monoclonal Anti-TNF-α Antibody (cA2) in the Treatment of RA

Monoclonal antibodies that block TNF-α prevent the development of symmetrical, chronic inflammatory polyarthritis, resembling RA, in transgenic mice that express large amounts of TNF-α *(41)*. Furthermore in CIA anti-TNF-α mAbs ameliorate established joint disease when administered in multiple doses of 10–12 mg/kg *(42)*.

The use of anti-TNF-α mAbs in human RA patients has provided the first evidence that TNF-α is a potential therapeutic target in this disease. It has also provided a means for human in vivo testing of the hypothesis, formulated on the basis of in vitro studies; namely that in RA, TNF-α is an important pathogenic agent and regulator of other proinflammatory mediators.

The first antibody to be used in clinical trials was cA2 (from Centocor, Malvern, PA), a chimerized (human IgG1/mouse Fv) mAb shown to bind TNF-α with high affinity (1.8×10^{-9} M) and neutralizing various biological activities in vitro *(43)*. The rationale for the use of chimerized antibodies was twofold; an attempt to reduce immunogenicity as compared to a murine mAb (cA2 is 75% human immunoglobulin) and to increase the half-life of murine antibodies *(44)*.

Anti-TNF-α mAb (cA2) was first administered to RA patients by intravenous infusion in an open label study initiated in May 1992 *(45)*. The dose regimen and schedule were derived by extrapolation from studies utilizing analogous anti-TNF-α antibody reagents in the treatment of collagen-induced arthritis *(42)*. Twenty patients with chronic, erosive RA and evidence of active joint disease despite a history of treatment with multiple DMARDs (such as gold, methotrexate, and salazopyrin) received a total dose of 20 mg/kg cA2 by

2–4 intravenous infusions over a 2-wk period. In order to assess the effects of cA2 infusion without any introduction of bias by concomitantly administered DMARD or other anti-inflammatory therapy, prior to administration of cA2 patients underwent a washout period of at least 4 wk, during which DMARDS were withdrawn and doses of nonsteroidal anti-inflammatory drugs and/or corticosteroids were fixed.

Preclinical safety tests on primates and human volunteers (in dose ranges predicted to be therapeutic in RA) showed cA2 to be nontoxic. The primary aims of the open-label study were to evaluate safety and tolerability of cA2 in RA patients. Patients were found to be free of adverse effects during the timeframe of the trial and antibody infusions were well tolerated without alteration in cardiorespiratory function or body temperature.

Clinical responses in the open-label study were also encouraging. Patients showed marked and statistically significant improvement in all measures of clinical disease activity assessed. These included duration of early morning stiffness, tender and swollen joint count, and pain scores. The improvements in clinical status were accompanied by large and statistically significant falls in measures of acute phase response, such as CRP and serum amyloid A. The magnitude and consistency of both clinical and serological measures strongly suggested that cA2 has a therapeutic effect.

To confirm the impression of a clinical benefit to RA patients following administration of cA2, a placebo-controlled trial of short-term administration of this antibody was conducted at four European centers with 73 participating patients *(1)*. The trial design included randomization of patients to one of three treatment limbs, consisting of a single infusion of placebo (0.1% human serum albumin), or cA2 (at a dose or 1 or 10 mg/kg) and standardized means of evaluating clinical response. In common with the open-label trial, entry criteria to the first placebo-controlled trial of cA2 in RA included the requirement of long-standing disease refractory to conventional therapy, and the need for a washout period for withdrawal of existing DMARD treatment and stabilization of doses of other concomitant anti-inflammatory medications. The primary outcome measure of this study, assessed at wk 4, was the attainment of a standardized improvement in a composite index of disease activity incorporating six independent variables as defined by Paulus et al. *(46)*. The Paulus criteria define a positive outcome as a significant improvement in at least four of six variables as follows:

1. At least 20% improvement in the four continuous variables: tender and swollen joint count, duration of morning stiffness, and ESR;
2. At least two-grade improvement in the patient's and observer's assessment of disease severity.

At the predetermined 4-wk endpoint, clear differences in outcome, as judged by the Paulus 20% criteria, became evident in the three treatment limbs. Nineteen out of 24 patients (79%) in the high-dose group and 11 out of 25 patients (44%) in the low-dose group responded to therapy, compared with only 2 out of 24 (8%) of patients treated with placebo. By arbitrarily raising the threshold of response to 50% improvement in the continuous variables comprising the Paulus index, it was found that 58% of patients benefited at the higher dose of cA2 and 28% at the lower dose. Given that the participating patients had previously received an average of three different DMARDs without adequate long-term disease suppression, these results seem even more impressive.

Secondary outcome measures in the placebo-controlled trial *(1)* included several individual clinical assessments of disease activity, such as tender and swollen joint counts, pain and fatigue scores, patient and clinician assessment of overall disease activity, grip strength, and duration of early morning stiffness. A highly significant improvement was observed in each of these measures in recipients of both high- and low-dose anti-TNF-α groups compared with recipients of placebo.

Over the first 2 wk following cA2 infusion the proportion of patients responding as defined by the Paulus 20% criteria was broadly similar in recipients of either the low-dose (1 mg/kg) or high-dose (10 mg/kg) regimen. Similarly, the magnitude of improvement in various clinical parameters was comparable in the two groups at this early stage, generally 60–70% change from baseline. However, the two groups differed with respect to duration of response. A clear dose–response relationship with time became apparent when participants in the blinded phase of the trial were followed to relapse of disease and further information concerning magnitude and duration of responses to an intermediate dose of cA2 (3 mg/kg) became available in an open-label, follow-up phase of this trial. In this follow-up phase, recipients of placebo became eligible for treatments with one of several cA2 doses. Pooled analysis of the data from 14 recipients of 3 mg/kg cA2, together with data from the recipients of placebo, 1 mg/kg, or 10 mg/kg cA2 in the blinded phase of the study, permitted construction of dose-response curves over time (**Fig. 4**).

The median duration of clinical response, assessed by the Paulus 20% criteria, was 3, 6, and 8 wk in the 1, 3, and 10 mg/kg cA2 dose regimens.

In RA joint cell cultures the effects of TNF-α are inhibited by concentrations of cA2 between 1 and 5 µg/mL. It is likely that duration of clinical response is directly related to maintenance of serum concentrations above approx 1 µg/mL. This would also explain why the proportion of responders and magnitude of responses are much the same at all three treatment doses in the first 2 wk after administration of cA2. Following a single infusion of 1 and

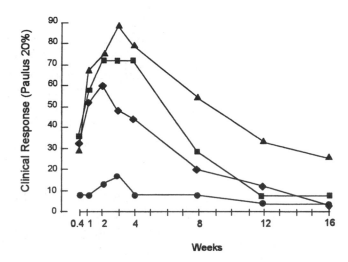

Fig. 4. Duration of clinical response assessed by the Paulus disease activity index following placebo, 0.1 HAS, $n = 24$ (●); and cA2, anti-TNF MAb at 1 mg/kg, $n = 25$ (♦); 3 mg/kg, $n = 14$ (■); and 10 mg/kg, $n = 24$ (▲).

10 mg/kg cA2, concentrations (C_{max}) of 23 and 277 μg/mL are achieved. The terminal half-life of the chimerized antibody at the 10 mg/kg dose is 9–10 d, a time intermediate between the 1–2 d elimination half-life for most intact murine immunoglobulin and the 23 d half-life reported for human IgG1 gammaglobulin *(47)*.

The clinical improvements observed in the first placebo-controlled trial of anti-TNF-α antibody treatment in RA were paralleled by improvements in various laboratory measures. There was significant improvement in the acute-phase proteins CRP, serum amyloid A, fibrinogen, and haptoglobin *(47)*. A dose-dependent increase in hemoglobin levels was observed as compared to placebo, accompanied by reductions in both erythropoietin and IL-6 levels. These observations implicate TNF-α in the pathogenesis of anemia of chronic disease by a mechanism independent of erythropoietin suppression *(48)*, perhaps acting directly on erythroid precursors in bone marrow. Thrombocytosis was also observed to be significantly reduced by cA2 in RA patients *(1)*, possibly by downregulation of IL-6.

The results of the first randomized double-blind study utilizing chimeric anti-TNF-α mAbs to treat RA represents compelling evidence that selected cytokine blockade is of unequivocal therapeutic benefit in human chronic inflammatory disease. Nonetheless, despite impressive disease amelioration in the majority of patients following a single pulse of antibody treatment, the disease invariably relapsed. The important question to ask, therefore, is whether repeated antibody treatments result in long-term suppression of inflammation and in particular, modification of long-term disease outcomes. Although many of the standard drugs used in the treatment of RA are termed "disease modifying," it cannot be unequivocally stated that use of these drugs results in a more favorable long-term outcome. As yet, it is unknown whether cA2, or other antibody treatments targeting TNF-α, are disease modifying. However, there is evidence that repeated administration of anti-TNF-α mAbs can result in longer term suppression of inflammation.

The first experience of repeat administration of cA2 was with a small cohort of patients originally enrolled in the open-label trial. A total of 7 patients received between 2 and 4 complete treatment cycles as a single infusion of 10 mg/kg in cycles 2–4, following an initial dose of 20 mg/kg. After the initial treatment, the timing of the 10 mg/kg infusions was determined by the point of disease relapse, defined as loss of the Paulus 20% response measure consequent upon the proceeding treatment cycle *(49)*. A reproducibly beneficial clinical response of similar magnitude was observed after each retreatment with anti-TNFα mAb, suggesting that there is no TNF-α-independent pathway responsible for maintaining chronic joint inflammation. However, there was considerable variation in response duration between patients, with a trend (although not statistically significant) toward shorter beneficial responses to successive antibody administrations. In the first treatment cycle, at a dose of 20 mg/kg, the median response duration was 12 wk. By the fourth cycle, at a dose of 10 mg/kg, the median duration of benefit was 7.7 wk, a figure not statistically different from an 8 wk median response time reported following a single 10 mg/kg infusion in the placebo-controlled trial.

The murine-variable region of the chimeric anti-TNF-α mAb used in the study might be expected to stimulate antimurine antibody responses after repeated administration. Half the patients receiving retreatment cycles developed antimurine antibodies, mostly at low titer, as compared to only one recipient of cA2 participating in the original open-label trial *(50)*.

The feasibility of long-term suppression of inflammation in RA and a potential strategy for induction of immunological tolerance to cA2 were recently investigated in a multicenter placebo-controlled trial of repeated treatment cycles of cA2, given either as monotherapy or combined with methotrexate *(51)*. In this study, five infusions of placebo or cA2 at 1, 3, or 10 mg/kg were administered over a 14 wk period either with or without concomitant methotrexate therapy at a dose of 7.5 mg/kg once weekly. Responses were sustained through to 26 wk in about 60% of patients and the frequency of human anti-cA2 antibody responses (HACA) was reduced in recipients of combination therapy. Thus, there is evidence that low-dose methotrexate induces immunological tolerance to chimeric mAbs. Current phase III trials have been designed to investigate long-term treatment of RA with low-dose methotrexate and cA2 combination therapy.

4.2. Other Antibody Treatments for RA-Targeting TNF-α

A number of anti-TNF-α biologic agents have now been shown to be effective in RA, confirming that TNF-α is a good choice of therapeutic target in this disease. Other anti-TNF-α mAbs include the humanized antibody CDP571, consisting of hypervariable regions from a mouse mAb, grafted onto a human IgG4 with κ light chains. CDP571 has a similar binding affinity to soluble TNF-α (K_D approx 100 picomolar), as does cA2. Like cA2, in a randomized placebo-controlled trial *(52)*, CDP571 was reported to be effective in reducing the early acute phase response in RA. The published data *(52)* would suggest that CDP571 is less effective than cA2 in amelioration of clinical disease assessment. A 10 mg/kg iv infusion of CDP571 induced some improvement in swollen joint count but without achieving statistical significance. The magnitude of response was less than the change from baseline observed in similar patients receiving the same dose of cA2 *(47)*. There is comparable downregulation of the acute phase protein CRP following administration of cA2 or CDP571 at the same dosage, as might be predicted given that IgG1 and IgG4 isotypes neutralize soluble antigen with similar efficiency. Once possible explanation for the observed differences in clinical efficacy of cA2 and CDP571 is that isotype-dependent cell lysis, mediated by IgG1, may contribute to amelioration of joint inflammation.

A different approach for targeting TNF-α in inflammatory disease would be to infuse exogenous-soluble TNF receptor proteins (sTNFR). To increase the half-life, affinity, and biovaliability of the sTNFR, DNA encoding the soluble portion of human TNFRp75 was linked to DNA encoding the Fc portion of human IgG1 and the combined DNA was then expressed in a mammalian cell line to form a recombinant fusion protein (sTNFR:Fc). This protein, an immunoglobulin-like dimer, consists entirely of human amino acid sequences and acts as a competitive inhibitor of TNF-α. Unlike mAb, with specificity for TNF-α, sTNFR:Fc can also bind lymphotoxin-α (TNF-β). In a multicenter, double-blind trial, 180 patients with refractory RA were randomly assigned to receive twice weekly subcutaneous injections of placebo, or 1 of 3 doses of TNFR:Fc for a 3 mo time period *(53)*. The three treatment groups comprise doses of 0.25, 2, or 16 mg/m² body surface area. Clinical responses were measured by change in a composite index of disease activity as defined by the American College of Rheumatology (ACR) criteria. Administration of sTNFR:Fc induced a dose-dependent reduction in disease activity, 75% of patients in the high-dose group responding at the 20% ACR level at 3 mo, a highly significant finding compared with a 14% response in the placebo group. The mean percentage reduction in the number of tender or swollen joints at 3 mo was 61%, as compared with 25% in the placebo group. As reported in the case of anti-TNF-α mAb therapy, sTNR:Fc treatment was associated with significant reduction in measures of acute phase response, such as ESR and CRP. Cessation of therapy was associated with an increase of disease activity toward the pretrial base line. No dose-limiting toxic effects were observed in this study, and no antibodies to TNF:Fc were detected in serum samples. Adverse events thought to be related, or potentially related, to administration of the fusion protein included mild injection site reactions and upper respiratory tract symptoms.

4.3. Antibodies to TNF-α in the Treatment of Other Inflammatory Conditions

4.3.1. Sepsis

The largest clinical trial of anti-TNF-α mAb for the treatment of sepsis included 994 patients. In a retrospective analysis of a subgroup considered to have had septic shock, there was a 45% reduction in mortality 3 d after the antibody (*54*). However, there was no significant reduction in mortality in the antibody-treated cohort of the 28-d primary endpoint of this study. The findings of this large study are consistent with a number of others using anti-TNF-α mAbs or TNFR-IgG fusion protein constructs (*47*), in which little or no clinical benefit was observed. In the case of a murine anti-TNF-α mAb (CD006: Celltech), only a subgroup of recipients with elevated circulating TNF-α appeared to benefit from antibody infusion, but there was no overall improvement in survival (*55*).

A recently reported phase II study suggests a possible advance in characterizing a subgroup of patients for sepsis syndrome who may potentially benefit from TNF-α (*56*). In this study, 122 patients were randomized to receive different doses of anti-TNF-α antibody fragment (MAK195F) or placebo. As in earlier trial, no overall increase in survival was observed in recipients of the antibody fragment as compared to placebo. Retrospective re-examination of the data following the stratification of patients according to plasma IL-6 concentrations suggested a dose-dependent benefit of the antibody fragments in those patients with IL-6 concentrations, exceeding 1000 pg/mL. Since TNF-α induces IL-6 production identification of patients with this level of plasma, IL-6 may select a group with high cumulative TNF-α exposure. Follow-up trials are underway to further investigate this particular subgroup.

4.3.2. Jarisch-Herxheimer Reaction

Antibiotic treatment of patients with louse-borne relapsing fever is often complicated by acute fever, rigors, and hypotension, a syndrome termed the Jarisch-Herxheimer reaction. This syndrome is associated with elevated plasma levels of TNF-α, IL-6, and IL-8 *(29)*. Anti-TNF-α pretreatment has been shown to markedly attenuate this sepsis syndrome-like condition in patients with louse-borne relapsing fever *(57)*. In a double-blind, placebo-controlled trial, the frequency of reaction was reduced to 50% in patients pretreated with sheep anti-TNF-α Fab as compared to 90% of patients receiving placebo prior to antibiotic therapy.

4.3.3. Inflammatory Bowel Disease

Crohn's disease is characterized by the classic triad of diarrhea, abdominal pain, and weight loss. TNF-α is believed to be an important mediator of inflammatory lesions, which can occur in any portion of the alimentary tract. In support of this hypothesis, rapid and sustained improvements following anti-TNF-α mAb therapy were first observed in patients with steroid-dependent Crohn's disease in open-label studies involving single infusion of between 1 and 20 mg/kg cA2 *(58,59)*. These observations were confirmed in a double-blind, placebo-controlled trial in which 108 patients with active Crohn's disease were randomized to receive placebo of three different doses of cA2 (5, 10, or 20 mg/kg) as a single intravenous dose *(60)*. Of the placebo-treated patients, a degree of clinical response was observed in 17%, and 4% achieved remission. By contrast, 65% of the anti-TNF-α-treated groups achieved clinical responses. The response was sustained for 8 wk in 80% of patients and beyond 12 wk in 63%.

Similar therapeutic benefits have been reported at 2 wk in phase III trials with humanized anti-TNF-α CDP571. However, there was no beneficial effect in the treated groups at later time points *(61)*.

4.4. Mechanisms of Action of Anti-TNF-α Antibodies in the Treatment of RA

The clinical trials of therapy for RA directed at TNF-α, including the use of antibodies or soluble receptor fusion proteins that bind TNF-α and block its biological activity, demonstrate marked dose-dependent improvement in both clinical and laboratory measures of inflammation. As previously discussed, this outcome was anticipated on the basis of known multiple biological effects of TNF-α. However, it remains to be established which of these activities, interrupted by TNF-α blockade, are of central importance in the observed amelioration of disease. Evidence to date support the hypothesis that there are two particularly important mechanisms of action; deactivation of the proinflammatory cytokine cascade at the site of inflammation and diminished recruitment of inflammatory cells from blood to the rheumatoid joint.

The first indirect evidence to suggest that TNF-α blockade in vivo has an effect on the cytokine network was the marked reduction in acute phase proteins, such as CRP, within days of administration of anti-TNF-α antibody. Elevated serum concentrations of CRP in RA reflect production by hepatocytes under the regulation of cytokines signaling via the gp130 receptor, in particular, IL-6. Since circulating IL-6 is detectable in the majority of patients with active RA, it has been possible to directly confirm that changes in CRP are accompanied by changes in IL-6 *(45,62)*, maximum reductions occurring within 24 h of cA2 infusion. In contrast, IL-1 is either undetectable or present in very low concentrations in peripheral blood of most patients, so it is not possible to directly test the prediction, based on the in vitro studies discussed earlier *(10)*, that TNF-α blockade regulates IL-1 production. Dose-dependent reductions in serum concentrations of the chemokines IL-8 and MCP1 have also been observed after administration of cA2 (Paleolog et al., unpublished data).

There is clear evidence that the therapeutic benefit of anti-TNF antibody treatment is not mediated by an upregulation of endogenous proinflammatory cytokine inhibitors, since circulating IL-1ra and soluble TNF receptor levels fall after cA2 infusion *(47)*. Histological examination of multiple synovial biopsies obtained during arthroscopic examination of knee joints of RA patients immediately prior to and 4 wk after a single infusion of 10 mg/kg cA2 revealed significant reduction in synovial cellularity after treatment. In particular, there was significant reduction in synovial CD3 cells and a trend to diminished macrophage infiltration *(63,64)*. Given that these cell types are relatively long-lived, these findings may underestimate the maximum effect of TNF-α blockade on synovial cellularity. There was a significant reduction in synovial endothelial E-selectin expression after cA2 and also tissue expression of VCAM-1. There was a down trend in ICAM-1 expression in both the lining and sublining layers *(63,64)*.

Soluble forms of the adhesion molecules ICAM 1, VCAM-1, and E-selectin are derived from the corresponding cell surface forms by proteolytic cleavage *(65)*. The release of shed adhesion molecules correlates with changes in expression of the corresponding cell surface molecules on cultured endothelial cells following activation with TNF-α or IL-1 *(66)*. Serum samples from RA patients participating in the first placebo-controlled trial of cA2 *(1)* were assayed by enzyme-linked immunosorbent assay (ELISA) for all three soluble adhesion molecules. Median baseline concentrations were markedly elevated, and significant dose-dependent reduction in soluble E-selectin and ICAM-1 were observed 4 wk after cA2 administration *(67)*. The magnitude of change was generally greatest in those patients assessed as having a good clinical response. Levels of soluble VCAM-1 were unchanged. These findings are consistent with the hypothesis that TNF-α blockade downregulates adhesion molecule expression with consequent reduction in inflammatory cell migration to the joint.

Downregulation of endothelial adhesion molecule expression following TNF-α blockade would be predicted to reduce margination and migration to all leukocyte classes to sites of inflammation, with a consequent increase in circulating cell counts. In keeping with this prediction, peripheral blood lymphocyte counts were found to rise to a maximum level within 24 h of anti-TNF-α infusion *(67)*.

In contrast, numbers of peripheral blood granulocytes, which have a circulating half-life measured in hours, decrease after cA2 with maximal changes within 24 h. This observation may reflect reduced myeloid cell production as a consequence of downregulation of GM-CSF since TNF-α induces GM-CSF production by cultured RA synovial cells *(68,69)*. As a consequence of the short circulating half-life of the granulocyte, it seems likely that a diminished rate of cell production will dominate the peripheral blood picture at the time point sampled. However, by studying the kinetics of autologous granulocytes, separated and labeled with ^{111}In, we now have evidence of reduction in the marginating granulocyte pool after a single 10 mg/kg infusion of cA2 *(70)*. Analysis of images of knee, hand, and wrist joints after bolus injection of autologous ^{111}In granulocytes confirm that TNF-α blockade results in significantly reduced granulocyte traffic to inflamed joints.

Histologic assessment of synovial biopsies obtained during arthroscopic knee joint examination at baseline and 2 wk after administration of anti-TNF-α demonstrate a significant reduction in expression of the chemokines IL-8 and MCP-1 *(70)*. Thus, TNF-α blockade reduces both endothelial adhesiveness and chemotactic gradients with corresponding reduction in inflammatory cell margination and migration in to RA joints.

Sustained synovial inflammation in RA also depends on a neovascular network to promote the delivery of cells and nutrients. Vasculoendothelial growth factor (VEGF) is a particularly important promoter of neovascularization that is expressed in synovial membrane and elevated in the serum of RA patients relative to nonarthritic controls. A single 10 mg/kg infusion of cA2 significantly reduces serum VEGF, and combination therapy with methotrexate and multiple infusions of anti-TNF-α antibody enhance the magnitude of reduction to a maximum of 50% of baseline concentrations *(71)*. It might be speculated that the rapid improvements in clinical measures, such as early morning stiffness, joint swelling, and effusion, observed after anti-TNF-α antibody therapy may be the result of reduced vascular permeability consequent to down-regulation of VEGF.

4.5. Potential Limitations of Anti-TNF-α Antibody Therapy in RA

4.5.1. General

One potential limitation of the anti-TNF-α antibody agents discussed is the need for parentral administration. Alternative means of targeting TNF-α include the use of small molecules, effective by oral administration, inhibiting the proteases that process the membrane-bound cytokine or the protein kinases regulating TNF-α synthesis.

A particularly important question, as yet unanswered, is whether TNF-α blockade is simply anti-inflammatory or whether it can actually halt the destructive process responsible for erosion of cartilage, bone, and soft tissue. Although the clinical trials using the anti-TNF-α agents previously discussed demonstrate a marked symptomatic benefit in a high proportion of patients with long established RA, the responses are all transient. Nonetheless, clinical benefit is reproducibly observed after repeated antibody administration, indicating the joint inflammation remains TNF-α dependent. That therapy is palliative, rather than curative, is presumably because such intervention does not permanently reset the homeostatic balance of the cytokine network. The chronic synovitis of RA has both inflammatory and invasive elements that can be mediated by distinct mechanisms *(72)*. The many biological activities of TNF-α in RA include promotion of cell proliferation and production of destructive metalloproteinase (MMP) enzymes by fibroblasts and other synoviocytes. However, a large body of evidence from animal models of arthritis indicates that TNF-α plays a central role in joint inflammation but is subservient to IL-1 in the destructive process *(73)*. If a parallel dichotomy applies in RA, then retardation or abolition of disease progression may depend on whether TNF-α blockade in vivo downregulates IL-1 production, as has been demonstrated in RA synovial cell cultures. If not, inhibition of IL-1, in addition to TNF-α, may be required for disease modification. Dose-related, significant reductions in serum MMP1 (collagenase) and MMP3 (stromelysin 1) have been demonstrated following infusion of cA2 but not placebo *(74)*, although it is not yet known how peripheral blood MMP levels relate to those in the joints.

4.5.2. Safety Issues

Given that TNF-α evolved to serve specific biological functions, the near elimination of this factor by specific antibody treatment raised the concern that any benefits of therapy might be accompanied by side effects related to defective immune surveillance. In fact, neither opportunistic infections nor increased neoplasia have been observed and there is little evidence of defective responses to infectious diseases in recipients of cA2 (reviewed in detail in Feldmann [47]). Where infections have been observed in patients with Crohn's disease or RA treated with anti-TNF-α antibody they have been typical of the infections commonly occurring in these disease groups. In a placebo-controlled trial in which cA2 was administered to patients with presumed sepsis, there was a trend toward mortality benefit at 4 wk in recipients of cA2, no opportunistic infections were observed, and adverse events were similar in the anti-TNF-α and placebo-treated groups (47).

An unexpected side effect reported in RA trials of several anti-TNF-α biologics was the development of antibodies to double-stranded DNA (anti-ds-DNA). IgM class anti-ds-DNA antibodies were observed several weeks after cA2 infusion in 7 of 69 (6%) patients treated in early trials (1,45,49). Three of these individuals received a subsequent cA2 infusion. In one patient, the anti-ds-DNA became undetectable after the second cA2 infusion; in a second, the titer remained unaltered; and in the third, titers rose after the second cA2 infusion. None of these patients developed any signs or symptoms of a lupus-like syndrome. In a multidose study of cA2 in RA, one patient developed worsening arthritis, dyspnea, and pleuritic chest pain 4 wk after a fourth dose of 3 mg/kg cA2. These symptoms abated and a further 3 mg/kg infusion was given, followed 3 wk later by more severe and persistent symptoms. Serial serum analysis revealed that ANA and antibodies to ds-DNA appeared for the first time 6 wk into the study, suggesting that cA2 administration may have precipitated a lupus-like syndrome in this individual (47). The symptoms resolved with oral steroid treatment. The pathogenesis of induction of anti-ds-DNA antibodies in a minority of RA patients treated with anti-TNF-α therapy remains unknown, although other antirheumatic drugs, such as sulfasalazine, can also induce such autoantibodies.

5. Concluding Remarks

The development of anticytokine therapy represents an important advance in both treatment and understanding of basic disease mechanisms in chronic inflammation. In the example of RA, TNF-α is the most extensively studied target to date, but others, such as IL-1 and IL-6, are also under evaluation. Alternatives to antibody treatment include the use of naturally occurring anti-inflammatory cytokines, for example, IL-4, IL-10, and IL-11. Given the now compelling evidence of proinflammatory cytokine involvement in the pathogenesis of RA, and the marked clinical benefit of TNF-α blockade in established disease, it may well be that enhanced long term benefit will be derived by anticytokine intervention earlier in the evolution of disease.

It remains to be determined how anticytokine antibody treatment will be used in clinical practice. In the case of RA, short courses of anti-TNF-α treatment could be used to induce remission, or to control disease flares, thus allowing conventional medication to exert its beneficial effect. Long-term monotherapy with anti-TNF-α antibodies alone seems less likely than combination therapy using both conventional drugs and anticytokine agents. In established murine collagen-induced arthritis, for example, addition of a lytic anti-CD4 antibody to a treatment regimen with anti-TNF-α antibody was noted to have synergistic benefit with histological evidence of reduced erosion of bone and cartilage *(76)*. It is predicted that inhibition of T-cell function and TNF-α blockade will be a particularly useful combination strategy in RA.

References

1. Elliott, M. J., Maini, R. N., Feldmann, M., Kalden, J. R., Antoni, C., Smolen, J. S., Leeb, B., Breedveld, F. C., Macfarlane, J. D., Bijl, H., and Woody, J. N. (1994) Randomised double-blind comparison of chimeric monoclonal antibody to tumour necrosis factor α (cA2) versus placebo in rheumatoid arthritis. *Lancet* **344**, 1105–1110.
2. Pincus, T. and Callahan, L. F. (1993) What is the natural history of rheumatoid arthritis? *Rheum. Dis. Clin. North Am.* **19**, 123–151.
3. Sharp, J. T., Wolfe, F., Mitchell, D. M., and Bloch, D. A. (1991) The progression of erosion and joint space narrowing scores in rheumatoid arthritis during the first twenty-five years of disease. *Arthritis Rheum.* **34**, 660–668.
4. Janossy, G., Panayi, G., Duke, O., Bofill, M., Poulter, L. W., and Goldstein, G. (1981) Rheumatoid arthritis: a disease of T-lymphocyte/macrophage immunoregulation. *Lancet* **ii**, 839–841.
5. Cush, J. J. and Lipsky, P. E. (1988) Phenotypic analysis of synovial tissue and peripheral blood lymphocytes isolated from patients with rheumatoid arthritis. *Arthritis Rheum.* **31**, 1230–1238.
6. Firestein, G. S. and Zvaifler, N. J. (1990) How important are T cells in chronic rheumatoid synovitis? *Arthritis Rheum.* **33**, 768–773.
7. Miossec, P., Naviliat, M., D'Angeac, A. D., Sany, J., and Banchereau, J. (1990) Low levels of interleukin-4 and high levels of transforming growth factor β in rheumatoid synovitis. *Arthritis Rheum.* **33**, 1180–1187.
8. Feldmann, M., Brennan, F. M., and Maini, R. N. (1996) Role of cytokines in rheumatoid arthritis. *Ann. Rev. Immunol.* **14**, 397–440.
9. Buchan, G., Barrett, K., Turner, M., Chantry, D., Maini, R. N., and Feldmann, M. (1988) Interleukin-1 and tumour necrosis factor mRNA expression in rheumatoid arthritis: prolonged production of IL-1α. *Clin. Exp. Immunol.* **73**, 449–455.
10. Brennan, F. M., Chantry, D., Jackson, A., Maini R., and Feldmann, M. (1989) Inhibitory effect of TNF α antibodies on synovial cell interleukin-1 production in rheumatoid arthritis. *Lancet* **2**, 244–247.

11. Butler, D., Maini, R. N., Feldmann, M., and Brennan, F. M. (1995) Modulation of proinflammatory cytokine release in rheumatoid synovial membrane cell cultures. Comparison of monoclonal anti TFN-alpha antibody with the interleukin-1 receptor antagonist. *Eur. Cytokine Netw.* **6(4),** 225–230.

12. Dayer, J. M., Beutler, B., and Cerami, A. (1985) Cachectin/tumor necrosis factor stimulates collagenase and prostaglandin E2 production by human synovial cells and dermal fibroblasts. *J. Exp. Med.* **162,** 2163–2168.

13. Katsikis, P. D., Chu, C. Q., Brennan, F. M., Maini, R. N., and Feldmann, M. (1994) Immunoregulatory role of interleukin 10 in rheumatoid arthritis. *J. Exp. Med.* **179,** 1517–1527.

14. Fava, R., Olsen, N., Keski-Oja, J., Moses, H., and Pincus, T. (1989) Active and latent forms of transforming growth factor β activity in synovial effusions. *J. Exp. Med.* **169,** 291–296.

15. Wahl, S. M. (1994) Transforming growth factor β: The good, the bad, and the ugly. *J. Exp. Med.* **180,** 1587–1590.

16. Cope, A. P., Aderka, D., Doherty, M., Engelmann, H., Gibbons, D., Jones, A. C., Brennan, F. M., Maini, R. N., Wallach, D., and Feldmann, M. (1992) Increased levels of soluble tumor necrosis factor receptors in the sera and synovial fluid of patients with rheumatoid diseases. *Arthritis Rheum.* **35,** 1160–1169.

17. Coley, W. (1893) The treatment of malignant tumours by repeated inoculations of erysipelas: with a report of ten original cases. *Am. J. Med. Sci.* **105,** 487–511.

18. Aggarwal, B. B., Kohr, W. J., Hass, P. E., Moffat, B., Spencer, S. A., Henzel, W. J., Bringman, T. S., Nedwin, G. E., Goeddel, D. V., and Harkins, R. N. (1985) Human tumor necrosis factor. Production, purification, and characterization. *J. Biol. Chem.* **260,** 2345–2354.

19. Pennica, D., Nedwin, G. E., Hayflick, J. S., Seeburg, P.H., Derynck, R., Palladino, M. A., Kohr, W. J., Aggarwal, B. B., and Goeddel, D. V. (1984) Human tumor necrosis factor: precursor structure expression and homology to lymphotoxin. *Nature* **312,** 724–729.

20. Shirai, T., Yamaguchi, H., Ito, H., Todd, C. W., and Wallace, R. B. (1985) Cloning and expression in *Escherichia coli* of the gene for human tumour necrosis factor. *Nature* **313,** 803–809.

21. Wang, A. M., Creasey, A. A., Ladner, M. B., Lin, L. S., Strickler, J., Van Arsdell, J. N., Yamamoto, R., and Mark, D. F. (1985) Molecular clongin of the complementary DNA for human tumor necrosis factor. *Science,* **228,** 149–154.

22. Beutler, B. and Cerami, A. (1986) Cachectin and tumour necrosis factor as two sides of the same biological coin. *Nature* **320,** 584–588.

23. Jones, E. Y., Stuart, D. I., and Walker, N. P. C. (1989) Structure of tumour necrosis factor. *Nature* **338,** 225–228.

24. Bazzoni, F. and Beutler, B. (1996) The tumor necrosis factor ligand and receptor families (review). *N. Engl. J. Med.* **334,** 1717–1725.

25. Engelmann, H., Aderka, D., Rubinstein, M., Rotman, D., and Wallach, D. (1989) A tumor necrosis factor-binding protein purified to homogeneity from human urine protects cells from tumor necrosis factor toxicity. *J. Biol. Chem.* **264,** 11,974–11,980.

26. Seckinger, P., Isaaz, S., and Dayer, J. M. (1988) A human inhibitor of tumor necrosis factor α. *J. Exp. Med.* **167,** 1511–1516.
27. Poltorak, A., Peppel, K., and Beutler, B. (1994) Receptor-mediated label-transfer assay (RELAY): a novel method for the detection of plasma tumor necrosis factor at attomolar concentrations. *J. Immunol. Methods* **169,** 93–99.
28. Tracey, K. J. and Cerami, A. (1994) Tumor necrosis factor: a pleiotropic cytokine and therapeutic target. *Ann. Rev. Med.* **45,** 491–503.
29. Negussie, Y., Remick, D. G., DeForge, L. E., Kunkel, S. L., Eynon, A, and Griffin, G. E. (1992) Detection of plasma tumor necrosis factor, interleukins 6, and 8 during the Jarisch-Herxheimer reaction of relapsing fever. *J. Exp. Med.* **175,** 1207–1212.
30. Chatenoud, L., Ferran, C., Reuter, A., Legendre, C., Gevaert, Y., Kreis, H., Franchimont, P., and Bach, J. F. (1989) Systemic reaction to the anti-T-cell monoclonal antibody OKT3 in relation to serum levels of tumor necrosis factor and interferon-gamma. *N. Engl. J. Med.* **320,** 1420,1421.
31. Dayer, J. M. and Burger, D (1994) Interleukin-1, tumor necrosis factor and their specific inhibitors. *Eur. Cytokine Netw.* **5,** 563–571.
32. Marchant, A., Bruyns, C., Vanderabeele, P., Ducarme, M., Gerard, C., Delvaux, A., De Groote, D., Abramowicz, D , Velu, T , and Goldman, M. (1994) Interleukin-10 controls interferon-gamma and tumor necrosis factor production during experimental endotoxemia. *Eur. J. Immunol.* **24,** 1167–1171.
33. Espevik, T., Figari, I. S., Shalaby, M. R., Lackides, G. A., Lewis, G. D., Shepard, H. M., and Palladino, M. A. J. (1987) Inhibition of cytokine production by cyclosporin A and transforming growth factor beta. *J. Exp. Med.* **166,** 571–576.
34. Han, J., Thompson, P., and Beutler, B. (1990) Dexamethasone and pentoxifylline inhibit endotoxin induced TNF synthesis at separate points in their signaling pathway. *J. Exp. Med.* **172,** 391–394.
35. Parmely, M. J., Zhou, W. W., Edwards, C. K., Borcherding, D. R., Silverstein, R., and Morrison, D. C. (1993) Adenosine and a related cabocyclic nucleoside analogue selectively inhibit tumor necrosis factor-alpha production and protect mice against endotoxin challenge. *J. Immunol.* **151,** 389–396.
36. Bouma, M. G., Stad, R. K., van den Wildenberg, F. A., and Buurman, W. A. (1994) Differential regulatory efffects of adenosine on cytokine release by activated human monocytes. *J. Immunol.* **153,** 4159–4168.
37. Vannier, E., Miller, L C , and Dinarello, C. A. (1991) Histamine suppressess gene expression and synthesis of tumor necrosis factor alpha via histamine H2 receptors. *J. Exp. Med.* **174,** 281–284.
38. Florquin, S., Amraoui, Z., Dubois, C., Decuyper, J., and Goldman, M. (1994) The protective role of endogenously synthesized nitric oxide in staphylococcal enterotoxin B-induced shock in mice. *J. Exp. Med.* **180,** 1153–1158.
39. Eigler, A., Moeller, J., and Endres, S. (1995) Exogenous and endogenous nitric oxide attenuate tumor necrosis factor synthesis in the murine macrophage cell line RAW 264.7. *J. Immunol.* **154,** 4048–4054.

40. Moreira, A. L., Sampaio, E. P., Zmuidzinas, A., Frindt, P., Smith, K. A., and Kaplan, G. (1993) Thalidomide exerts its inhibitory action on tumor necrosis factor alpha by enhancing mRNA degradation. *J. Exp. Med.* **177,** 1675–1680.
41. Keffer, J., Probert, L., Cazlaris, H., Georgopoulos, S., Kaslaris, E., Kioussis, D., and Kollias, G. (1991) Transgenic mice expressing human tumour necrosis factor: a predictive genetic model of arthritis. *EMBO J.* **10,** 4025–4031.
42. Williams, R. O., Feldmann, M., and Maini, R. N. (1992) Anti-TNF ameliorates joint disease in murine collagen-induced arthritis. *Proc. Natl. Acad. Sci. USA* **89,** 9784–9788.
43. Knight, D. M., Trinh, H., Le, J., Siegel, S., Shealy, D., McDonough, M., Scallon, B., Moore, A. M., Vilcek, J., Daddona, P., and Ghrayeb, J. (1993) Construction and initial characterization of a mouse-human chimeric anti-TNF antibody. *Mol. Immunol.* **30,** 1443–1453.
44. Winter, G. and Harris, W. J. (1993) Humanized antibodies. *Immunol. Today* **14,** 243–246.
45. Elliott, M. J., Maini, R. N., Feldmann, M., Long-Fox, A., Charles, P., Katsikis, P., Brennan, F. M., Walker, J., Bijl, H., Ghrayeb, J., and Woody, J. N. (1993) Treatment of rheumatoid arthritis with chimeric monoclonal antibodies to tumor necrosis factor α. *Arthritis Rheum.* **36,** 1681–1690.
46. Paulus, H. E., Egger, M. J., Ward, J. R., Williams, H. J., and The Cooperative Systemic Studies of Rheumatic Diseases Group (1990) Analysis of improvement in individual rheumatoid arthritis patients treated with disease-modifying antirheumatic drugs, based on the findings in patients treated with placebo. *Arthritis Rheum.* **33,** 477–484.
47. Feldmann, M., Elliott, M. J., Woody, J. N., and Maini, R. N. (1997) Anti-tumor necrosis factor-α therapy in rheumatoid arthritis. *Adv. Immunol.* **64,** 283–350.
48. Davis, D., Charles, P. J., Potter, A., Feldmann, M., Maini, R. N., and Elliott, M. J. (1997) Anaemia of chronic disease in rheumatoid arthritis: in vivo effects of tumour necrosis factor α. *Br. J. Rheum.* **36,** 950–956.
49. Elliott, M. J., Maini, R. N., Feldmann, M., Long-Fox, A., Charles, P., Bijl, H., and Woody, J. N. (1994) Repeated therapy with monoclonal antibody to tumour necrosis factor α (cA2) in patients with rheumatoid arthritis. *Lancet* **344,** 1125–1128.
50. Maini, R. N., Elliott, M. J., Brennan, F. M., Williams, R. O., Chu, C. Q., Paleolog, E., Charles, P. J., Taylor, P. C., and Feldmann, M. (1995) Monoclonal anti-TNFα antibody as a probe of pathogenesis and therapy of rheumatoid disease. *Immunol. Rev.* **144,** 195–223.
51. Maini, R. N., Breedveld, F. C., Kalden, J. R., Smolen, J. S., Davis, D., MacFarlane, J. D., Antoni, C., Leeb, B., Elliott, M. J., Woody, J. N., Schaible, T. F., and Feldmann, M. (1997) Low dose methotrexate (MTX) suppresses anti-globulin responses and potentiates efficacy of a chimeric monoclonal anti-TNFα antibody (cA2) given repeatedly in rheumatoid arthritis (RA). *Arthritis Rheum.* **40,** S126.
52. Rankin, E. C. C., Choy, E. H. S., Kassimos, D., Kingsley, G. H., Sopwith, S. M., Isenberg, D. A., and Panayi, G. S. (1995) The therapeutic effects of an engineered

human anti-tumour necrosis factor alpha antibody (CDP571) in rheumatoid arthritis. *Br. J. Rheumatol.* **34,** 334–342.

53. Moreland, L. W., Baumgartner, S. W., Schiff, M. H., Tindall, E. A., Fleischmann, R. M., Weaver, A. L., Ettlinger, R. E., Cohen, S., Koopman, W. J., Mohler, K., Widmer, M. B., and Blosch, C. M. (1997) Treatment of rheumatoid arthritis with a recombinant human tumor necrosis factor receptor (p75)-Fc fusion protein. *N. Engl. J. Med.* **337,** 141–147.

54. Abraham, E., Wunderink, R., Silverman, H., Perl, T. M., Nasraway, S., Levy, H., Bone, R., Wenzel, R. P., Balk, R., Allred, R., et al. (1995) Efficacy and safety of monoclonal antibody to human tumor necrosis factor alpha in patients with sepsis sydrome. A randomized, controlled, double-bline, multicenter, clinical trial. TNF-alpha mAb Sepsis Study Group. *JAMA* **273,** 934–941.

55. Fischer, C. J. Jr., Opal, S. M., Dhainaut, J.-F., Stephens, S., Zimmerman, J. L., Nightingale, P., Harris, S. J., Schein, R. M. H., Panacek, E. A., Vincent, J.-L., Foulke, G. E., Warren, E. L., Garrard, C., Park, G., Bodmer, M. W., Cohen, J., Van Der Linden, C., Cross, A. S., Sadoff, J. C., and The Cooperative Systemic Studies of Rheumatic Diseases Group (1993) Influence of an anti-tumor necrosis factor monoclonal antibody on cytokine levels in patients with sepsis. *Crit. Care Med.* **21,** 318–327.

56. Reinhart, K., Wiegand-Lohnert, C., Grimminger, F., Kaul, M., Withington, S., Treacher, D., Eckart, J., Willatts, S., Bouza, C., Krausch, D., Stockenhuber, F., Eiselstein, J., Daum, L., and Kempeni, J. (1996) Assessment of the safety and efficacy of the antibody-fragment, MAK 195F, in patients with sepsis and septic shock: a multicenter, randomized, placebo-controlled, dose-ranging study. *Crit. Care Med.* **24,** 733–742.

57. Fekade, D., Knox, K., Hussein, K., Melka, A., Lalloo, D. G., Coxon, R. E., and Warrell, D.A. (1996) Prevention of Jarisch-Herxheimer reactions by treatment with antibodies against tumor necrosis factor alpha. *N. Engl. J. Med.* **335,** 311–315.

58. Van Dullemen, H. M., Van Deventer, S. J. H., Hommes, D. W., Bijl, H. A., Jansen, J., Tytgat, G. N. J., and Woody, J. (1995) Treatment of Crohn's disease with anti-tumor necrosis factor chimeric monoclonal antibody (cA2). *Gastroenterology* **109,** 129–135.

59. McCabe, R. P., Woody, J. N., van Deventer, S., Targan, S. R., Mayer, L., van Hogezand, R., Rutgeerts, P., Hahauer, S. B., Podolsky, D., and Elson, C. O. (1996) A multicenter trial of cA2 anti-TNF chimeric monoclonal antibody in patients with active Crohn's disease. *Gastroenterology* **110(Suppl.),** A962.

60. Targan, S. R., Hanauer, S. B., van Deventer, S. J., Mayer, L., Present, D. H., Braakman, T., DeWoody, K. L., Schaible, T. F., and Rutgeerts, P. J. (1997) A short-term study of chimeric monoclonal antibody cA2 to tumor necrosis factor alpha for Crohn's disease. Crohn's Disease cA2 Study Disease. *N. Engl. J. Med.* **337,** 1029–1035.

61. Stack, W. A., Mann, S. D., Roy, A. J., Heath, P., Sopwith, M., Freeman, J., Holmes, G., Long, R., Forbes, A., and Kamm, M. A. (1997) Randomised con-

trolled trial of CDP571 antibody to tumour necrosis factor-alpha in Crohn's disease. *Lancet* **349,** 521–524.

62. Charles, P., Potter, A., Elliott, M., Cope, A., Woody, J., Feldmann, M., and Maini, R. N. (1995) Regulation of sTNF-R and IL-6 following TNF blockade in RA: *in vivo* evidence for a cytokine cascade. *Arthritis Rheum.* **38,** S342.

63. Tak, P. P., Taylor, P. C., Breedveld, F. C., Smeets, T. J. M., Daha, M. R., Kluin, P. M., Meinders, A. E., and Maini, R. N. (1996) Decrease in cellularity and expression of adhesion molecules by anti-tumor necrosis factor α monoclonal antibody treatment in patients with rheumatoid arthritis. *Arthritis Rheum.* **39,** 1077–1081.

64. Taylor, P. C., Maini, R. N., Tak, P. P., Breedveld, F. C., Smeets, T. J. M., Daha, M. R., Kluin, P. M., and Meinders, A. E. (1997) Reply to Decrease in cell adhesion molecules by treatment with anti-tumor necrosis factor α monoclonal antibody. *Arthritis Rheum.* **4,** 789–790.

65. Gearing, A. J. H. and Newman, W. (1993) Circulating adhesion molecules in disease. *Immunol. Today* **14,** 506–512.

66. Leeuwenberg, J. F. M., Smeets, E. F., Neefjes, J. J., Shaffer, M. A., Cinek, T., Jeunhomme, T. M. A. A., and Buurman, W. A. (1992) E-selectin and intercellular adhesion molecule-1 are released by activated human endothelial cells *in vitro*. *Immunology* **77,** 543–549.

67. Paleolog, E. M., Elliott, M. J., Woody, J. N., Feldmann, M., and Maini, R. N. (1996) Deactivation of vascular endothelium by monoclonal anti-tumour necrosis factor α antibody in rheumatoid arthritis. *Arthritis Rheum.* **39,** 1082–1091.

68. Alvaro-Gracia, J. M., Zvaifler, N. J., Brown, C. B., Kaushansky, K., and Firestein, G. S. (1991) Cytokines in chronic inflammatory arthritis. *J. Immunol.* **146,** 3365–3371.

69. Haworth, C., Brennan, F. M., Chantry, D., Turner, M., Maini, R. N., and Feldmann, M. (1991) Expression of granulocyte-macrophage colony-stimulating factor in rheumatoid arthritis: regulation by tumor necrosis factor-α. *Eur. J. Immunol.* **21,** 2575–2579.

70. Taylor, P. C., Chapman, P., Elliott, M. J., Schaible, T. F., Peter, A. M., Feldmann, M., and Maini, R. N. (1997) Reduced granulocyte traffic and chemotactic gradients in rheumatoid joints following anti-TNFα therapy. *Arthritis Rheum.* **40,** S80.

71. Paleolog, E. M., Young, S., Stark, A. C., McCloskey, R. V., Feldmann, M., and Maini, R. N. (1998) Modulation of angiogenic vascular endothelial growth factor (VEGF) by TNFα and IL-1 in rheumatoid arthritis. *Arthritis Rheum.* **41,** 1258–1265.

72. Gay, S., Gay, R. E., and Koopman, W. J. (1993) Molecular and cellular mechanisms of joint destruction in rheumatoid arthritis: Two cellular mechanisms explain joint destruction? *Ann. Rheum. Dis.* **52,** S39–S47.

73. Vanlent, P. L. E. M., Vandeloo, F. A. J., Holthuysen, A. E. M., Vandenbersselaar, A. M., Vermeer, H., and Vandenberg, W. B. (1995) Major role for interleukin 1 but not for tumor necrosis factor in early cartilage damage in immune complex arthritis in mice. *J. Rheumatol.* **22,** 2250–2258.

74. Brennan, F. M., Browne, K. A., Green, P. A., Jasper, J.-M., Maini, R. N., and Feldmann, M. (1997) Reduction of serum matrix metalloproteinase 1 and matrix: metalloproteinase 3 in RA patients following anti-TNFα (cA2) therapy. *Br. J. Rheumatol.* **36,** 643–650.

75. Wolfe, F., Mitchell, D. A., Sibley, J. T., Fries, J. F., Bloch, D. A., Williams, C. A., Spitz, P. W., Haga, M., Kleinheksel, S. M., and Cathey, M. A. (1994) The mortality of rheumatoid arthritis. *Arthritis Rheum.* **37,** 481–494.

76. Williams, R. O., Mason, L. M., Feldmann, M., and Maini, R. (1994) Synergy between anti-CD4 and anti-tumor necrosis factor in the amelioration of established collagen-induced arthritis. *Proc. Natl. Acad. Sci. USA* **91,** 2762–2766.

10

Antibodies for Transplantation

Denise L. Faustman

1. Introduction

The use of antibodies in transplantation has become a clinical reality. Antibodies have been used to both dampen the recipient's immune response and to obscure the immunogenicity of the donor graft. Traditionally, antibodies have been administered to the transplant recipient to transiently inactivate the host's T cells, the lymphocytes responsible for recognizing and attacking foreign proteins, cells, and tissues. Antibodies can also be used to eliminate any highly immunogenic passenger cells from a donor graft prior to transplantation, and antibodies can mask or conceal antigens present on donor cells that might trigger rejection.

In addition to enhancing the survival of grafts in the clinic, antibodies are adding to our basic understanding of the molecular mechanisms responsible for transplant rejection. Antibodies designed to recognize various components of the immune system have helped to clarify the role that host T cells and cells in donor transplant play in the rejection cascade.

2. A Host of Antibodies; Meet the Antibodies

Systemically administered antibodies have been used for decades to promote the survival of transplanted tissues and organs. The first preparations, given to the recipients of kidney transplants, contained polyclonal antisera directed against lymphocytes. Administered in conjunction with immunosuppressive drugs, the antibodies temporarily deplete the lymphocytes in the recipient, allowing the graft to take hold before the immune system kicked in. However, these antibodies were nonspecific, and combined with pharmacologic immunosuppression would leave recipients susceptible to infections.

From: *Methods in Molecular Medicine, Vol. 40: Diagnostic and Therapeutic Antibodies*
Edited by: A. J. T. George and C. E. Urch © Humana Press Inc., Totowa, NJ

More recently monoclonal antibodies (mAbs) have been directed against specific proteins on the surface of T cells. The most famous commercial preparation, OKT3 made by Ortho (Raritan, NJ), targets the CD3 receptor on T cells, which has allowed better quality control and fewer side effects. Administered to the recipient prior to transplantation or during a rejection episode, this antibody depletes the host's cytotoxic T lymphocytes. The large-scale production of pure mAbs, such as OKT3, was made possible by the development of hybridoma technology, which allowed the fusion of immortalized lymphoma cells with antibody-producing spleen cells *(1)*.

Generally speaking, polyclonal antibody preparations react most strongly with host lymphocytes because they recognize more cell types and a larger number of markers per cell. At the same time, polyclonal antibodies show greater batch-to-batch variability. Monoclonal antibodies, on the other hand, are restricted in that they recognize only one type of marker on a cell, but they are more uniform in their properties and show less variability then polyclonal preparations.

In addition to choosing between polyclonal versus monoclonal antibodies, investigators can also use antibody fragments for treating transplant recipients or donor graft tissues. Antibodies are composed of a dimeric antigen-binding region, called the F(ab), and a tail, or Fc, region that can bind to cells via Fc receptors. The Fc portion of the antibody can also bind to serum complement proteins, an interaction that promotes lysis of any cell bound to the F(ab) region. Whole antibodies are used when cell lysis is desired—to deplete host T cells, for example. To block or mask an antigen without lysing the cell, a Fab fragment can be used in place of whole antibodies. Such antibody fragments are used to conceal antigenic proteins present on donor grafts. At the other end of the spectrum, antibodies can also be engineered to kill target cells with greater efficiency. In this case, an antibody can be linked to a cellular toxin, such as cholera or diphtheria toxin.

Most antibodies are murine in origin. Because these proteins contain many species-related differences, humans receiving such antibody preparations often mount an immune response against the antibodies themselves. Such a reaction obviously lessens the efficacy of the antibody preparation. Considerable commercial efforts have been directed toward "humanizing" murine mAbs to diminish the host immune reactions that could inactivate the protein. Other chapters in this book address the types of methods used to generate antibodies that can bind human antigens but that lack the foreign amino acid sequences present in the mouse protein.

As mentioned earlier, mAbs can be directed against a number of markers or epitopes on the surface of T cells—the lymphocytes that recognize and destroy donor grafts (**Table 1**). Some of these antibody preparations may also interfere

Table 1
Systemically Administered mAb Target to Host

Target	Expression Pattern
CD3	Expressed on all T cells
TCR	Expressed on all T cells
CD25	IL-2R-IL2 receptor antibody
CD4	Expressed only helper T cells
CD8	Expressed only on cytotoxic suppressor T cells
CD5	T-cell marker
CD45	T-cell marker
LFA	Adhesion epitope; increased expression with activation
ICAM	Adhesion epitope; increased expression with activation

with the host's inflammatory response. Antibodies against interleukin (IL)-2 receptors, or against IL-2 itself, may help to alleviate transplant damage caused by inflammation.

3. Multiple Mechanisms

For transplantation, antibodies that target T cells have been routinely administered systemically to the host at the time of the transplant. However, other applications exist (**Table 2**). As mentioned, anti-T-cell antibodies can be administered to the host during acute rejection episodes. Lytic antibodies can also be used to treat donor grafts prior to transplantation to remove immunogenic passenger cell populations. Nonlytic antibody fragments can be designed to mask donor antigens prior to transplantation. Cloaking donor cell antigens, particularly HLA class I molecules, can prolong the life of the graft. Each of these treatments will be discussed in detail below. In the future, donor cells may be induced to express antibodies internally prior to transplantation. Antibodies inside the cell might then sequester antigenic proteins, preventing them from being displayed on the cell surface. Such experiments have been performed in cultured cells with some success.

To date, most antibodies administered systemically have been used to enhance the survival of allografts—transplants between two unrelated members of the same species. Transplantation of xenografts—tissues from different species—represents a more challenging problem. Because the supply of donor organs and tissues is limited, xenografts offer some advantages for transplantation. Further, using xenografts will permit investigators to select donors of a particular age or with certain desired characteristics. Recently, antibodies that mask donor class I antigens have shown success in enhancing the survival of xenografts even in the human setting. In fact, the ablation of class I molecules

Table 2
Methods of Antibody Administration

	Mechanism	Timing	Examples
Administered to recipient	Usually directed against T-cell determinants	At time of transplantation or during rejection episodes	OKT3
Administered to donor cells, tissues, or organs	Directed against passenger lymphocytes	Pretransplantation	α class II
	Directed toward masking antigenic proteins on surface of cells	Pretransplantation	α HLA class I, α ICAM
	Directed toward preventing the expression of antigenic proteins on the cell surface		α HLA class I

may allow the development of animals that can be considered "universal donors." These and other studies on antibodies and transplantation are discussed more fully below.

4. Using Antibodies to Inactivate Host's T Cells

Conventional wisdom dictates that treating the transplant recipient with some type of immunosuppressive drug will hamper graft rejection (**Table 3**). Sir Peter Medawar first formulated the premise that immunosuppressive drugs could be used to prevent immune rejection when donor organs or cells of identical genetic origin are not available *(2)*.

Traditionally, immunosuppressive medications, such as azathioprine (Imuran), prednisone (steroids), cyclophosphamide, Cyclosporin A, and FK506, have pharmacologically inactivated the immune system of the transplant recipient. Many of these drugs are targeted against T cells as well as all lymphoid cells. Although these drugs effectively control rejection, they also leave the host susceptible to infections.

Antibodies were developed as an attempt to get around the lack of specificity of immunosuppressive drugs. Although there is variation between different antibody preparations, a great deal of data suggests antibodies are very effective at inhibiting transplant rejection when administered to the host *(3)*.

With the advent of hybridoma technology, it became possible to produce large amounts of homogeneous mAb in vitro. Such pure and reproducible

Table 3
Contrasting Immunologic Targets to Prevent Rejection

Target	Route	Goal	Approaches
Recipient T cells	In vivo	Destroy or inactivate	Drugs: Steroid, aziothoprine, FK506, Cyclosporin A Antibodies: polyclonal serum, OKT3, CD3, CD4, ICAM, HLA Class II
Donor passenger lymphocytes	In vitro	Destroy or inactivate	Culture: 24°C, 37°C, hyperbaric oxygen Antibodies: HLA class II antibodies, CD45 antibodies UV Irradiation of donor cells
Donor tissue	In vitro	Camouflage, mask	Antibodies: Nonlytic masking antibodies to eliminate donor antigen, e.g., HLA class I Genetic engineering: β_2-microglobulin gene ablation

antibody preparations are useful for transplantation. Further, investigators could now produce antibodies directed against specific lymphoid cell lineages.

OKT3 remains the most common mAb used in transplantation research. The antibody is directed against CD3, a protein linked to the T-cell antigen receptor. In culture, OKT3 prevents cytotoxic human T lymphocytes from attacking the transplant tissue. In vivo, OKT3 promotes the removal of T cells from the circulation (*4–7*).

Although many other mAbs directed to other T-cell epitopes have been used to prevent transplant rejection (**Tables 1** and **3**), OKT3 mAb therapy is the most effective. Even with the added specificity of OKT3, the antibody still elicits adverse reactions and shows limitations in clinical effectiveness. OKT3 is a murine antihuman antibody, so host immune responses to the murine protein are common, particularly with prolonged or repeated infusions. Other side effects include pulmonary edema, fever, and a lessening of effectiveness with repeated dosages. The side effects and the dwindling efficacy are presumably attributable to the host antibodies to the murine hybridoma as well as host anti-idiotype responses to the antigen-binding regions of the antibody.

At present, clinical pancreatic islet transplantation programs rely on monoclonal and polyclonal antibody treatments of the recipient rather than the use of immunosuppressive drugs. The use of antibodies over drugs may be the result, in part, of the realization that such drugs as Cyclosporin A and steroids are toxic to islet grafts. This discovery allowed physicians to turn to antilymphocyte antibody treatment of the recipient as a major mode of therapy. In the case of Cyclosporin A, the drug may be directly toxic to islet cells. In addition, the drug appears to accumulate in the portal veins of the liver prior to detoxification (8,9). Because many islet transplants lie ectopically in the terminal portal vessels of the liver, the cells may receive a high "first pass" dose of Cyclosporin A. Steroids, on the other hand, have long been known to induce diabetes. Thus, two of the most common drugs used to prevent transplant rejection—Cyclosporin A and steroids—are poorly suited for use in islet transplants.

For islet cell transplants, infusion of monoclonal or polyclonal antibodies into the transplant host is an effective therapy for suppressing graft rejection. According to Federlin and his colleagues at the International Islet Transplantation Registry, polyclonal antiserum or monoclonal OKT3 therapy, in the absence of Cyclosporin A, resulted in better successes in early clinical trials of islet transplants (10).

The success of antibody therapies confirms the importance of the host T cell in the rejection circuit. The development of antibodies with restricted target specificities has paved the way for the design of a specific "bullet" for preventing transplant rejection. Perhaps generating antibodies to alternative targets would alleviate some of the toxic side effects seen with some preparations.

5. Using Antibodies to Eliminate Passenger Lymphocytes from Donor Cell Preparations

In 1957, George Snell proposed a theory of transplant rejection that was in direct contrast to Medawar's T-cell theory. He suggested that passenger lymphocytes present in donor cell transplants are highly immunogenic and trigger rejection. If the theory were correct, it suggested that grafts could be modified prior to transplantation to deplete the passenger lymphocytes. This was a dramatic conceptual departure from the belief that only treatment of the recipient could successfully control transplant rejection. Because antibodies could be used to target and eliminate passenger lymphocytes from the donor grafts, they eventually became an important tool for demonstrating that donor lymphoid cells are major triggers of immunologic rejection.

But before antibodies were used to test the theory, several different groups noted that culturing donor organs or tissues prior to transplant could enhance the survival of the graft. For example, Jacobs demonstrated that culturing ovaries prior to transplantation prolonged their survival (11). Lafferty et al. (11a) demonstrated a marked extension of survival of a thyroid allograft after pretransplantation culturing for 3–5 wk at 95% oxygen. Lacy and colleagues found that using rat islet cells cultured in vitro for 4 d at 24°C, combined with antilymphocyte treatment of the recipient, yielded 85% survival of the allograft

100 d after transplantation *(12)*. Naji et al. similarly demonstrated prolonged survival of parathyroid allografts after culturing at 95% oxygen *(13)*. Similar culture procedures appeared to decrease the immunogenicity of many other allogeneic tissues and to xenografts as well.

Why did culturing transplant grafts change their immunogenicity? The conditions were thought to eliminate passenger lymphocytes (**Table 3**). At the time, investigators believed that passenger lymphocytes were more susceptible to death or inactivation in cell culture than the graft's parenchymal cells. Culture of organs caused rapid degeneration of the vascular bed and release of free-floating blood elements and lymphocytes. These transplants showed decreased immunogenicity, particularly after culture at low temperatures (25°C). The methodology was highly effective for lengthening the survival of islet allografts *(14)*. In addition, Opelz and Terasaki *(15)* demonstrated that lymphocytes cultured at 24°C for 4 d would lose their ability to stimulate allogenic lymphocytes in vitro.

At the time these experiments were being conducted, it was unclear whether islet cells expressed the classic transplantation antigens, such as HLA class I and class II molecules. Although it was initially reported that islets lacked class I and class II antigens, this observation may have resulted from the use of improper fixation techniques that caused stripping of the antigens *(16)*. Subsequent studies in the mouse *(17)* and human *(18)* demonstrated that islets selectively express HLA class I but not HLA class II antigens.

This observation led the way to experiments designed to specifically and selectively remove the passenger lymphocytes from donor grafts—a direct test of Snell's hypothesis—and these methods again employed antibodies in a new transplantation setting. Because all lymphoid cells bear HLA class II antigens, freshly isolated islets were briefly treated with antibodies specific for HLA class II molecules and complement prior to transplantation. This treatment specifically eliminates possible passenger lymphocytes without harming the donor parenchymal cells, which lack class II molecules.

Transplantation of pretreated islets resulted in no immunosuppression in the recipient *(19)*. Further, these established pretreated allogenic islet transplants were rejected when the recipients were injected with donor lymphocytes *(19)*. These experiments reinforced the idea that in the absence of passenger lymphocytes, the class I antigens present on donor parenchymal cells were not necessarily triggers of immune rejection. Rather, donor passenger lymphocytes appeared to trigger the rejection cascade.

Experimental data confirming the role of donor passenger lymphocytes in immunogenic rejection continued to accumulate. In 1982, researchers in the Batchelor laboratory found that immunologically enhanced, long-term surviving kidney transplants could be moved from a primary to a secondary host without eliciting rejection (20). This result offered indirect support that a loss of passenger lymphocytes inhibited rejection. Furthermore, the passage of donor tissue through an athymic mouse as a way of eliminating short-lived passenger lymphocytes in vivo prior to transplantation in an allogenic host may also allow prolonged acceptance.

Hart and Fabre were the first to visually demonstrate that cells expressing HLA class II molecules exist in parenchymal tissues, such as kidney (21). The presence of HLA class II-positive dendritic cells in parenchymal tissue was demonstrated in 1984 (22). Further, detailed characterization of these scattered lymphoid cells using subset-specific antibodies revealed that they are, in part, dendritic cells, which are highly immunogenic and excellent antigen-presenting cells. As predicted, selective removal of donor dendritic cells with dendritic-cell-specific antiserum prior to transplantation allowed long-term islet allograft survival in the absence of any immunosuppressive drug treatment of the recipient (22). Taken together, these results suggest that donor dendritic cells are important passenger lymphocytes in the rejection circuit.

Lymphocyte-specific antibodies were also used to selectively remove passenger lymphocytes from a number of different parenchymal tissues and cellular transplants. Donor rat cardiac transplants, donor pancreas transplants, and canine renal allografts pretreated with lytic antibodies directed against donor lymphocytes showed significantly prolonged survival compared to untreated grafts (23–25). More importantly, pretreatment of renal grafts with lymphocyte-specific antibodies decreased the incidence of kidney allograft rejection episodes in humans (26). Clinical trials were conducted in the United Kingdom to expand these results in the setting of tough recurrent graft rejection of kidneys. In this higher species model, impressive graft prolongation was not observed. In part, this may be because of the simultaneous use of immunosuppression, which may deplete the passenger lymphocytes remaining. This is a long-held theory of Starzl and colleagues.

The use of antibodies to specifically deplete passenger lymphocytes from grafts prior to transplantation validated the role these cells play in allograft rejection. Further, the data demonstrated that antibody treatment to delete passenger cells from grafts could, in and of itself, enhance the long-term survival of transplants, even when no immunosuppressive drugs were administered to the recipient (19,22).

6. Using Antibodies to Camouflage, Mask, or Genetically Eliminate Donor Transplant Antigens

Throughout the 1980s, investigators worked on defining the mechanisms by which cytotoxic T lymphocytes (CTLs) kill cells bearing target antigens. Both CTL activation and lysis of the target were thought to involve a lock-and-key type interaction between proteins on the surface of the CTL and its target *(27)*. In the first step, the CTL and target cells interact via adhesion molecules, such as LFA-3, ICAM-1, and LFA-1. This step appears to be reversible: Separation of the cells at this point yields no damage to the target, no T-cell activation, and no T-cell memory. The second step involves the T-cell receptor (TCR), CD3 protein, and CD8 protein complex on the CTL binding to the HLA class I molecule on the target cell. This interaction occurs after the first binding step and CTLs retain immunologic memory of the event. Finally, the CTL lyses and kills the target cell.

The delineation of the interactions between CTLs and target cells provided an alternative means of averting transplant rejection (**Table 3**). As discussed earlier, systemic injections of OKT3—the mAb that stimulates lysis of cells bearing CD3—could effectively prolong the life of kidney transplants. Presumably this antibody therapy, administered to the transplant recipient, interfered with the second step of CTL killing by eliminating the attacking T cell.

We hoped to use a similar strategy to alter donor cells in vitro prior to transplantation, rather than depleting the T lymphocytes in the host. To accomplish this goal, we set out to define the dominant antigens on the surface of islet cells. Although adhesion molecules were common on the vascular endothelium of whole organs, we found that freshly isolated islets were virtually devoid of determinants, such as ICAM-1, LFA-3, and LFA-1 *(28)*. As we had demonstrated 10 yr previously, the prominent protein on the surface of islets and other parenchymal cells was HLA class I.

Studies in the literature at the time suggested that donor HLA class I would be a poor target for modifications that could block CTL killing. In fact, many studies concluded that donor HLA class I was not immunogenic. For instance, donor islets or thyroid transplants depleted of passenger lymphocytes were easily rejected by recipients following injections of donor lymphocytes, indicating that HLA class I had been present on the stably transplanted tissue and, with the proper trigger, was available for immune attack. Injections of isolated donor HLA class I antigens, however, were either weakly immunogenic or enhanced the growth of tumor transplants. Further, donor-specific immunologic responsiveness could be induced by pretransplant injections of donor cells transfected with HLA class I genes or class I enriched donor cells.

Despite the discouraging nature of the literature, we decided to press ahead and design antibodies that could immunologically disguise or eliminate donor HLA class I antigens. To maintain the molecular specificity of the antibody but eliminate its lytic function (which would destroy the donor cell), we removed the tail of the antibody by enzymatic treatment with papain. This digestion yielded specific target binding antibody $F(ab')_2$ fragments lacking the Fc region that activates the complement system.

Table 4
Masking Approaches to Transplantation[a]

Tissue	Methods	Reference
Islets/liver	Masking donor HLA class I	*28*
Islets	Polyclonal serum masking all donor antigens	*28*
Heart	Masking donor LFA-1 with lytic ICAM-1 to recipient	*30*
Skin	Masking donor HLA class I-associated β_2-microglobulin	*29*

[a]Masking refers to coating donor cells with nonlytic antibody or antibody fragments generated by $F(ab')_2$ production.

The "masking" of freshly isolated donor human islets with these nonlytic HLA class I antibodies allowed long-term survival and function of xenografts in mice that were not treated with immunosuppressive drugs. This methodology worked in a tough islet xenograft model as well as in a liver xenograft model. Importantly, the antibody enhanced xenograft survival in the absence of immunosuppressive regimens administered to the recipient. The successfully transplanted recipients even developed graft-specific tolerance.

Although masking all donor surface molecules with nonlytic polyclonal serum also allowed survival of islet and liver xenografts, each marker did not play an equal role in promoting graft survival. The less dense surface proteins, such as LFA-3 and ICAM-1, failed to produce extended xenograft survival when masked prior to transplantation *(28)*. Further, masking only the passenger lymphocytes did not prolong xenograft survival. Although high-affinity HLA class I masking antibodies are difficult to produce, these experiments demonstrated that modifying donor parenchymal structures avert graft rejection (**Table 4**).

Further experiments demonstrated that other treatments that mask class I proteins and adhesion proteins could enhance survival of different transplanted tissues *(29,30)*. For example, Wu and colleagues demonstrated that skin allografts survived longer after masking with HLA class I-associated β_2-microglobulin antibodies. For cardiac transplants, using a nonlytic antibody against donor LFA-1 combined with a lytic ICAM-1 antibody against recipient T cells allowed impressive survival or whole heart allografts *(30)*.

If HLA class I is an important protein involved in immune rejection, then permanent ablation of donor class I seemed like an attractive means of generating nonimmunogenic graft tissue. In fact, such a "universal donor" animal was generated by the transgenic elimination of HLA class I-associated

Table 5
Use of HLA Class I-Deficient Mice as Organ Donors

Tissue	Method	Success/failure	Reference
Skin	β_2-Microglobulin ablation	Failure	*36*
Liver	β_2-Microglobulin ablation	Partial	*35*
Kidney	β_2-Microglobulin ablation	Success	*34*
Islets	β_2-Microglobulin ablation	Success	*45*

β_2-microglobulin *(31,32)*. In the absence of β_2-microglobulin, HLA class I cannot easily fold into the correct three-dimensional structure required to allow the protein to exit the endoplasmic reticulum and reach the cell surface. These transgenic mice therefore have tissue that expresses extraordinarily low levels of class I antigens.

In 1992, Markmann and colleagues demonstrated that islets isolated from these class I-deficient mice survive indefinitely in nonimmunosuppressed, fully allogenic recipients *(33)*. These results confirmed that eliminating or masking donor class I antigens promotes prolonged graft survival. Although the grafts were resistant to transplant rejection, they were fully susceptible to recurrent autoimmunity when transplanted into autoimmune NOD mice *(33)*. Whole kidney transplants from the class I-deficient mice also had long-term survival *(34)*.

Interestingly, the survival of grafts from the β_2-microglobulin-deficient mice varied, depending on the type of tissue being transplanted (**Table 5**). Allogenic liver cells from class I deficient mice only demonstrated partial survival *(35)*. Skin allografts showed no prolonged survival *(36)*, but liver xenografts from class I-deficient mice survived and showed long-term survival in frog recipients *(35)*. These results clashed with the generally accepted belief that allografts survive better than xenografts and cellular transplants fare better than whole organ transplants.

Why was there a disparity between allografts and xenografts? The answer may lie in the β_2-microglobulin of the host. β_2-microglobulin is one of the most plentiful proteins in the serum of all species, and it appears that the host's β_2-microglobulin may rapidly infiltrate the graft after transplantation, thus restoring the expression of class I donor antigens. Experiments in culture have confirmed that serum containing β_2-microglobulin or media specifically supplemented with β_2-microglobulin can rapidly reconstitute the β_2-microglobulin in deficient tissues.

The rate at which the reconstitution occurs varies with the transplant tissue in question and correlates with the varying transplant survival times; e.g., liver is reconstituted rapidly, islet and kidney cells more slowly. The reconstitution can be traced by observing the reappearance of class I in cultured tissues *(35)*. Further, in vitro and in vivo evidence confirms that transplantation of β_2-microglobulin-deficient murine cells into discordant xenogenic species with nonidentical β_2-microglobulin correlates well with the ability of these discordant forms of β_2-microglobulin to reconstitute the transgenic graft and restore donor class I *(35)*. The divergence of β_2-microglobulin between distantly related species may explain the enhanced survival of xenografts over allografts in this transgenic model of donor class I ablation.

Currently in the United States, human clinical trials are underway examining the efficacy of class I grafts in nonimmunosuppressed hosts. Clinically, improvements in Parkinson's patients receiving fetal pig neurons appears evident. Expansion of donor class I ablation to other types of cellular xenografts using nonlytic antibody fragments appears within the scope of the technology.

These experiments confirm the critical role that donor MHC class I antigens play in stimulating the rejection cascade by serving as a critical target for the host rejection response. Further, these studies suggest that masking of donor class I antigen or genetic interference with class I expression can prolong the survival of allografts and xenografts. Because matching MHC class I antigens between donor and recipient is virtually impossible, concealing or eliminating these models may serve as a feasible means of suppressing transplant rejection. Some data even suggests that culturing donor cells prior to transplantation may enhance graft survival by downregulation of class I antigen, rather than by passenger lymphocyte elimination *(37,38)*.

In the future, transgenic animals with permanent modifications to their donor antigens will continue to play an important role in studying organ and cellular transplantation. In addition, new ways to genetically eliminate class I antigens—including mutations of Tap 1 and 2, proteins important for antigen processing, and direct interruption of the genes for class I molecules themselves—may lead the way to new universal donor animals.

Making a tissue less immunogenic by masking or eliminating its class I antigen by antibodies is a relatively new concept in the transplantation field, but Mother Nature appears to have known this trick all along. Malignant tumors frequently lack class I molecules, a deficiency that may allow them to escape elimination from recognition and destruction by CTLs *(39–43)*. Further, some studies suggest that hosts may actually protect their tumors by generating nonlytic antibodies that prevent CTLs from destroying the malignant growth *(44)*.

7. Summary

The use of antibodies in transplantation has allowed the delineation of three different pathways of immunologic rejection and the identification of new targets that can help enhance graft survival. The ability of intravenous mono-clonal and polyclonal anti-T-cell antibodies to suppress graft rejection has con-firmed the central role of host T cells in triggering transplant destruction. Experimental and clinical data with lytic antibodies directed against donor pas-senger lymphocytes reinforces the theory that these immunogenic cells can trigger graft rejection. Finally, the use of antibodies that camouflage or elimi-nate donor HLA class I antigen substantiates the role that class I molecules play in stimulating the rejection cascade.

Whether antibodies will remain a central drug for enhancing the survival of transplanted tissue—both allografts and xenografts—remains to be seen. What is certain is that antibodies will remain a critical immunologic reagent for studying the mechanisms of rejection and developing novel approaches for prolonging the survival of transplants.

References

1. Köhler, G. and Milstein, C. (1975) Continuous culture of fused cells secreting antibody of predefined specificity. *Nature* **256,** 495–497.
2. Medawar, P. B, (1957) *The Uniqueness of the Individual,* Basic Books, New York.
3. Russell, P. S. (1977) Antilymphocyte sera for immunosuppression, in *Human Diagnosis and Therapy* (Haber, E. and Krause, R., eds.), Raven, New York, pp. 303–355.
4. Anonymous (1985) A randomized clinical trial of OKT3 monoclonal antibody for acute rejection of cadaveric renal transplants. Ortho Multicenter Transplant Study Group. *New Engl. J. Med.* **313,** 337–342.
5. Thurlow, P. J., Lovering, E., d'Apice, A. J., and McKenzie, I. F. (1983) A mono-clonal antipan-T cell antibody: *in vitro* and *in vivo* studies. *Transplantation* **36,** 293–298.
6. Takahashi, H., Okazaki, H., Terasaki, P. I., Iwaki, Y., Kinukawa, T., Taguchi, Y., Chia, D., Hardiwidjaja, S., Miura, K., and Ishizaki, M. (1983) Reversal of trans-plant rejection by monoclonal antiblast antibody. *Lancet* **2,** 1155–1158.
7. Kirkman, R. L., Araujo, J. L., Busch, G. J., Carpenter, C. B., Milford, E. L., Reinherz, E. L., Schlossman, S. F., Strom, T. B., and Tilney, N. L. (1983) Treat-ment of acute renal allograft rejection with monoclonal anti-T12 antibody. *Trans-plantation* **36,** 620–626.
8. Kneteman, N. M., Marchetti, P., Tordjman, K., Bier, D. M., Santiago, J. V., Swanson, C. J., Olack, B. J., and Scharp, D. W, (1992) Effects of cyclosporine on insulin secretion and insulin sensitivity in dogs with intrasplenic islet autotransplants. *Surgery* **111,** 430–437.
9. Metrakos, P., Hornby, L., and Rosenberg, L. (1993) Cyclosporine and islet mass—implications for islet transplantation. *J. Surg. Res.* **54,** 375–380.
10. Hering, B. J., Browatzki, C. C., Schultz, A., Bretzel, R. G., and Federlin, K. F. (1993) Clinical islet transplantation-registry report, accomplishments in the past and future research needs. *Cell Transplant.* **2,** 269–282.

11. Jacobs, B. B. (1974) Ovarian allograft survival. Prolongation after passage in vitro. *Transplantation* **18,** 454–457.

11a. Lafferty, K., Cooley, M., Woolnough, J., and Walker, K. (1975) Thyroid allograft immunogenicity is reduced after a period of organ culture. *Science* **188,** 259–261.

12. Lacy, P. E., Davie, J. M., and Finke, E. H. (1979) Prolongation of islet allograft survival following in vitro culture (24°C) and a single injection of ALS. *Science* **204,** 312,313.

13. Naji, A., Silvers, W. K., and Barker, C. F. (1979) Effect of culture in 95% O_2 on the survival of parathyroid allografts. *Surg. Forum* **30,** 109–111.

14. Parr, E. L., Bowen, K. M., and Lafferty, K. J. (1980) Cellular changes in cultured mouse thyroid glands and islets of Langerhans. *Transplantation* **30,** 135–141.

15. Opelz, G. and Terasaki, P. I. (1974) Lymphocyte antigenicity loss with retention of responsiveness. *Science* **184,** 464–466.

16. Parr, E. L. (1979) The absence of H-2 antigens from mouse pancreatic β-cells demonstrated by immunoferritin labeling. *J. Exp. Med.* **150,** 1–9.

17. Faustman, D., Hauptfeld, V., Davie, J., Lacy, P., and Shreffler, D. (1980) Murine pancreatic β cells express H-2K and H-2D but not Ia antigens. *J. Exp. Med.* **151,** 1563–1569.

18. Baekkeskov, S., Kanatsuna, T., Klareskog, L., Nielsen, D. A., Peterson, P. A., Rubenstein, A. H., Steiner, D. F., and Lernmark, A. (1981) Expression of major histocompatibility antigens on pancreatic islet cells. *Proc. Natl. Acad. Sci. USA* **78,** 6456–6460.

19. Faustman, D., Hauptfeld, V., Lacy, P., and Davie, J. (1981) Prolongation of murine islet allograft survival by pretreatment of islets with antibody directed to Ia determinants. *Proc. Natl. Acad. Sci. USA* **78,** 5156–5159.

20. Lechler, R. I. and Batchelor, J. R. (1982) Restoration of immunogenecity to passenger cell-depleted kidney allografts by the addition of donor strain dendritic cells. *J. Exp. Med.* **155,** 31–41.

21. Hart, D. N. and Fabre, J. W. (1981) Demonstration and characterization of Ia-positive dendritic cells in the interstitial connective tissue of rat heart and other tissues, but not brain. *J. Exp. Med.* 154, 347-361.

22. Faustman, D., Steinman, R., Gebel, H., Hauptfeld, V., Davie, J., and Lacy, P. (1984) Prevention of rejection of murine islet allografts by pre-treatment with anti-dendritic cell antibody. *Proc. Natl. Acad. Sci. USA* **81,** 3864–3868.

23. Sone, Y., Sakagami, K., and Orita, K. (1987) Effect of ex vivo perfusion with anti-IA monoclonal antibodies on rat cardiac allograft survival. *Transplant. Proc.* **19,** 599–604.

24. Lloyd, M., Buckingham, M., Stuart, F., and Thistlethwaite, J. R. (1989) Does depletion of donor dendritic cells an allograft lead to prolongation of graft survival in transplantation? *Transplant. Proc.* **21,** 482–483.

25. Otsubo, O., Sakai, A., Watanabe, T., and Inoi, T. (1983) Effect of anti-mouse Ia monoclonal antibody on canine renal allograft survival. *Transplant. Proc.* **15,** 797–799.

26. Brewer, Y., Palmer, A., Taube, D., Welsh, K., Bewick, M., Bindon, C., Hale, G., Waldmann, H., Dische, F., Parsons, V., and Snowden, S. (1989) Effect of graft perfusion with two CD45 monoclonal antibodies on incidence of kidney allograft rejection. *Lancet* **2,** 935–937.
27. Spits, H., van Schooten, W., Keizer, H., van Seventer, G., van de Rijn, M., Terhorst, C., and de Vries, J. E. (1986) Alloantigen recognition is preceded by nonspecific adhesion of cytotoxic T cells and target cells. *Science* **232,** 403–405.
28. Faustman, D. and Coe, C. (1991) Prevention of xenograft rejection by masking donor HLA class I antigens. *Science* **252,** 1700–1702.
29. Wu, J., Menapace, L., Barisoni, D., and Armato, U. (1992) An anti-beta-2-microglobulin monoclonal antibody prevents the reactive proliferation of lymphocytes elicited by allo-human epidermal cells. *J. Immunol. Res.* **4,** 21–25.
30. Isobe, M., Yagita, H., Okumura, K., and Ihara, A. (1992) Specific acceptance of cardiac allograft after treatment with antibodies to ICAM-1 and LFA-1. *Science* **255,** 1125–1127.
31. Koller, B. H. and Smithies, O. (1989) Inactivating the beta-2 microglobulin locus in mouse embryonic stem cells by homologous recombination. *Proc. Natl. Acad. Sci. USA* **86,** 8932–8935.
32. Zijlstra, M., Bix, M., Simister, N. E., Loring, J. M., Raulet, D. H., and Jaenisch, R. (1990) Beta 2-microglobulin-deficient mice lack CD4-8+ cytolytic T cells. *Nature* **344,** 742–746.
33. Markmann, J. F., Bassiri, H., Desai, N. M., Odorico, J. S., Kim, J. I., Koller, B. H., Smithies, O., and Barker, C. F. (1992) Indefinite survival of MHC class I-deficient murine pancreatic islet allografts. *Transplantation* **54,** 1085–1089.
34. Coffman, T., Geier, S., Ibrahim, S., Griffiths, R., Spurney, R., Smithies, O., Koller, B., and Sanfilippo, F. (1993) Improved renal function in mouse kidney allografts lacking MHC class I antigens. *J. Immunol.* **151,** 425–435.
35. Li, X. and Faustman, D. (1993) Use of donor β2-microglobulin-deficient transgenic mouse liver cells for isografts, allografts, and xenografts. *Transplantation* **55,** 940–946.
36. Zijlstra, M., Auchincloss, H., Loring, J. M., Chase, C. M., Russell, P. S., and Jaenisch, R. (1992) Skin graft rejection by beta 2-microglobulin-deficient mice. *J. Exp. Med.* **175,** 885–893.
37. Markmann, J. F., Jacobson, J. D., Kiumura, H., Choti, M. A., Hickey, W. F., Fox, I. J., Silvers, W. K., Barker, C. F., and Naji, A. (1989) Modulation of the major histocompatibility complex antigen and the immunogenicity of islet allografts. *Transplantation* **48,** 478–486.
38. Barker, C. F., Markmann, J. F., Posselt, A. M., and Naji, A. (1991) Studies of privileged sites and islet transplantation. *Transplant. Proc.* **23,** 2138–2142.
39. Doherty, P. C., Knowles, B. B., and Wettstein, P. J. (1984) Immunological surveillance of tumors in the context of major histocompatibility complex restriction of T-cell function. *Adv. Cancer Res.* **42,** 1–65.

40. Hui, K., Grosveld, F., and Festenstein, H. (1984) Rejection of transplantable AKR leukaemia cells following MHC DNA-mediated cell transformation. *Nature* **311,** 750–752.

41. Rees, R. C., Buckle, A. M., Gelsthorpe, K., James, V., Potter, C. W., Rogers, K., and Jacob, G. (1988) Loss of polymorphic A and B locus HLA antigens in colon carcinoma. *Br. J. Cancer* **57,** 374–377.

42. Karre, K., Ljunggren, H. G., Piontek, G., and Kiessling, R. (1986) Selective rejection of H-2-deficient lymphoma variants suggests alternative immune defense strategy. *Nature* **319,** 675–678.

43. Smith, M. E., Marsh, S. G., Bodmer, J. G., Glesthorpe, K., and Bodmer, W. F. (1989) Loss of HLA-A,B,C allele products and lymphocyte function-associated antigen 3 in colorectal neoplasia. *Proc. Natl. Acad. Sci. USA* **86,** 5557–5561.

44. Manson, L. A. (1991) Does antibody-dependent epitope masking permit progressive tumour growth in the face of cell-mediated cytotoxicity? *Immunol. Today* **12,** 352–355.

45. Osorio, R. W., Ascher, N. L., Jaenisch, R., Freise, C. E., Roberts, J. P., and Stock, P. G. (1993) Major histocompatibility complex class I deficiency prolongs islet allograft survival. *Diabetes* **42,** 1520–1527.

11

Antibody-Based Therapies in Infectious Diseases

H. Barbaros Oral and Cezmi A. Akdiş

1. Introduction

Before antibiotics, sera from immune animals and humans were used to treat a variety of infectious diseases, often with successful results. In the beginning of the 20th century, serum therapy had taken a place in standard treatment protocols for several infectious diseases, such as meningitis, diphtheria, tetanus, and lobar pneumonia. As early as 1906, antimeningococcal serum was intravenously used as a treatment for meningitis, since it was proved to cross the blood–brain barrier. However, treatment with meningococcal antiserum was shown to be ineffective, because available antiserum was only effective against type A meningococcus, whereas type C was a more common cause of meningococcal meningitis *(1)*. Several trials demonstrated that application of type-specific antipneumococcal serum reduced mortality in patients with lobar pneumonia by about 50%, from 30–40% to 10–20% *(2)*. Several successes with immune serum were observed in treatment and prevention of other infectious diseases, which include *Haemophilus influenzae* meningitis, measles, diphtheria, hepatitis A and B, poliovirus infection, and cytomegalovirus (CMV) infection *(1)*. However, numerous problems have been observed with immune sera, including lot-to-lot variations characterized with variable amounts of specific antibodies, occurrence of serum sickness as a complication, and some hazards in transmission of some infectious diseases *(3,4)*.

After the discovery of antimicrobial chemotherapy in the mid-1930s, serum therapy for some bacterial infections was rapidly forsaken *(5)*. However, today antibody-based therapy for infectious diseases is still routinely used in few situations, including replacement therapy in patients with immunodeficiency, prophylaxis against various viruses (rabies, measles, hepatitis A and B, varicella, mumps, cytomegalovirus) following exposure, and toxin neutralization (diphtheria, tetanus, and botulism).

From: *Methods in Molecular Medicine, Vol. 40: Diagnostic and Therapeutic Antibodies*
Edited by: A. J. T. George and C. E. Urch © Humana Press Inc., Totowa, NJ

In the last two decades, problems with treatment of newly emerged, re-emerged, or persistent infectious diseases necessitated researchers to develop new and/or improved immune therapeutic approaches. The development of monoclonal antibody (mAb) technology by Köhler and Milstein was the most important forward step in this area *(6)*. Since then, mAbs have been used for diagnostic purposes and they are applicable to immunotherapy of human diseases. They have been applied clinically against various specific microorganisms, such as *Escherichia coli, Klebsiella pneumonia, Pseudomonas aeruginosa*, CMV, Varicella Zoster Virus (VZV), and Respiratory Syncytial Virus (RSV) *(7,8)*. In several multicenter clinical trials, mAbs raised against specific epitopes or cellular components of microorganisms, against microorganisms themselves, or against some host factors responsible for the pathogenesis of infectious diseases, such as proinflammatory cytokines, complement components, and tissue factors, have been tested to evaluate the efficacy, safety, tolerance, and pharmacokinetics in antibody-based therapy of infectious diseases *(8–11)*.

In this chapter, we summarize information on the in vivo use of antibodies for the treatment of infectious disease, with special reference to the most seminal discoveries and current advances as well as available treatment approaches in this field.

2. How Can Antibodies Prevent or Treat Infectious Diseases?

Antibodies mediate antimicrobial function through a variety of mechanisms, which can be categorized as follows *(12,13)*:

1. Neutralization: Antibodies can prevent virus infectivity by a variety of mechanisms, especially following attachment of the virus to the host cell. This could be internalization by the cell and/or interference with the uncoating process of the viral particles. Antibodies also combine with the microbial surface and prevent them from attaching to susceptible cells or tissues, and prevent microbial penetration into deep tissues. In addition, they can neutralize microbial toxins and impedins.*
2. Phagocytosis: Antibodies may act as cytophilic molecules or opsonins and promote phagocytosis at the site of infection (*see also* **items 5** and **6**).
3. Complement activation and microbial lysis: Activation of complement by antigen–antibody or microorganism–antibody complex can induce inflammatory responses and attract phagocytes and serum antibodies to the site of infection. On the other hand, by combining with the surface of bacteria, enveloped viruses, and so forth, antibodies can activate the complement cascade and lead to lysis of the infectious agent or the infected cells.

---

*Microbial factors that inhibit the operation of host defense mechanisms without doing any damage.

4. Antibody-dependent cellular cytotoxicity: Antibodies allow certain effector leukocytes, which include monocytes, neutrophils, and natural killer (NK) cells, to kill infected host cells bearing microbial antigens on their surface. These effector cells bear receptors for the Fc region of IgG (FcγR) that recognizes IgG Ab specifically bound to the infected cell surface.

5. Agglutination: Antibodies that attach to the surface of microorganisms can cause agglutination. This may lessen the number of separate infectious units and also make them more easily phagocytosed since the mass of particles becomes larger in size.

6. Restriction or inhibition of microbial motility: Antibodies, when attached to the surface of motile microorganisms, may make them nonmotile, and so improve the opportunities for phagocytosis.

7. Inhibition of microbial metabolism and growth: Antibodies targeting an essential transport molecule on a bacterial surface can prevent the uptake of a particular nutritional factor, such as iron, and inhibit its metabolism and growth.

8. Attenuation of the effects of proinflammatory mediators: Proinflammatory mediators, such as bacterial endotoxin (lipopolysaccharide; LPS) and cytokines (interleukin [IL]-6, IL-1 and tumor necrosis factor [TNF]-α), locally induce rapid elimination of pathogens, enhance neutrophil activity, and increase binding of leukocytes to endothelium. However, excessive production of these mediators is implicated in the injury observed in several infectious conditions, including septic shock, tuberculosis, and cerebral malaria. Use of antibodies against proinflammatory mediators should, therefore, be a beneficial strategy to prevent their deleterious effects.

3. Commercially Available Immunoglobulins Used in Infectious Diseases

Human immunoglobulin (IG) has been widely used both for prevention and treatment of infectious diseases. At the moment, three kinds of human IGs commercially exist in the market. Standard IG is a polyvalent immunoglobulin produced from human placenta or plasma by fractionation with alcohol, and is composed almost exclusively of IgG. It can only be used intramuscularly, since its aggregates have anticomplement activity. So, it is preferred when a small amount of antibody is needed. However, when large amounts of antibody are required, it cannot be intramuscularly administered because of local reactions and pain. To overcome this problem new IG preparations have been developed for intravenous use. Intravenous IG (IVIG) provided an important advantage for long-term usage in high doses with good tolerability. Specific IGs are purified from individuals rendered hyperimmune by vaccination or natural infection. Immunoglobulins effectively prevent or treat many diseases caused by bacteria (tetanus, *H. influenzae* infections, and so forth) or viruses (measles, rubella, varicella, mumps, hepatitis A and B, CMV infections, and so forth) (reviewed in **ref. *14***).

3.1. Viral Infections

1. Measles: 16.5% standard IG (0.25–0.30 mL/kg) provides short-term sero-prevention when given within 5 d following exposure, whereas administration between d 6 and 10 leads to seroattenuation *(15)*.
2. Rubella: Indications for the use of IG for rubella prophylaxis are quite few, because IG may not prevent viremia though it represses the symptoms. Use of standard IG or specific rubella IG preparations are restricted to pregnant suscep-tible women who are exposed to rubella and decline to have an abortion *(16)*.
3. Hepatitis A and B: The most common indication in recent years for the use of IG preparations is hepatitis A and B. The mainstay of hepatitis A immunoprophylaxis is passive immunization with standard IG. A single intramuscular injection of IG at a dose of 0.02–0.06 mL/kg is effective for 2–6 mo *(17)*. With this protocol minimal effective titer is unclear, but very low levels of neutralizing antibodies seem to provide considerable protection. In addition, even if IG does not always prevent hepatitis, it reduces the severity of disease resulting in active and definite immunity (passive-active immunity) *(18,19)*. Prophylaxis of hepatitis B includes pre-exposure and postexposure passive immunization. For pre-exposure passive immunization, either hyperimmune serum globulin (HBIG) or standard IG has been administered to risk groups, such as hemodialysis patients, medical staff, and institutionalized children *(20,21)*. In addition, no significant difference between HBIG and standard IG has been found in terms of efficacy. However, because of the availability of an effective vaccine, pre-exposure passive immuni-zation is recommended for individuals who fail to respond to vaccine or patients with disorders that preclude a response, such as agammaglobulinemia. Postexposure passive immunization is widely used within 7 d as recommended by the Public Health Service Advisory Committee on Immunisation Practices *(22)*. However, administration of HBIG as soon as possible following exposure seems to be important for maximum protection. HBIG appears to be superior to standard IG for postexposure immunization, since standard IG may not contain sufficient amounts of anti-HB_s. The dose of HBIG for effective postexposure immunization is not known, but 0.07 mL/kg is a reasonable dose for treatment in accordance with two different controlled trials *(23,24)*. Another important indi-cation for postexposure immunization is for neonates born of HBsAg-positive mothers. It is recommended that HBIG and vaccine be given intramuscularly in the delivery room at the same time *(25)*. Use of this immunization protocol has been shown to achieve 94% protection *(26)*.
4. Varicella-zoster virus (VZV) infections: Chickenpox is usually a benign disease. However, it may cause severe disease in children with immune deficiency or in immunocompromised patients. It has been shown that the administration of vari-cella immunoglobulin (VZIG) or varicella-zoster immune plasma (ZIP) to the immunocompromised individual who has not been previously exposed to chickenpox is useful for both prevention and attenuation of chickenpox infec-tion *(27)*.

5. Mumps: Indication for the use of IG is restricted to adult men because of disease severity. Intramuscular administration of mumps-specific IG has been shown to reduce the incidence of orchitis from 27.4 to 7.8% *(28)*. Because specific IG is no longer commercially available, 0.5 mL/kg standard IG may be recommended to be used instead.

6. Rabies: For postexposure therapy, human rabies immunoglobulin (HRIG) (20 IU/kg) is simultaneously administered with vaccine to the host who has not been vaccinated previously. Since infiltration of serum into the exposure site has provided more protection than systemic injection alone, it is recommended that a portion of the HRIG be injected into the site of exposure *(29)*. If HRIG is unavailable, antirabies sera of equine origin may be used after considering the severity of the exposure and individual skin test sensitivity to the antiserum *(30)*.

7. CMV: Passive immune prophylaxis for the CMV infection may be undertaken in seronegative transplant recipients. The administration of hyperimmune plasma or globulin has been shown to significantly reduce primary infection rates and lessen disease severity *(31,32)*. However, passive immune prophylaxis against CMV after transplantation should remain the decision of the clinician, and needs further studies.

3.2. Bacterial Infections

1. Tetanus: Passive immune prophylaxis and therapy for tetanus has been reviewed in detail *(33)*. Briefly, patients with dirty wounds who have not been actively immunized in the past 5 yr should receive passive immunization with human tetanus immunoglobulin (HTIG) (250–500 IU, intramuscularly) in addition to active immunization *(34)*. Passive immunization can also be used in large doses (3000–6000 U) for therapeutic purpose, since it can shorten the course of disease and reduce the severity of symptoms *(33)*.

2. Diphtheria: Diphtheria antitoxin (DAT), which is a hyperimmune serum produced in horses, is a key component of therapy for diphtheria. Administration of DAT as soon as possible following diagnosis is essential, because antitoxin can only neutralize toxin before entry into cells. It is recommended that 20,000–40,000 U of antitoxin for pharyngeal or laryngeal disease of 48 h, 40,000–60,000 U for nasopharyngeal lesions, and 80,000–100,000 U for extensive disease of three or more days be administered intravenously over 60 min to inactivate the toxin as rapidly as possible *(35)*.

4. Recent Advances in Pathogen-Specific Antibody-Based Therapies

Antibody-based therapies may allow new therapeutic opportunities to prevent or treat diseases caused by specific pathogens. For a number of infections caused by these pathogens for which preventive or therapeutic approaches are imperfect or unavailable, such as *Cryptosporidium parvum*, vancomycin-resistant enterococcus, *Bordetella pertussis*, HIV, drug-resistant *M. tuberculosis*, and

RSV infections, antibody-based therapy should be at least considered as alternative or adjunct therapy. Recent advances in antibody-based therapy in infectious diseases have been discussed in detail by leading researchers in an antibody workshop held on June 4–6, 1996 in Washington, DC and reviewed by Krause et al. *(1)*, and further studies since that date have been published.

RSV is the most common cause of childhood infections of the lower respiratory tract. Premature infants, as well as those with bronchopulmonary dysplasia (BDP) and congenital heart disease have a particular tendency to severe disease from RSV infection. Recently, intramuscular use of a humanized mAb raised against the fusion protein of RSV (MEDI-493), which is broadly reactive to numerous subtype A and B clinical isolates and 50–100 times more active than a polyclonal IVIG enriched for RSV, has been found to prevent approx 50% of RSV infections in premature neonates and those with bronchopulmonary dysplasia *(1)*. In a recent clinical trial, it has been shown that this antibody is safe, well tolerated in a high-risk pediatric population, and induces no specific anti-MEDI-493 antibody *(8)*. Further studies considering the clinical outcome are undergoing.

In recent years, incidence of invasive infections caused by group A streptococci (GAS), which includes streptococcal toxic shock syndrome (STSS) and necrotizing fasciitis, have been increasingly reported by several countries. Despite the availability of effective antibiotic treatment, early mortality rate in STSS is thought to be approx 50% *(36)*. This suggests a requirement for adjunctive therapy to lessen the potent systematic inflammatory response. Since IVIG has been shown to contain neutralizing antibodies against a broad variety of streptococcal toxins and superantigens, such as opsonic antibodies against the surface M protein *(37)*, it can be used for an adjunctive therapeutic approach. As a matter of fact, IVIG has been used in patients with STSS as an adjunctive therapeutic approach and has provided an approximate 50% decrease in mortality rates of patients *(38,39)*. Recent efforts are now underway to optimize the doses and timing of the IVIG administration in STSS.

In addition to the aforementioned infections, some infectious diseases caused by new pathogens (e.g., *Cryptosporidium parvum* and HIV) cannot be cured with available antimicrobial chemotherapeutics. In the last 10 years, several experimental approaches have been investigated to treat *C. parvum* infections using passive immunotherapy. These studies include the use of colostral antibodies produced from bovine colostrum *(40)*, mAbs *(41,42)*, and orally given human plasma antibodies *(43)*. Most of these studies have demonstrated some degree of efficacy and usefulness in animals and humans.

Humoral immune response is thought to play an important role in HIV infection, since studies in the past indicated that there is a significant correlation between progression of HIV infection and decreasing neutralization activity. Thus, antibodies could be employed to prevent or treat this infection with several antibody-based approaches. Several studies have shown that using HIV-immune human plasma reduces antigenemia and the frequency of polymerase chain reaction (PCR) positivity and delays the onset of the AIDS-defining event *(44–47)*. Because of safety and difficulties in standardization of plasma, it is reasonable to use mAbs or mAb cocktails for the treatment of HIV infections. A phase I trial in which anti-V3 mAb, a mAb raised against one of five gp120 variable loops, was administered to the HIV-infected volunteers with late-stage disease over 22 wk at escalating doses showed a reduction in plasma HIV DNA and viral antigenemia *(48)*. Neutralizing capacities of both an anti-CD4 binding-site mAb and an anti-V2 mAb have also been observed *(49,50)*. A combination of anti-V3 , anti-V2, and anti-CD4 binding site antibodies showed highly significant synergy in neutralization of HIV-1 *(51)*. Therefore, it should be beneficial to combine several epitope-specific mAbs to achieve high suprathreshold neutralization titers and to select an optimal spectrum of HIV target epitopes that would not only include conserved protective epitopes stable to neutralization escape but would also exclude infection-enhancing epitopes. This can be fulfilled by using phage display libraries with epitope masking techniques to supress selection of immunodominant epitopes for identification of several valuable antibodies *(52–54)*.

5. Antibodies in Sepsis and Septic Shock

Despite broad-spectrum antimicrobial therapy and aggressive intensive care measures, such as mechanical ventilation, use of vasoactive drugs, and hemodialysis, sepsis still remains a highly life-threatening disease. Endotoxin (LPS), which is present in the outer membrane of gram-negative bacteria, plays a key role in triggering the development of the clinical and laboratory manifestations of gram-negative septicemia *(55)*. Endotoxemia initiates the rapid biosynthesis and release of several proinflammatory cytokines, including TNF-α, IL-1, and IL-6 *(56,57)*. These cytokines mediate a variety of biological effects, invoking inflammatory response and activation of coagulation pathways, which result in the development of end-organ failure *(57)*.

Because the endotoxin molecule is presumed to have phylogenetically conserved antigenics among the variety of gram-negative bacteria, antibodies directed against these regions are thought to provide crossprotection against heterologous gram-negative bacteria *(58,59)*. Encouraging initial results in animal models caused the development and release of antiendotoxin antibodies, such as HA-1A (Centoxin, Centocor, Malvern, PA) in Europe in 1991 *(59)*. HA-A1, a humanized monoclonal IgM antilipid A antibody, has been widely tested in phase III human clinical trials. Both animal studies and human clinical trials gave conflicting observations regarding the protective efficacy of HA-1A in gram-negative bacteremia (GNB) (9,10,58,59). Early studies in murine and rabbit models revealed that HA-1A increased the survival rate in sepsis (58). However, later studies in mice and canine models produced contrary data (10,60). In a canine model, HA-1A did not influence the severity of bacteremia or endotoxemia and actually decreased the survival (10). These conflicting results may be caused by differences in sensitivity to endotoxin among distinct species (10).

In the first human clinical trial, a single 100 mg dose of HA-1A was administered to patients who were presumed to have gram-negative sepsis (59). HA-1A reduced the mortality rate from 48% in patients receiving placebo to 24% in those receiving HA-1A 14 d after its administration. The mortality rate was reduced from 56% in the placebo group to 33% in the HA-1A at d 28 (59). In another clinical trial examining the reproducibility of the first study, 14 d after giving the same dose of HA-1A to the patients with GNB, mortality rates between placebo and HA-1A groups were similar, with 32 and 33%, respectively (9). In the same and study, use of HA-1A treatment in the patients without GNB, interestingly, seemed to cause a higher mortality rate compared to the patients receiving placebo (9). A similar finding was demonstrated in a cohort study by another group in France (11). This may be explained by the fact that the group of patients without gram-negative bacteria infection was heterogenous, having sepsis of other causes, some of which had a worse prognosis than gram-negative infections, and also included patients with noninfectious causes of sepsis syndrome who may poorly respond to conventional therapy (61). The other possibility, suggested by Quezado et al., is that HA-1A could worsen cardiovascular performance by binding nonspecifically endothelial structures (10,60). As a matter of fact, the epitope specificity of this antibody has been questioned by some researchers. H1-1A has been defined by some authors as a lipid A-specific mAb (62,63), whereas others observed that this antibody crossreacted with antigens found on cord erythrocytes, a ligand on human B lymphocytes, and some anionic polymers, such as ssDNA, chondroitin sulfate, and cardiolipin (64,65). This has recently been explained by the fact that this polyreactivity of HA-1A is caused by its binding ability to a wide variety of hydrophobic ligands (66). HA-1A was withdrawn by the manufacturer because of excess mortality in patients without GNB (67).

Release of proinflammatory cytokines into the bloodstream occurs in humans with serious GNB. Because cytokines have been considered important mediators of sepsis, it should be reasonable to devise ways to interrupt or mitigate their actions on target cells (68). For this purpose, antibodies directed toward either the cytokine (TNF-α or IL-6) or the cytokine receptor (IL-1r) have been employed in several animal models. The first report by Beutler et al. *(69)* demonstrated that anti-TNF-α antibodies prevented the lethal effect of endotoxemia in mice. In baboons, use of anti-TNF-α mAb prior to treatment with live *E. coli* for 2 h protected against septic shock and multiple-system organ failure *(70)*. Fong et al. *(71)* showed that it is possible to attenuate the release of proinflammatory cytokines, including TNF-α, IL-1β, and IL-6, by passive immunization of baboons with TNF-α antibodies. Bagby et al. *(72)* demonstrated that use of anti-TNF-α antibodies improved survival from 8 to 75% in rats treated with intravenous endotoxin. However, in these studies there was no clear relationship between the in vitro binding of the TNF-α antibodies to TNF-α and in vivo efficacy *(73)*. In a study by Eskandari et al. *(74)*, it has been shown that use of anti-TNF-α antibody fails to extend survival following induction of sepsis in mice by cecal ligation and puncture (CLP) or intravenous or intraperitoneal administration of endotoxin, although TNF activity is reduced to undetectable levels. These data suggest that blockade of TNF activity is not sufficient to prevent lethality. O'Riordain et al. *(75)* used a different strategy to induce sepsis. In their study, mice were exposed to a full thickness burn or sham burn followed by CLP on d 10. Administration of anti-TNF-α Ab (1×10^4 neutralizing unit (nu)/kg) at d 7 following the burn significantly improved the survival, whereas no benefit was provided when administered at d 0 or 4 or at the time of CLP. In addition, high doses of antibody (3.2×10^5 nu/kg) were not only unbeneficial but also deleterious *(75)*. Therefore, the timing of administration and dose of the antibody may be critical to the clinical outcome.

In an international, multicenter, placebo-controlled trial, safety and efficacy of a murine mAb directed to human TNF-α, BAY × 1351, was evaluated in patients with sepsis *(76)*. There was no significant difference in 28-d mortality rates between placebo and treatment groups with sepsis, whereas there was a significant delay in the time of onset of first organ failure in patients suffering from septic shock and surviving 28 d. These data provided additional clinical data implicating TNF-α as one of the key mediators of septic shock, and anti-TNF-α antibody may be feasible for adjunctive therapy in septic shock. Another anti-TNF α antibody fragment, MAK 195F, was examined in a phase II trial in patients with severe sepsis in terms of its biological effects, efficacy, and safety *(77)*. This study demonstrated that patients with baseline serum IL-6 concentrations of >1000 pg/mL seemed to gain benefit from this antibody in a dose-dependent manner. Significant decreases in circulating IL-6 concentrations were seen during the first 24 h of treatment in the patients receiving anti-TNF-α antibody treatment but not in the placebo group. However, there was no improvement in survival from sepsis for the patients treated with anti-TNF-α antibody. In addition, although this antibody was well tolerated by all patients, 40% of patients developed human antimurine antibodies *(77)*.

Interleukin-6 is, indeed, another important mediator of sepsis syndrome. In one of the early studies, the effect of anti-IL-6 Ab pretreatment was assessed in mice subsequently challenged with lethal doses of ip *E. coli* or iv TNF-α. In this study, rat antimouse IL-6 mAb was administered intravenously 2 h before the challenge, and it neutralized specifically mouse IL-6 but not other factors, including TNF-α, and partially abrogated the in vivo effects of GNB *(78)*. Actually, treatment with anti-IL-6 mAb paradoxically increased circulating TNF-α levels, and using anti-TNF-α caused a significant decrease in serum IL-6 levels. According to these data, TNF-α seems to elevate the synthesis of IL-6, whereas IL-6 decreases the production of TNF-α *(78)*. In a more recent report, Höpken et al. *(79)* demonstrated that pretreatment of pigs with a mAb directed against complement 5a (C5a) led to a significant decrease in IL-6 levels in animals subsequently challenged with *E. coli*. These data indicated a role of C5a in the induction of IL-6 production in GNB.

Anticytokine receptor antibodies are thought to bind to the cytokine receptors on the surface of responding cells and prevent the binding of cytokines. The efficacy of anti-IL-1 receptor (L-1r) antibodies in sepsis syndrome have been widely assessed in animal models. Antibodies directed against IL-1r has been shown to be effective in blocking stress hormones induced by endotoxin *(80)* and preventing IL-6 stimulation by IL-1 *(81)*. McIntyre et al. *(82)* demonstrated that anti-IL-1r antibodies led to increases in peripheral blood neutrophil numbers and also blocked endotoxin-induced peritonitis in mice. Although all these studies performed in animal models seem to indicate that the biological effects of IL-1 can be prevented by an antibody directed toward the IL-1r, these still remain to be tested in well designed, randomized, placebo-controlled clinical trials in well defined clinical populations.

In sepsis syndrome, antibodies alone do not seem to be feasible therapeutically, and administration of a cocktail of mAbs with different specificities, perhaps also in the presence of antimicrobial drugs, could provide much better outcome.

6. Advantages and Problems of Antibody-Based Therapies

6.1. Spectrum of Activity

Advantages and problems of antibody-based therapies in infectious diseases have been previously reviewed in detail *(5,7,83)*. Antibodies can modify bacterial, fungal, parasitic, and viral infections with broad antimicrobial activity against diverse pathogens. Antibody-based therapies are usually pathogen-specific and have the theoretical advantage that they should not affect the normal flora of the patient or select for resistance in nontargeted microorganisms. The narrow specificity needed for this purpose is a disadvantage in some cases because mixed infections may not be treated by a single antibody preparation. Pneumonia attributable to *S. pneumoniae* with more than one serotype recognized as a reason for the failure of type-specific serum therapy is an example *(84)*. The use of cocktails of mAbs against common antigenic types designed to include mAbs with multiple isotypes will certainly enhance the efficacy of antibody-based treatments. Given the large array of diversity of pathogens, the pathogen-specific nature of antibody therapies, and the cost, of development of such therapies for most pathogens at present would be impractical. However, for selected pathogens, antibody-based therapies could provide new therapeutic options. Opportunities for the development of antibody-based strategies include pathogens for which there is no available antimicrobial therapy, such as *C. parvum* and vancomycin-resistant enterococcus. In addition, pathogens that affect primarily immunocompromised patients in whom antimicrobial therapy is not very effective, such as invasive fungal infections, and pathogens for which drug-resistant variants are rapidly spreading, such as *Pseudomonas aeruginosa*, are targets for developing antibody-based strategies. Furthermore, highly virulent pathogens for which few effective antimicrobial agents are available, such as methicillin-resistant *S. aureus*, are goals for future antibody-based therapies.

6.2. Mechanism of Action

Antibodies function through a variety of mechanisms, whereas conventional antimicrobial chemotherapy kills or inhibits the replication of microorganisms. Direct antibody mechanisms of action include inhibition of attachment, agglutination, immobilization, viral neutralization, toxin neutralization, antibody-mediated cellular cytotoxicity, complement activation, and opsonization (*see* **Subheading 2.**) *(13)*. Antibody therapy has the potential to enhance immune function in immunosuppressed hosts. However, since the mechanism of action of many antibodies involves promoting microbial clearance through nonspecific cellular immunity, antibody-based therapies may be less effective in individuals with defective macrophage, neutrophil, and natural killer cell function. In this respect, it is encouraging that antibodies are effective against *P. aeruginosa* in neutropenic mice *(85)* and that they can reduce the number of infections in AIDS patients *(86)*.

Numerous pathologic situations may benefit from a specific means of antagonizing cytokine response by mAbs in vivo, such as septic shock, acute inflammatory diseases, cytokine-dependent tumor growth, neopathic disease, and organ transplantation *(87,88)*. The phenomenon of stabilization of a cytokine and accumulation of monomeric immune complexes are encountered during cytokine neutralization therapies. This problem was solved in the particular case of IL-6 neutralization treatment by using a cocktail of three different mAbs directed to different epitopes on IL-6 that enhance the clearance of the molecule *(88)*.

Antibodies are usually considered to be protective effector mechanisms of the immune system. However, antibody responses to pathogens are not all protective and some may be detrimental to the host. For example, some viral-specific antibodies are capable of enhancing infection *(89)*. Thus, antibody molecules being considered for clinical development will require extensive testing in vitro and in vivo. Studies of the mechanisms of antibody action are important for understanding the mode of protection and for designing clinical trials.

Although intracellular pathogens are commonly believed to be outside the reach of antibody immunity, several reports have suggested that some mAbs are active against some intracellular micro-organisms. This has been shown by intracellular virus neutralization *(90)* and inhibition of intracellular *Toxoplasma gondii* replication by antibodies *(91)*. Engineering of antibodies in the future should also allow a reliable cell wall accessibility and better tissue penetration. Recent advances in antibody engineering now allow the manipulation of the genes encoding specific antibodies and provide intracellular expression of the antigen-binding domain within target cells *(92)*.

6.3. Pharmacokinetics

The pharmacokinetics of human IgG suggests several useful characteristics for its role as an anti-infective agent. Depending on the IgG subtype, half life, tissue penetration, and the ability to cross the placenta or to be excluded by the placental barrier can be controlled. Mouse mAbs have shorter half-lives in humans, but chimeric and humanized mAbs have longer half-lives than their precursors. To modulate pharmacokinetics mAbs can be engineered by altering the regions of the constant domain that regulate clearance.

A disadvantage of antibody-based therapies for infectious diseases is the need for systemic administration. Oral administration is unlikely to be effective, with the possible exception of therapy for enteric pathogens *(93)*. The blood–brain barrier is a potential obstacle for antibody therapy for infections of the central nervous system (CNS). However, in inflammation caused by meningitis, the blood–brain barrier enables antibody penetration, as shown in the treatment of meningococcal meningitis by antibodies *(94)*. Antibodies can also be administered directly into the subarachnoid space, as has been done for the treatment of meningococcal and *H. influenzae* meningitis *(94,95)*.

Enhanced penetration of the brain can be achieved by modifying the charge of the molecule *(96)* or by linking it to carrier proteins that cross the blood–brain barrier *(97)*. Antibody treatment of CNS infections is likely if the antibody used penetrates the blood–brain barrier. Complex pharmacokinetics and penetration problems have to be further evaluated by sophisticated research tools for the use of antibodies in infections *(98)*.

6.4. Toxicity

Although immunoglobulin treatment is generally accepted as safe, severe side effects have been reported. Toxicities described with high-dose serum therapy may not be relevant for mAb-based therapies. For example, 0.7 mg of two antitetanus toxin human mAbs provides the same activity as 100–170 mg of horse serum antitetanique *(99)*. Nevertheless, renal failure, aseptic meningitis, and thromboembolic events have been reported with high-dose immunoglobulin therapy *(100,101)*. Murine mAbs against T-cell CD3 molecules to prevent graft rejection in transplantation *(102)* and antiendotoxin murine IgM *(103)* are two examples for the use of murine mAbs in the treatment of human diseases. Administration of murine mAbs is generally well tolerated in humans. Allergic reactions occur in 1–2% of patients but most patients develop antibody responses to the mAbs that may interfere with their therapeutic function *(104)*. Mouse–human chimeric and humanized mAbs are less immunogenic than their murine precursors and they are relatively safe compounds *(105)*, but anti-idiotypic responses occur after repeated treatments *(106)*.

6.5. Antigenic Variation and Antibody Resistance

The efficacy of antibody-based therapies may be diminished by antigenic changes in the pathogen. In a manner analogous to that of antibiotic resistance, large-scale use of antibody-based therapies may result in antibody resistance. Antibody-resistant mutants can be generated in the laboratory and it is possible that the same can occur in patients *(107)*. Widespread antibody use may lead to selection of resistant micro-organisms, such as mutations that change the antigenic site and protease production *(108)*. The increasing incidence of resistant organisms resulting from the use of broad-spectrum antibiotic regimens could make pathogen-specific drugs attractive to pharmaceutical companies, since the narrow specificity reduces the potential market for the drug. High diversity of antibody compounds may overcome these problems. An antibody-resistant strain can be treated by a new antibody directed toward the mutated epitope or another antigenic target. Furthermore, antiprotease antibodies can be used in combination to inhibit the proteases of a resistant micro-organism. In addition, designing antibodies without protease cleavage sites can be used to resist protease-producing resistant strains.

6.6. Cost

The major obstacle for the development of passive antibody therapies is likely to be cost effectiveness. In the past, serum therapy was used despite its high cost because it was believed to be effective. The cost of prevention of infection in immunocompromised patients by antibodies has always been questioned. Antibody prophylaxis for CMV infections can cost $4000–9000 per patient *(109)*. Cost effectiveness of mAbs to gram-negative endotoxin in the treatment of gram-negative sepsis was calculated in the case of HA-1A mAb, which reduced the 28 d mortality by 39% in the first human trial *(87)*. The annual total cost was expected to reach to £100m in the United Kingdom and $1.6 billion in the United States. However, if it had proved to be actually effective in subsequent human trials, in the United Kingdom HA-1A could have saved between 5000 and 10000 lives per year at a cost of about $5000 per life saved. This is a very favorable amount in comparison to other widely accepted medical interventions *(110)*. In addition, the present production of mAbs in tissue culture is costly, but mAbs produced in yeast and bacteria is less expensive and further development of new techniques will decrease the production costs.

7. Conclusion and Future Directions

For every pathogen an antibody that will modify the course of infection for the benefit of the host can be produced. Such antibodies are candidates to develop new antimicrobial options to prevent or treat infectious diseases caused by pathogens for which there are no or few antimicrobial therapy strategies available or that threaten immunocompromised patients in whom existing antimicrobial drugs are inefficient. In the future it should also be possible to produce mAbs against several toxic products of infecting organisms, as well as other components of inflammatory cascade. In addition, treatment with a combination of mAbs will be feasible. Thus, immunotherapy of infectious diseases with antibodies will bring a new perspective for the treatment of infectious diseases.

Acknowledgments

The authors gratefully thank Prof. K. Kılıçturgay and Prof. G. Göral (Uludağ University, Turkey) for continuous support and many useful discussions on the subject.

References

1. Krause, R. M., Dimmock, N. J., and Morens, D. M. (1997) Summary of antibody workshop: the role of humoral immunity in the treatment and prevention of emerging and extant infectious diseases. *J. Infect. Dis.* **176,** 549–559.

2. Casadevall, A. and Schraff, M. D. (1994) "Serum therapy" revisited: animal models of infection and the development of passive antibody therapy. *Antimicrob. Agents Chemother.* **38,** 1695–1702.
3. Felton, L. D. (1928) The units of protective antibody in anti-pneumococcus serum and antibody solution. *J. Infect. Dis.* **43,** 531–542.
4. Slade, H. B. (1994) Human immunoglobulins for intravenous use and hepatitis C viral transmission. *Clin. Diagn. Lab. Immunol.* **1,** 613–619.
5. Casadevall, A. (1996) Antibody-based therapies for emerging infectious diseases. *Emerging Infect. Dis.* **2,** 200–208.
6. Köhler, G. and Milstein, C. (1975) Continuous cultures of fused cells secreting antibody of predefined specificity. *Nature* **256,** 495–497.
7. Waldmann, T. A. (1991) Monoclonal antibodies in diagnosis and therapy. *Science* **252,** 1657–1662.
8. Subramannian, K. N. S., Weisman, L. E., Rhodes, T., Ariagno, R., Sanchez, P. J., Steichen, J., Givner, L. B., Jennings, T. L., Top, F. H., Jr., Carlin, D., and Connor, E. (1998) Safety, tolerance and pharmacokinetics of a humanized monoclonal antibody to respiratory syncytial virus in premature infants and infants with bronchopulmonary dysplasia. *Pediatr. Infect. Dis. J.* **17,** 110–115.
9. McCloskey, R. V., Straube, R. C., Sanders, C., Smith, S. M., Smith, C. R., and the CHESS Trial Study Group (1994) Treatment of septic shock with human monoclonal antibody HA-1A. *Ann. Intern. Med.* **121,** 1–5.
10. Quezado, Z. M. N., Natanson, C., Alling, D. W., Banks, S. M., Koev, C. A., Elin, R. J., Hosseini, J. M., Bacher, J. D., Danner, R. L., and Hoffman, W. D. (1993) A controlled trial of HA-1A in a canine model of gram-negative septic shock. *JAMA* **269,** 2221–2227.
11. The National Committee for the Evaluation of Centoxin. (1994) The French National Registry of HA-1A (Centoxin) in Septic Shock. *Arch. Intern. Med.* **154,** 2484–2491.
12. Mims, C. A., Dimmock, N. J., Nash, A., and Stephen, J. (1995) The immune response to infection, in *Mims' Pathogenesis of Infectious Disease* (Mims, C. A., ed.), Academic, London, UK, pp. 136–167.
13. Heinzel, F. P. (1995) Antibodies, in *Principles and Practice of Infectious Diseases* (Mandel, G. L., Bennett, J. E., and Dolin, R., eds.), Churchill Livingstone, New York, pp. 36–57.
14. Mandel, G. L., Bennett, J. E., and Dolin, R., eds. (1995) *Principles and Practice of Infectious Diseases.* Churchill Livingstone, New York.
15. Stiehm, E. R. (1979) Standard and special human immune serum globulins as therapeutic agents. *Pediatrics* **63,** 301.
16. Schiff, G. M. (1969) Titered lots of immune globulin. Efficacy in the prevention of rubella. *Am. J. Dis. Child.* **118,** 322.
17. Green, M. S. and Dotan, K. (1988) Eficacy of immune serum globuline in an outbreak of hepatitis A virus infection in adults. *J. Infect. Dis.* **17,** 265–270.
18. Stokes, J., Jr. and Neefe, J. R. (1945) The prevention and attenuation of infectious hepatitis by gamma globulin. *JAMA* **127,** 144,145.

19. Winokur, P. L. and Stapleton, J. T. (1992) Immunoglobulin prophylaxis for hepatitis A. *Clin. Infect. Dis.* **14,** 580–586.

20. Desmyter, J., Bradbourne, A. F., Vermylen, C., Daneels, R., and Boelaert, J. (1975) Hepatitis B immunoglobulin in prevention of HB_s antigenemia in haemodialysis patients. *Lancet* **2,** 376,377.

21. Iwarson, S., Kjellman., H., Ahlmén, J., Ljunggren, C., Eriksson, E., Selander, D., and Hermodsson, S. (1975) Hepatitis B immune serum globulin and standard gamma globulin in prevention of hepatitis B infection among hospital staff: a preliminary report. *Am. J. Med. Sci.* **270,** 385–389.

22. Centers for Disease Control and Prevention (1977) Immune globulins for protection against viral hepatitis. *MMWR* **26,** 425.

23. Hoofnagle, J. H., Seeff, L. B., Bales, Z. B., Wright, E. C., and Zimmerman H. J. (1979) Passive-active immunity from hepatitis B immune globulin. Reanalysis of a Veterans Administration cooperative study of needle-stick hepatitis. The Veterans Administration Cooperative Study Group. *Ann. Intern. Med.* **91,** 813–818.

24. Grady, G. F., Lee, V. A., Prince, A. M., Gitnick, G. L., Fawaz, K. A., Vyas, G. N., Levitt, M. D., Senior, J. R., Galambos, J. T., Bynum, T. E., Singleton, J. W., Clowdus, B. F., Akdamar, K., Aach, R. D., Winkelman, E. I., Schiff, G. M., and Hersh, T. (1978) Hepatitis B immune globulin for accidental exposures among medical personnel: final report of a multicenter controlled trial. *J. Infect. Dis.* **138,** 625–638.

25. Advisory Committee for Immunization Practices (1990) Recommendation for protection against viral hepatitis. *MMWR* **38(Suppl.).**

26. Beasley, R. P., Hwang, L. Y., Lee, G. C., Lan, C. C., Roan, C. H., Huang, F. Y., and Chen, C. L. (1983) Prevention of perinatally transmitted hepatitis B virus infections with hepatitis B immunoglobulin and hepatitis B vaccine. *Lancet* **2,** 1099–1102.

27. Centers for Disease Control and Prevention (1984) Varicella zoster immune globulin for the prevention of chickenpox: recommendations of the immunization practices advisory committee. *Ann. Intern. Med.* **100,** 859–865.

28. Gellis, S. S., McGuiness, A. C., and Peters, M. (1945) A study on the prevention of mumps orchitis with gamma globulin. *Am. J. Med. Sci.* **210,** 661.

29. Dean, D. J. (1963) Pathogenesis and prophylaxis of rabies in man. *NY State J. Med.* **63,** 3507–3513.

30. Wilde, H., Chomchey, P., Punyaratabandhu, P., Phanupak, P., and Chutivongse, S. (1989) Purified equine rabies immune globulin: a safe and affordable alternative to human rabies immune globulin. *Bull. WHO* **67,** 731–736.

31. Winston, D. J., Ho, W. G., Lin, C. H., Bartoni, K., Budinger, M. D., Gale, R. P., and Champlin, R. E. (1987) Intravenous immune globulin for prevention of cytomegalovirus infection and interstitial pneumonia after bone morrow transplantation. *Ann. Intern. Med.* **106,** 12–18.

32. Snydman, D. R., Werner, B. G., Dougherty, N. N., Griffith, J., Rubin, R. H., Dienstag, J. L., Rohrer, R. H., Freeman, R., Jenkins, R., and Lewis, W. D. (1993) Cytomegalovirus immune globulin prophylaxis in liver transplantation. A ran-

domized, double-blind, placebo-controlled trial. The Boston Center for Liver Transplantation CMVIG Study Group. *Ann. Intern. Med.* **119,** 984–991.

33. Bleck, T. P. (1995) Clostridium tetani, in *Principles and Practice of Infectious Diseases* (Mandel, G. L., Bennett, J. E., and Dolin, R., eds.), Churchill Livingstone, New York, pp. 2173–2178.

34. Brand, D. A., Acampora, D., Gottlieb, L. D., Glancy, K. E., and Frazier, W. H. (1983) Adequacy of antitetanus prophylaxis in six hospital emergency rooms. *N. Engl. J. Med.* **309,** 636 640.

35. MacGregor, R. R. (1995) Corynebacterium diphtheriae, in *Principles and Practice of Infectious Diseases* (Mandel, G. L., Bennett, J. E., and Dolin, R., eds.), Churchill Livingstone, New York, pp. 1865 1872.

36. Davies, H. D., McGeer, A., Schwartz, B., Green, K., Cann, D., Simor, A. E., and Low, D. E., and Ontario Streptococcal Study Group (1996) Invasive group A streptococcal infections in Ontario, Canada. *N. Engl. J. Med.* **335,** 547–554.

37. Basma, H., Norrby-Teglund, A., McGeer, A., Low, D. E., El-Ahmedy, O., Dale, J. B., Schwartz, B., and Kotb, M. (1998) Opsonic antibodies to the surface of group A streptococci in pooled normal immunoglobulins (IVIG): potential impact on the clinical efficacy of IVIG therapy for severe invasive group A streptococcal infections. *Infect. Immun.* **66,** 2279–2283.

38. Barry, W., Hudgins, L., Donta, S. T., and Pesanti, E. I. (1992) Intravenous immunoglobulin therapy for toxic shock syndrome. *JAMA* **267,** 3315,3316.

39. Stegmayer, B., Björck, S., Holm, S., Niseli, J., Rydvalt, A., and Settergren, B. (1992) Septic shock induced by group A streptococcal infection: clinical and therapeutic aspects. *Scand. J. Infect. Dis.* **24,** 589–597.

40. Nord, J., Ma, P., DiJohn, D., Tzipori, S., and Tacket, C. O. (1990) Treatment with bovine hyperimmune colostrum of cryptosporodial diarrhea in AIDS patients. *AIDS* **4,** 581–584.

41. Langer, R. C. and Riggs, M. W. (1997) Neutralizing monoclonal antibody protects against *Cryptosporidium parvum* infection by inhibiting sporozoite attachment and invasion. *J. Eukaryot. Bicrobiol.* **43,** 76S,77S.

42. Riggs, M. W., Stone, A. L., Yount, P. A., Langer, R. C., Arrowood, M. J., and Bentley, D. L. (1997) Protective monoclonal antibody defines a circumsporozoite-like glycoprotein exoantigen of *Cryptosporidium parvum* sporozoites and merazoites. *J. Immunol.* **158,** 1787–1795.

43. Kuhls, T. L., Orlicek, S. L., Mosier, D. A., Crawford, D. L., Abrams, V. L., and Greenfield, R. A. (1995) Enteral human serum immunoglobulin treatment of cryptosporidosis in mice with severe combined immunodeficiency. *Infect. Immun.* **63,** 3582 3586.

44. Jackson, G. G., Perkins, J. T., Rubenis, M., Paul, D. A., Knigge, M., Despotes, J. C., and Spencer, P. (1988) Passive immunoneutralization of human immunodeficiency virus in patients with advanced AIDS. *Lancet* **8612,** 647–652.

45. Karpas, A., Hill, F., Toule, M., Cullen, V., Gray, J., Byron, N., Hayhoe, F., Tenant-Flowers, M., Howard, L., and Gilgen, D (1988) Effect of passive immunization in patients with the acquired immunodeficiency syndrome-related complex

and acquired immunodeficiency syndrome. *Proc. Natl. Acad. Sci. USA* **85,** 9234–9237.

46. Karpas, A., Hewlett, I. K., Hill, F., Gray, J., Byron, N. Gilgen, D., Bally, V., Oates, J. K., Gazzard, B., and Epstein, J. E. (1990) Polymerase chain reaction evidence for human immunodeficiency virus 1 neutralization by passive immunization in patients with AIDS and AIDS-related complex. *Proc. Natl. Acad. Sci. USA* **87,** 7613–7617.

47. Vittecoq, D., Chevret, S., Morand-Joubert, L., Heshmati, F., Audat, F., Bary, M., Dusautoir, T., Bismuth, A., Viard, J. P., and Barre-Sinoussi, F. (1995) Passive immunotherapy in AIDS: a double-blind randomized study based on transfusions of plasma rich in anti-human immunodeficiency virus 1 antibodies vs. transfusions of seronegative plasma. *Proc. Natl. Acad. Sci. USA* **92,** 1195–1199.

48. Günthard, H. F., Gowland, P. L., Schüpbach, J., Fung, M. S., Böni, J., Liou, R. S., Chang, N. T., Grob, P., Graepel, P., and Braun, D. G. (1994) A phase I/IIA clinical study with a chimeric mouse-human monoclonal antibody to the V3 loop of human immunodeficiency virus type 1 gp120. *J. Infect. Dis.* **170,** 1384–1393.

49. Tilley, S. A., Honnen, W. J., Racho, M. E., Hilgartner, M., and Pinter, A. (1991) A human monoclonal antibody against the CD4-binding site of HIV1 gp120 exhibits potent, broadly neutralizing activity. *Res. Virol.* **142,** 247–259.

50. Warrier, S. V., Pinter, A., Honnen, W. J., Girard, M., Muchmore, E., and Tilley, S. A. (1994) A novel, glycan-dependent epitope in the V2 domain of human immunodeficiency virus type 1 gp120 is recognized by a highly potent, neutralizing chimpanzee monoclonal antibody. *J. Virol.* **68,** 4636–4642.

51. Vijh-Warrier, S., Pinter, A., Honnen, W.J., and Tilley, S. A. (1996) Synergistic neutralization of human immunodeficiency virus type-1 by a chimpanzee monoclonal antibody against the V2 domain of gp120 in combination with monoclonal antibodies against the V3 loop and the CD4-binding sites. *J. Virol.* **70,** 4466–4473.

52. Burton, D. R., Barbas, C. F., 3rd, Persson, M. A., Koenig, S., Chanock, R. M., and Lerner, R. A. (1991) A large array of human monoclonal antibodies to type 1 human immunodeficiency virus from combinatorial libraries of asymptomatic seropositive individuals. *Proc. Natl. Acad. Sci. USA* **88,** 10,134–10,137.

53. Burton, D. R. and Barbas, C. F., 3rd (1993) Human antibodies to HIV-1 by recombinant DNA methods. *Chem. Immunol.* **56,** 112–126.

54. Ditzel, H. J., Binley, J. M., Moore, J. P., Sodroski, J., Sullivan, N., Sawyer, L. S., Hendry, R. M., Yang, W. P., Barbas, C. F., 3rd, and Burton, D. R. (1995) Neutralizing recombinant human antibodies to a conformational V2- and CD4-binding site-sensitive epitope of HIV-1 gp120 isolated by using an epitope-masking procedure. *J. Immunol.* **154,** 893–906.

55. Danner, R. L., Elin, R. J., Hosseini, J. M., Wesley, R. A., Reilly, J. M., and Parrillo, J. E. (1991) Endotoxemia in human septic shock. *Chest* **99,** 169–175.

56. Michie, H. R., Manogue, K. R., Spriggs, D. R., Revhaug, A., O'Dwyer, S., Dinarello, C. A., Cerami, A., Wolff, S. M., and Wilmore, D. W. (1988) Detection of circulating tumor necrosis factor after endotoxin administration. *N. Engl. J. Med.* **318,** 1481–1486.

57. van Deventer, S. J. H., Büller, H. R., ten Cate, J. W., Aarden, L. A., Hack, C. E., and Sturk, A. (1990) Experimental endotoxemia in humans: analysis of cytokine release and coagulation, fibrinolytic, and complement pathways. *Blood* **76,** 2520–2526.

58. Teng, N. N. H., Kaplan, H. S., Hebert, J. M., Moore, C., Douglas, H., Wunderlich, A., and Braude, A. I. (1985) Protection against gram-negative bacteraemia and endotoxemia with human monoclonal IgM antibodies. *Proc. Natl. Acad. Sci. USA* **82,** 1790–1794.

59. Ziegler, E. J., Fisher, C. J., Jr., Sprung, C. L., Straube, R. C., Sadoff, J. C., Foulke, G. E., Wortel, C. H., Fink, M. P., Dellinger, R. P., Teng, N. N. H., Allen, I. E., Berger, H. J., Knatterud, G. L., Lobuglio, A. F., Smith, C. R., and the HA-1A Study Group (1991) Treatment of gram-negative bacteraemia and septic shock with HA-1A human monoclonal antibody against endotoxin. *N. Engl. J. Med.* **324,** 429–436.

60. Baumgartner, J. D., Heumann, D., Gerain, J., Weinbreck, P., Grau, G. E., and Glauser, M. P. (1990) Association between protective efficacy of anti-lipopolysaccharide (LPS) antibodies and suppression of LPS-induced tumour necrosis alfa and interleukin-6. *J. Exp. Med.* **171,** 889–896.

61. Sprung, C. L., Eidelmen, L. A., Pizov, R., Fisher, C. S., Jr., Ziegler, E. J., Sadoff, J. C., Straube, R. C., and McCloskey, R. V. (1997) Influence of alterations in foregoing life-sustaining treatment practice on a clinical sepsis trial. The HA-1A Sepsis Study Group. *Crit. Care Med.* **3,** 283–287.

62. Bogard, W. C., Siegel, S. A., Leone, A. O., Damiano, E., Shealy, D. J., Ely, T. M., Frederick, B., Mascelli, M. A., Siegel, R. C., Machielse, B., Naveh, D., Kaplan, P. M., and Daddona, P. E. (1993) Human monoclonal antibody HA-1A binds to endotoxin via an epitope in the lipid A domain of lipopolysaccharide. *J. Immunol.* **150,** 4438–4449.

63. Fujihara, Y., Lei, M., and Morrison, D. C. (1993) Characterization of specific binding of a human immunoglobulin M monoclonal antibody to lipopolysaccharide and its lipid A domain. *Infect. Immun.* **61,** 910–918.

64. Bhat, N. M., Bieber, M. M., Chapman, C. J., Stevenson, F. K., and Teng, N. N. H. (1993) Human antilipid A monoclonal antibodies bind to human B cells and the i antigen on cord red blood cells. *J. Immunol.* **151,** 5011–5021.

65. Bieber, M. M., Bhat, N. M., and Teng, N. N. H. (1995) Anti-endotoxin human monoclonal antibody A6H4C5 (HA-1A) utilizes the VH4.21 gene. *Clin. Infect. Dis.* **21,** 186–189.

66. Helmerhorst, E. J., Maaskant, J. J., and Appelmelk, B. J. (1998) Anti-lipid A monoclonal antibody Centoxin (HA-1A) binds to a wide variety of hydrophobic ligands. *Infect. Immun.* **66,** 870–873.

67. Medicines Control Agency, Department of Health (1993) Drug Alert. *MDR* 13-1/93, Jan 20.

68. Christman, J. W., Wheeler, A., and Bernard, G. (1991) Cytokines and sepsis: What are the therapeutic implications? *J. Crit. Care* **6,** 172–182.

69. Beutler, B., Milsarek, I. W., and Cerami, A. C. (1985) Passive immunization against cachectin/tumor necrosis factor protects mice from lethal effect of endotoxin. *Science* **229,** 869–871.

70. Tracey, K. J., Fong, J. Y., Hesse, D. G., Manogue, K. R., Lee, A. T., Kuo, G. C., Lowry, S. F., and Cerami, A. (1987) Anti-cachectin/TNF monoclonal antibodies prevent septic shock during lethal bacteraemia. *Nature* **330**, 662–664.
71. Fong, Y., Tracey, K. J., Moldawer, L. L., Hesse, D. G., Manogue, K. B., Kenny, J. S., Lee, A. T., Kuo, G. C., Allison, A. C., Lowry, S. F., et al. (1989) Antibodies to cachetic/tumor necrosis factor reduce interleukin-1β and interleukin 6 appearance during lethal bacteraemia. *J. Exp. Med.* **170**, 1627–1633.
72. Bagby, G. J., Plesalla, K. J., Wilson, L. A., Thompson, J. J., and Nelson, S. (1991) Divergent efficacy of antibody to tumor necrosis factor a in intravascular and peritonitis models of sepsis. *J. Infect. Dis.* **163**, 83–88.
73. Christman, J. W. (1992) Potential treatment of sepsis syndrome with cytokine-specific agents. *Chest* **102**, 613–617.
74. Eskandari, M. K., Bolgos, G., Miller, C., Nguyen, D. T., DeForge, L. E., and Remick, D. G. (1992) Anti-tumor necrosis factor antibody therapy fails to prevent lethality after cecal ligation puncture or endotoxemia. *J. Immunol.* **148**, 2724–2730.
75. O'Riordain, M. G., O'Riordain, D. S., Molloy, R. G., Mannick, J. A., and Rodrick, M. L. (1996) Dosage and timing of anti-TNF-alpha antibody treatment determine its effect of resistance to sepsis after injury. *J. Surg. Res.* **64**, 95–101.
76. Cohen, J. and Carlet, J. (1996) INTERSEPT: an international, multicenter, placebo-controlled trial of monoclonal antibody to human tumor necrosis factor-alpha in patients with sepsis. *Crit. Care Med.* **9**, 1431–1440.
77. Reinhart, K., Wiegand-Löhnert, C., Grimminger, F., Kaul, M., Withington, S., Treacher, D., Eckart, J., Willatts, S., Bouza, C., Krausch, D., Stockenhuber, F., Eiselstein, J., Daum, L., and Kempeni, J. (1996) Assessment of the safety and efficacy of the monoclonal anti-tumor necrosis factor antibody fragment, MAK 195F, in patients with sepsis and septic shock: a multicenter, randomized, placebo-controlled, dose-ranging study. *Crit. Care Med.* **24**, 733–742.
78. Starnes, H. F., Jr., Pearce, M. K., Tewari, A., Yim, J. H., Zou, J.-C., and Abrams, J. S. (1990) Anti-IL-6 monoclonal antibodies protect against lethal *Escherichia coli* infection and lethal tumor necrosis factor-α challenge in mice. *J. Immunol.* **145**, 4185–4191.
79. Höpken, U., Mohr, M., Strüber, A., Montz, H., Burchardi, H., Götze, O., and Oppermann, M. (1996) Inhibition of interleukin-6 synthesis in an animal model of septic shock by anti-C5a monoclonal antibodies. *Eur. J. Immunol.* **26**, 1103–1109.
80. Rivier, C., Chizzonite, R., and Vale, W. (1989) In the mouse the activation of the hypothalamic-pituatary-adrenal axis by lipopolysaccharide is mediated through interleukin-1. *Endocrinology* **185**, 2800–2805.
81. Neta, R., Vogel, S. N., Plocinski, J. M., Tare, N. S., Benjamin, W., Chizzonite, R., and Pilcher, M. (1990) In vivo modulation with interleukin-1 receptor antibody 35F5 of the response to IL-1: the relationship of radioprotection, colony stimulating factor, and IL-6. *Blood* **76**, 57–62.
82. McIntyre, K. W., Stephan, G. J., Kolinskyu, K. D., Benjamin, W. R., Plocinski, N. M., Kaffka, K. L., Campen, C. A., Chizzonite, R. A., and Kilian, P. L. (1991)

Inhibition of interleukin 1 binding and bioactivity in vivo and modulation of acute inflammation in vivo by IL-1 receptor antagonists and anti-IL-1 receptor monoclonal antibody. *J. Exp. Med.* **173**, 931–939.

83. Casadevall, A. and Scharff, M. D. (1995) Return to the past: the case for antibody-based therapies for infectious diseases. *Clin. Infect. Dis.* **21**, 150–161.

84. Bullowa, J. G. M. (1937) *The Management of Pneumonias*. Oxford University Press, New York.

85. Oishi, K., Sonoda, F., Iwagaki, A., et al. (1993) Therapeutic effects of a human anti-flagella monoclonal antibody in a neutropenic murine model of *Pseudomonas aeruginosa* pneumonia. *Antimicrob. Agents Chemother.* **37**, 164–170.

86. Mofenson, L. M., Moye, J., Jr., Korelitz, J., Ethel, J., Hischhorn, R., and Nugent, R. (1994) Crossover of placebo patients to intravenous immunoglobulin confirms efficacy for prophilaxis of bacterial infections and reduction of hospitalizations in human immunodeficiency virus-infected children. *Paediatr. Infect. Dis.* **13**, 477–484.

87. Hinds, C. J. (1992) Monoclonal antibodies in sepsis and septic shock. *Br. Med. J.* **304**, 132,133.

88. Montero-Julian, F. A., Klein, B., Gautherot, E., and Brailly, H. (1995) Pharmacokinetic study of anti-interleukin-6 (IL-6) therapy with monoclonal antibodies: enhancement of IL-6 clearance by cocktails of anti-IL-6 antibodies. *Blood* **85**, 917–924.

89. Halstead, S. B. (1982) Immune enhancement of viral infection. *Prog. Allergy* **31**, 301–364.

90. Mazanec, M. B., Kaetzel, C. S., Lamm, M. E., Fletcher, D., and Nedrud, J. G. (1992) Intracellular neutralization of virus by immunoglobulin A antibodies. *Proc. Natl. Acad. Sci. USA* **89**, 6901–6905.

91. Mineo, J. R., Khan, I. A., and Kasper, L. H. (1994) A monoclonal antibody that inhibits intracellular replication. *Exper. Parasitol.* **79**, 351–361.

92. Marasco, W. A. (1997) Intrabodies: turning the humoral immune system outside in for intracellular immunization. *Gene Ther.* **4**, 11–15.

93. Barnes, G. L., Doyle, L. W., Hewson, P. H., Knoches, A. M., McLellan, J. A., Kitchen, W. H., and Bishop, R. F. (1982) A randomized trial of oral gammaglobulin in low-birth-weight infants infected with rotavirus. *Lancet* **8286**, 1371–1373.

94. Hoyne, A. L. (1936) Intravenous treatment of meningococcic meningitis with meningococcus antitoxin. *JAMA* **107**, 478–481.

95. Alexander, H. E. (1943) Treatment of *Haemophilus influenzae* infections and of meningococcic and pneumococcic meningitis. *Am. J. Dis. Child.* **66**, 172–187.

96. Triquero, D., Buciak, J. B., Yang, J., and Pardridge, W. M. (1989) Blood–brain barrier transport of cationized immunoglobulin G: enhanced delivery compared to native protein. *Proc. Natl. Acad. Sci. USA* **86**, 4761–4765.

97. Friden, P. M., Walus, L. R., Musso, G. F., Taylor, M. A., Malfroy, B., and Starzyk, R. M. (1991) Anti-transferrin receptor antibody and antibody drug conjugates cross the blood–brain barrier. *Proc. Natl. Acad. Sci. USA* **88**, 4471–4775.

98. Akdiş, C. A., Towbin, H., Libsig, P., Motz, J., and Alkan, S. S. (1995) Cytokine immunotrapping: an assay to study the kinetics of production and consumption or degradation of human interferon-γ. *J. Immunol. Methods* **182,** 251–261.

99. Lang, A. B., Cryz, S. J., Jr., Schurch, U., Ganss, M. T., and Brudere, U. (1993) Immunotherapy with human monoclonal antibodies fragment: a specificity of polyclonal and monoclonal antibodies is crucial for full protection against tetanus toxin. *J. Immunol.* **151,** 466–472.

100. Sekul, E. A., Cupler, E. J., and Dalakas, M. C. (1994) Aseptic meningitis is associated with high dose intravenous immunoglobulin therapy: frequency and risk factors. *Ann. Intern. Med.* **121,** 259–262.

101. Wolff, S. N., Fay, J. W., Herzig, R. H., Greer, J. P., Dummer, S., Brown, R. A., Collins, R. H., Stevens, D. A., and Herzig, G. P. (1993) High-dose weekly intravenous immunoglobulin to prevent infections in patients undergoing autologous bone marrow transplantation or severe myelosuppressive therapy: a study of the American Bone Marrow Transplantation Group. *Ann. Intern. Med.* **118,** 937–942.

102. Ortho Multicenter Transplant Study Group (1985) A randomized clinical trial of OKT3 monoclonal antibody for acute rejection of cadaveric renal transplants. *N. Engl. J. Med.* **313,** 337–347.

103. Greenman, R. L, Schein, R. M. H., Martin, M. A., et al. (1991) A controlled clinical trial of E5 murine monoclonal IgM antibody to endotoxin in the treatment of Gram-negative sepsis. *JAMA* **266,** 1097–1102.

104. Schroff, R. W., Foon, K. A., Beatty, S. M., Oldham, R. K., and Morgan, A. C., Jr. (1985) Human anti-murine immunoglobulin responses in patients receiving monoclonal antibody therapy. *Cancer Res.* **45,** 879–885.

105. LoBuglio, A. F., Wheeler, R. H., Trang, J., Haynes, A., Rogers, K., Harvey, E. B., Sun, L., Ghrayeb, J., and Khazaeli, M. B. (1989) Mouse/human chimeric monoclonal antibody in man: kinetics and immune response. *Proc. Natl. Acad. Sci. USA* **86,** 4220–4224.

106. Isaacs, J. D., Watts, R. A., Hazleman, B. L., Hale, G., Keogan, M. T., Cobbold, S. P., and Waldmann, H. (1992) Humanized monoclonal antibody therapy for rheumatoid arthritis. *Lancet* **8822,** 748–752.

107. Sadziene, A., Rosa, P. A., Thimpson, P. A., Hogan, D. M., and Barbour, A. G. (1992) Antibody-resistant mutants of *Borrelia burgdorferi*: *in vitro* selection and characterization. *J. Exp. Med.* **176,** 799–809.

108. Halter, R., Pohlner, J., and Meyer, T. F. (1989) Mosaic-like organization of IgA protease genes in *Neissseria gonorrhoeae* generated by horizontal genetic exchange *in vivo. EMBO J.* **8,** 2737–2744.

109. Conti, D. J., Freed, B. M., Gruber, S. A., and Lempert, N. (1994) Prophylaxis of primary cytomegalovirus disease in renal transplant recipients: a trial of gancyclovir vs. immunoglobulin. *Arch. Surg.* **129,** 433–437.

110. Schmidt, G. A. (1991) The HA-1A monoclonal antibody for gram negative sepsis. *N. Engl. J. Med.* **325,** 280,281.

12

Antibodies in Nuclear Medicine

A. Michael Peters

1. Introduction

Radiolabeled antibodies in nuclear medicine may be used for therapy or diagnosis. Diagnostic antibodies may be monoclonal antibodies (mAbs), directed against a specific disease, or polyclonal antibodies, which are used largely as intravascular reference markers or markers of vascular permeability in the imaging of inflammatory disease.

2. Diagnostic mAbs

Monoclonal antibodies may be labeled with a range of radionuclides, the choice of which is influenced by the anticipated duration of the study. Monoclonal antibodies are generally of mouse origin and can be radiolabeled and administered as the whole antibody, divalent F(ab')$_2$ fragment, or monovalent Fab fragment. Again, the choice to some extent depends on the intended application, although to promote antigen accessibility and reduce possible immunological effects, including the generation of human antimouse antibodies in the recipient, the smaller fragments tend to be favored. Because of the almost infinite range of antigens that can potentially be targeted with radiolabeled mAbs, there is a wide range of disease processes for which immuno-scintigraphy may be helpful. A useful way to approach mAbs for imaging is to categorize them according to antigen accessibility: thus, targeted antigens may be intravascular, extravascular extracellular, or intracellular or otherwise "hidden."

2.1. Intravascular

Diagnostic mAbs that target intravascular antigens have been radiolabeled for imaging blood cells, components of thrombus, and endothelial adhesion molecules.

From: *Methods in Molecular Medicine, Vol. 40: Diagnostic and Therapeutic Antibodies*
Edited by: A. J. T. George and C. E. Urch © Humana Press Inc., Totowa, NJ

2.1.1. Blood Cells

Two of the three major diseases that kill humans—thrombosis and inflammation (the third being cancer)—share, as a central constituent process, the recruitment of blood cells, namely platelets and leukocytes, respectively. A major advance in nuclear medicine was the development of cell labeling in 1975 *(1)*. It had been possible to label blood cells with radioactivity before then but only with feeble or non-gamma emitting radionuclides like ^{32}P and ^{51}Cr. The aim of incorporating an efficient gamma emitter into blood cells was to be able to image thrombosis and inflammation with the gamma camera. The two radionuclides in general use in blood cell labeling for imaging are ^{111}In and ^{99m}Tc. The principle underpinning cell labeling is that lipophilic metal-chelate complexes of ^{111}In and ^{99m}Tc readily penetrate blood cells and become irreversibly bound. ^{111}In can be complexed to hydroxyquinoline or tropolone, and ^{99m}Tc with hexamethylpropyleneamine oxime (HMPAO). These lipophilic complexes freely diifuse across the cell membrane: ^{111}In then binds to intracellular proteins, whereas ^{99m}Tc-HMPAO is converted to a secondary complex that, because it is hydrophilic, is unable to penetrate the lipid cell membrane and is therefore trapped inside the cell. Because of their lipophilic nature, complexes of ^{111}In and ^{99m}Tc-HMPAO label blood cells indiscriminately. It is therefore necessary to isolate the cell of interest in vitro prior to labeling and reinfusion to the patient. This requires a skilled technician and has resulted in the technique being relatively expensive, not as widely available as it should be, and an infection hazard to both the patient and the technician. Against this background there has been much interest in developing off-the-shelf radiopharmaceuticals, capable of selectively labeling blood cells in vivo. Monoclonal antibodies directed against cell-surface antigens are an attractive option for in vivo targeting of specific blood cells.

2.1.2. Thrombus

One of the first mAbs to be developed for imaging is directed against the IIBIIIA fibrinogen receptor on platelets *(2)*. Given intravenously, this mAb becomes 80% platelet bound by 30 min after injection and gives a gamma camera image that is very similar to that seen 30 min after injection of platelets labeled in vitro with ^{111}In. This mAb gives clear images of fresh thrombus, deep venous as well as pulmonary embolic, but only in situations in which it is already in the circulation during thrombogenesis *(3)*. Therapeutic embolization of pulmonary arteriovenous malformations (AVMs) provides a good human model for thrombosis, because the technique aims to produce a thrombus, in response to embolized materials, that then organizes to permanently occclude the AVM. Precirculating mAb was abundantly incorporated, but antibody given more than 24 h after embolization gave negative images *(4)*. Clinical interest in the antibody therefore declined. There is currently more interest in mAbs/agents that target platelets that have already been activated and incorporated into thrombus rather than targeting the entire circulating platelet population, as anti-IIBIIIA does. One such antibody recognizes P-selectin, a presynthesized adhesion molecule that is expressed on the surface of platelets as a result of activation (5), but it has not gained widespread use. Monoclonal antibodies have been raised against fibrin (6). Again, however, although clinical trials were at first encouraging, the approach has not lead to any clinically accepted agents. There is continuing interest, however, in radiolabeled peptides for targeting components of thrombus (7).

2.1.3. Inflammation

Imaging inflammation with labeled leukocytes has become far more widely used clinically than labeled agents for imaging thrombus (8,9). The impetus for developing agents for in vivo targeting of inflammation has therefore been greater than for imaging thrombus. Monoclonal antibodies directed against leukocyte surface epitopes were first investigated at about the same time as mAbs to platelets (10), but it was soon clear that images depicting inflammation based on such antibodies were less impressive than images of inflammation obtained with leukocytes labeled in vitro and thrombus obtained with antiplatelet antibodies. Of several potential reasons for this, one obvious problem is the efficient targeting of leukocyte antigens in bone marrow (10,11), wherein perhaps 90% of the whole body population of such antigens are present. A neutrophil spends about 15 d in bone marrow before release into the circulation, where it spends only 10 h. As a result of antibody equilibration between plasma and a huge pool of marrow antigens, generally <20% of circulating radioactivity is bound to leukocytes after injection of antileukocyte antibodies. Positive images of inflammation, however, are obtained and the clinical results have been generally well received (12). Targeting of leukocytes that have already migrated has been put forward as a factor contributing toward positive images in inflammation. Currently, antineutrophil mAbs approved for clinical use are available commercially in several countries, including the United Kingdom.

Antilymphocyte mAbs have been studied experimentally, but not in humans. Apart from the disadvantages of in vitro labeling, mAbs against surface lymphocyte antigens (13) offer the additional potential attraction of reduced radiotoxicity, since labeling with ^{111}In complexes and deposition of the radionuclide intracellularly close to the nucleus results in early lymphocyte cell death (14). Intracellular ^{111}In is also actively eliminated by lymphocytes (15) and this would presumably also occur if ^{111}In-labeled antilymphocyte antibodies were internalized following antigen binding. Imaging of graft rejection and of chronic inflammation are the main goals for labeled lymphocytes.

2.1.4. Endothelium

An alternative cell to target, and to which access is readily available from the circulation, is the endothelial cell. The major advances that have been made in vascular biology over the last few years have provided the opportunity to target a range of endothelial adhesion molecules expressed on the luminal surface of the endothelial cell. Clearly, adhesion molecules would provide a more attractive option for imaging if they were expressed only in disease, and not constitutively, otherwise the background signal could be a problem. One such adhesion molecule is E-selectin, which is expressed during inflammation. This is a cytokine-inducible adhesion molecule, synthesized *de novo* in response to an appropriate stimulus *(16)*, and is responsible physiologically for inducing granulocyte rolling on the postcapillary venular endothelial surface prior to immobilization, adherence, spreading, and ultimately transmigration. Haskard and his group have raised a mAb to E-selectin and, after preliminary studies in experimental models of inflammation, including iv interleukin-1 (IL-1) *(16)*, locally induced cutaneous inflammation *(17)*, and acute synovitis of the knee *(18)*, have demonstrated its potential value for imaging both acute and chronic inflammation in humans *(19,20)*. As a labeled specific protein, anti-E-selectin has been compared with nonspecific polyclonal immunoglobulin (HIG) for imaging synovitis *(18,21)*. In both experimental and clinical synovitis, the distribution of anti-E-selectin uptake in the knee is different from that of HIG, showing a significantly greater targeting of synovial tissue and less generalized periarticular uptake *(19)*. An interesting finding that supports the notion that HIG accumulates as a result of increased endothelial permeability is that joints showing uptake of specific antibody but not of HIG are, in general, painful but not swollen; i.e., HIG uptake seems particularly closely correlated with local edema. Another interesting finding to emerge from studies on experimental cutaneous inflammation is that E-selectin expression more closely reflects lymphocyte than neutrophil migration, suggesting that imaging with anti-E-selectin may be at least as effective in chronic as compared with acute inflammation *(17)*. This is a tantalizing observation, giving the ineffectiveness of current agents for imaging chronic inflammation.

Because of the potential for Fc-receptor-induced inflammation, the $F(ab')_2$ is preferable to the whole mAb for humans and has been used successfully to image rheumatoid synovitis *(19)* and active inflammatory bowel disease *(20)*. It gives very similar results to the whole antibody in porcine models of PHA-induced arthritis *(21)* and generalized systemic inflammation in response to iv IL-1 *(21)*. E-selectin has the advantage, in the context of imaging, of being internalized by the endothelial cell following binding to specific antibody, in contrast to other adhesion molecules, such as vascular cell adhesion molecule-1

(VCAM-1), which are shed into the circulation *(22)*. Another endothelial adhesion molecule that has been targeted for imaging is intercellular adhesion molecule-1 (ICAM-1) *(23,24)*, especially with respect to the pulmonary circulation. Angiotensin converting enzyme (ACE), which is also abundant in pulmonary endothelium and acessible to circulating anti-ACE mAbs, is a further example of an antigen through which endothelium can be directly imaged *(25,26)*. The potential value of targeting this molecule in disease is not clear, although it may be more within therapy than diagnosis, providing a means of directing therapeutic agents to the lung *(26)*.

2.2. Antibodies with Extravascular Extracellular Antigens

2.2.1. Antitumor mAbs

The main class of antibodies in this category are the antitumor mAbs, which target antigens either specific for tumor cells or exposed in malignant tissue as a result of tissue disruption. Tumor-associated antigens range in their specificity for individual cancers. A large literature exists on the subject of imaging and treating tumors with radiolabeled mAbs. Despite this, only one diagnostic antibody is available commercially, and no therapeutic radiolabeled mAbs can be said to be in routine use. In general, antitumor mAbs take several days to target tumors in sufficient quantities for imaging. There are several reasons for this, including slow penetration of tumor neovascular endothelium, inhomogeneity of tumor blood flow, relatively large interstitial distances for diffusion, and a relatively high interstitial fluid pressure, which opposes convective transport of macromolecules into the tumor *(27)*. Use of antibody fragments improves endothelial penetration and interstitial diffusion, although because diffusion rate is broadly proportional to the cube root of molecular size, not dramatically.

An interesting strategy proposed by Khawli and Epstein *(28)* is to increase local endothelial permeability by injecting proinflammatory cytokines, which selectively target the tumor as a result of prior conjugation to the same antibody (cold) subsequently used to image the tumor—so-called vasoactive conjugates. Tumor uptake of radiolabeled antibody in animal models of cancer was significantly increased by pretreatment with several vasoconjugates. Some vasoconjugates achieved this by increasing tumor blood flow, some by increasing tumor microvascular permeability, and some by both mechanisms. No systemic effects were recorded, presumably because the cytokines remained antibody-bound and only exerted their vasoactive effects following local dissociation from antibody. Cytokines conjugated to irrelevant antibody had no effect on uptake of radiolabeled-specific antibody or any systemic effects.

Other strategies to improve access include the biotin/streptavidin approach *(28,29)*. With this technique, streptavidin conjugated with unlabeled specific antitumor antibody is injected intravenously. After a preselected time interval, usually a few days, radiolabeled biotin is given intravenously. Biotin is a small diffusible molecule that is freely filtered at the glomerulus and excreted in urine and has a high binding affinity for streptavidin. The aim of the technique is to visualize the tumor with a high dose of a short-lived radionuclide, such as ^{99m}Tc, conjugated to biotin, which, because it is cleared rapidly, gives low background activity. An attractive approach that would completely circumvent problems of access would be to target exposed endothelial ligands and receptors specific for tumor vessel endothelium, generally called neovascular antigens *(30)*.

The value of mAbs for imaging tumors has to be viewed against the alternative agents available and the broader strategy of tumor diagnosis. There are potentially seven different ways in which tumor imaging with radiopharmaceuticals may be useful (assuming therapeutic options are available):

1. Screening healthy populations;
2. Primary diagnosis in a patient suspected of having a tumor;
3. Detection of local and metastatic spread and staging in a patient known to have a tumor;
4. Diagnosis of recurrence;
5. Prediction of response to treatment and treatment planning;
6. Abrogation of tumor uptake as a marker of response to treatment; and
7. In relation to research.

Radiopharmaceuticals in general, and antitumor antibodies in particular, have no role in cancer screening. Because they are designed to target specific tumors, mAbs have a limited role in patients suspected of having a tumor but lacking a tissue diagnosis—this would include the rather specific category of unknown primary. Staging, diagnosing recurrence, and use as a marker of treatment response are good applications for antitumor mAbs. However, in these circumstances, when the nature of the patient's tumor is known, antitumor antibodies will in the future have to compete with nonspecific tumor localizing agents, especially ^{99m}Tc-sestamibi *(31)* and [^{18}F]fluorodeoxyglucose (FDG), which, as an analog of glucose, becomes metabolically trapped in malignant cells and gives strikingly positive images of tumors on positron emission tomography (PET) *(32)*. Nevertheless, the high specificity offered by anticancer immunoscintigraphy may enable the identification of functional properties peculiar to a particular tumor that may contribute toward management; for example, prediction of response to therapy, in a way similar to the use of sestamibi, which is a substrate for the multidrug resistance mechanism, for identifying resistance to chemotherapeutic agents *(33)*. Furthermore, the nonspecificity of FDG is being increasingly appreciated, especially with respect to inflammatory disease, which may be surprisingly glucose-avid *(34)*.

Cancers to which antitumor mAbs have been most applied include colorectal *(35)*, ovarian *(36)*, breast *(37)*, prostate *(38)*, lymphoma *(39)*, and melanoma *(40)*. The antigens they target have varying degrees of tumor specificity, and in some cases are used as diagnostic serum markers for cancer, e.g., carcinoembryonic antigen in colorectal cancer. In general, as in imaging inflammation with antiendothelial antibodies, anticancer antibodies should be directed against antigens that are not shed into the blood; otherwise, immune complexes will form with subsequent uptake in the reticuloendothelial system. *Oncoscint* is the only radiolabeled mAb for diagnostic imaging that is commercially available and registered for use in the United Kingdom. It is an anticolorectal mAb that recognizes the tumor-associated antigen, TAG-72. Its main application is in the detection of pelvic recuurence, which because of fibrosis is often difficult to detect with computed tomography (CT) and magnetic resonance imaging (MRI). It is most effectively used in conjunction with serum markers, although such tumor-associated proteins must be released in high enough amounts to first overcome reticuloendothelial uptake before being detectable in the peripheral circulation. The main application of antiovarian mAbs is the characterization of a pelvic mass strongly suspected to be malignant on transvaginal ultrasound. Monoclonal antibodies to breast cancer have no role in the diagnosis of a primary breast tumor but may be useful for detecting axillary lymph node involvement. In prostate cancer, immunoscintigraphy may have a role in identifying local spread prior to surgery. Immunoscintigraphy has no useful role in lung cancer, which from an imaging point of view is likely to be managed more and more with FDG and PET.

2.2.2. Antibodies to Other Extravascular Extracellular Antigens

There are several other, predominantly nontumor pathologies, for which radiolabeled mAbs targeting extravascular antigens may have a role in diagnostic imaging. These include transplant rejection and bone marrow imaging. Imaging inflammation with antibodies that recognize activated leukocyte antigens and target migrated leukocytes in the interstitial space could be included here.

Rejecting allografts express class 1 and 2 major histocompatability antigens, which are potential targets for specific mAbs and could therefore be used to diagnose rejection *(41,42)*. The precise microanatomical site of expression of antigen and the permeability characteristics of the allograft endothelium are factors of some importance since they determine the chances of intravenously injected mAb targeting its intended antigen. For example, extravascular expression of antigens in the kidney is potentially of less importance with respect to access than in the myocardium since renal tubular capillaries have a permeability of at least 1000 times that of myocardial capillaries. Bone marrow and liver also have highly permeable endothelium. Pulmonary capillaries have a lower permeability but a large surface area available for exchange.

Bone marrow is particularly interesting with respect to mAb imaging since anti-neutrophil antibodies developed for imaging inflammation also image hemopoietic bone marrow; in fact, better than any other radiopharmaceutical apart possibly from the positron emitter ^{52}Fe *(11,43)*. Indeed, in order to improve in vivo labeling of circulating neutrophils with antineutrophil antibodies, ways to reduce bone marrow uptake will have to be addressed. The ease with which antibodies target antigens on immature bone marrow blood cells raises hopes for mAb imaging of pathology within the marrow, such as myeloma, although again one must keep in mind how well they perform in comparison with cheaper alternatives, ^{99m}Tc-sestamibi in the case of myeloma.

2.3. mAbs with Intracellular Antigens

Obviously, mAbs with intracellular antigens are generally of limited value for diagnostic imaging because of lack of access. On the other hand, injection of a mAb for targeting an intracellular antigen that has become extracellular, and exposed, as the result of tissue damage, is a different philosophical approach. One such mAb that has received much attention over the last few years is antimyosin, which portrays infarcted myocardium by accessing and binding antigen as a result of breakdown of the myocardial cellular barriers *(44)*. Localization of some antitumor mAbs relies on the principle of antigen exposure resulting from the disease itself *(37)*. Under these circumstances, the limited access of the antigen to a poorly diffusible macromolecule, access that the cancer enhances, can be perceived as an advantage in favor of the macromolecule, since a smaller more diffusible molecule, able to target antigen in intact tissue, might be less specific.

3. Diagnostic Polyclonal Antibodies

Apart from specific targeting of endothelium with monoclonal antibodies as a means of imaging inflammation, the endothelium is a crucial factor in the use of macromolecules for imaging inflammation. In several disease processes, including inflammatory disease, increased endothelial permeability is an important basis for imaging with macromolecules that enter the extravascular space. Radiolabeled nonspecific human immunoglobulin (HIG) is being increasingly used in this way *(45,46)*. HIG was at first thought to be locally concentrated in inflammation as a result of specific binding to local Fc receptors, but is now generally regarded as a nonspecific marker of increased vascular permeability. The use of macromolecules for imaging inflammation would be enhanced if either the intact labeled complex or the label itself was concentrated in the lesion. Otherwise, the extravascular concentration, at least of a protein, cannot be expected to exceed a level determined by the extravascular to intravascular concentration ratio of a similar-sized native protein, a ratio that is between about 1:5 and 1:10. Interestingly, but not unexpectedly insofar as synovial fluid represents the extravascular space, ^{99m}Tc-HIG concentration in the synovial fluid of rheumatoid knees does not exceed the concentration in plasma (47). Claessens et al. (46), on the other hand, suggest that the extravascular concentration of ^{111}In-HIG exceeds that of ^{99m}Tc-HIG, in relation to intravascular concentration, as a result of transchelation of ^{111}In from IgG to local protein. It has been demonstrated, however, that macromolecular transfer across the endothelium in inflammation is predominantly unidirectional and at the level of the postcapillary venule (48). Moreover, the mechanism of macromolecular transfer in inflammation is not simply an exaggeration of the mechanism in uninflamed tissue but results specifically from contraction and separation of postcapillary venular endothelial cells, a process inducible by proinflammatory mediators and that can be blocked by anti-inflammatory agents. Unidirectional transport of macromolecules from plasma to interstitial fluid becomes more predominant with increasing molecular size because convective transport rather than diffusion becomes more dominant with increasing molecular size. Under these circumstances, the higher target-to-background ratio achieved with ^{111}In-HIG compared with ^{99m}Tc-HIG could be explained by poorer stability of ^{99m}Tc binding and back-diffusion of pertechnetate.

For imaging inflammation with radiolabeled proteins, penetration of less accessible subcompartments of the interstitial space, such as the gel meshwork, which is occupied by huge molecules and which tend to exclude smaller molecules (49), may be a factor contributing to a positive image, in addition to increased endothelial permeability and increased tissue vascularity. Another important physiological factor in the production of a positive image is local lymph flow. If lymphatic flow was zero, the intravascular and extravascular concentrations of a macromolecule would ultimately equalize, and the permeability of the endothelium for the macromolecule would determine the time to equilibration. The balance between lymphatic flow and permeability determines the concentration gradient; thus, for a highly diffusible small solute, diffusion will overwhelm lymphatic flow, and equilibrium will soon be reached. If permeability is low, as for a protein like IgG, then lymphatic flow will maintain a low extravascular concentration, hence the normal vascular to extravascular albumin ratio of 5–10. Radiolabeled IgG will give a positive image if permeability is increased in the face of a lymphatic flow that is reduced relative to net capillary fluid transfer.

4. mAbs for Therapy

The approaches to tumor therapy with radiolabeled mAbs are obviously closely related to those for diagnostic imaging and depend on accessibility, antigen–antibody binding characteristics, and internalization of the antibody–antigen complex. A different class of radionuclides is used, i.e., those with highly damaging, short-range particulate emissions. Therapy is almost always preceded by an imaging study with the antibody complexed to a gamma-emitting radionuclide to determine the biodistribution and proportion of antibody taken up by the tumor. This is essential for dosimetric calculations. In therapy, routes of injection other than intravenous may be important options, such as intrathecal administration for gliomas *(50)* or intraperitoneal injection for ovarian cancer *(51)*.

The requirements for successful therapy are even more stringent than those for successful imaging and include minimization of uptake in nontumor tissue and uniform and complete penetration of the tumor. Thus, a tumor may be easily imaged with a diagnostic antibody even though the antibody may fail to completely and homogeneously penetrate the tumor.

Monoclonal antibodies may also be used as a vehicle for treatment, using their antigen binding capacity to deliver antitumor therapy and to direct particles, such as viruses and liposomes, for therapeutic applications. For example, a bifunctional antibody (i.e., an immunoglobulin composed of two mAbs of differing specificity joined at their Fc ends) that binds an epitope on E-selectin at one Fab end and an epitope on an adenovirus at the other, has been shown to direct adenovirus to endothelial cells. Because E-selectin-anti-E-selectin is internalized, so is the virus, which can then encode protein synthesis and modify the function of the endothelial cell (D. O. Haskard, personal communication).

5. Future

The main thrust of development of mAbs in nuclear medicine will be to develop methods to produce large amounts of "humanized" antibody cheaply by genetic engineering. The antigen recognizing, i.e., variable, portions of an antibody are the terminal peptide sequences of the Fab arms (sFv fragments), which have a molecular weight of 27 kDa (cf IgG, 150 kDa). Like the Fc arm, the peptide sequences in the Fab arm proximal to the sFv fragments are peculiar to the species, so their elimination reduces the risk of the recipient developing anti-antibody antibodies. Using recombinant techniques, the two sFv fragments corresponding to the double chain of the Fab can be joined by a short peptide tail, thereby maintaining their ability to recognize antigen. At the same time, a further short peptide sequence can be encoded for specific binding of a selected radionuclide. George et al., for example, furnished an sFv fragment with a four-residue sequence containing three glycine residues to enable it to firmly bind ^{99m}Tc *(52)*. The huge potential of this technology is easy to appreciate: large quantities of cheaply produced agent, toxin and viral free, "humanized" and in a form ready to label with the radionuclide of one's choice.

References

1. McAfee, J. G. and Thakur, M. L. (1976) Survey of radioactive agents for in vitro labelling of phagocytic leukocytes. I. Soluble agents. *J. Nucl. Med.* **17,** 480–487.
2. Peters, A. M., Lavender, J. P., Needham, S. G., Loutfi, I., Snook, D., Epenetos, A. A., Lumley, P., Keery, R. J., and Hogg, N. (1986) Imaging thrombus with a radiolabelled monoclonal antibody to platelets. *Br. Med. J.* **293,** 1525–1527.
3. Stuttle, A. W. J., Klosok, J., Peters, A. M., and Lavender, J. P. (1989) Sequential imaging of post-operative thrombus using the In-111 labelled platelet specific monoclonal antibody P256. *Br. J. Radiol.* **62,** 963–969.
4. Jackson, J. E., Stuttle, A. W. J., Henderson, B. L., Peters, A. M., Allison, D. J., and Lavender, J. P. (1990) Imaging pulmonary thrombus with indium-111 labelled antiplatelet monoclonal antibody. *Eur. J. Nucl. Med.* **16,** S142 (abstract).
5. Miller, D. D., Rivera, F. J., Garcia, O. J., Palmaz, J. C., Berger, H. J., and Weisman, H. F. (1992) Imaging of vascular injury with 99mTc-labeled monoclonal antiplatelet antibody S12. Preliminary experience in human percutaneous transluminal angioplasty. *Circulation* **85,** 1354–1363.
6. Rosebrough, S. F., Grossman, Z. D., McAfee, J. G., et al. (1987) Aged venous thrombi: radioimmunoimaging with fibrin specific monocloanl antibody. *Radiology* **162,** 575–577.
7. Lister-James, J., Knight, L. C., Maurer, A. H., Bush, L. R., Moyer, B. R., and Dean, R. T. (1996) Thrombus imaging with a technetium-99m-labeled, activated platelet receptor-binding peptide. *J. Nucl. Med.* **37,** 775–781.
8. Datz, F. L. (1994) Indium-111-labeled leukocytes for the detection of infection: current status. *Semin. Nucl. Med.* **24,** 92.
9. Peters, A. M. (1994) The utility of Tc-99m HMPAO labeled leukocytes for imaging infection. *Semin. Nucl. Med.* **24,** 110–127.
10. Lind, P., Langsteger, W., Kotringer, P., et al. (1990) Immunoscintigraphy of inflammatory processes with a technetium-99m-labeled monoclonal antigranulocyte antibody (Mab BW 250/183). *J. Nucl. Med.* **31,** 417–423.
11. Reske, S. N. (1994) Marrow scintigraphy, in *Nuclear Medicine in Clinical Diagnosis and Treatment* (Murray, I. P. C. and Ell, P.J., eds.), Churchill Livingstone, Edinburgh, UK, pp. 705–709.
12. Becker, W., Goldenberg, D. M., and Wolf, F. (1994) The use of monoclonal antibodies and antibody fragments in the imaging of infectious lesions. *Semin. Nucl. Med.* **24,** 142–153.
13. Loutfi, I., Chishom, P. M., Bevan, D., and Lavender, J. P. (1990) In vivo imaging of rat lymphocytes with an indium 111-labelled anti-T cell monoclonal antibody: a comparison with indium 111-labelled lymphocytes. *Eur. J. Nucl. Med.* **16,** 69–76.

14. Chisholm, P. M., Danpure, H. J., Healey, G., and Osman, S. (1979) Cell damage resulting from the labeling of rat lymphocytes and Hela S3 cells with In-111 oxine. *J. Nucl. Med.* **20**, 1308–1311.

15. Kuyama, J., McCormack, A., Heelan, B. T., George, A. J. T., Osman, S., Batchelor, J. R., and Peters, A. M. (1997) Indium-111 labeled lymphocytes: isotope distribution and cell division. *Eur. J. Nucl. Med.* **24**, 488–496.

16. Keelan, E., Licence, S. T., Peters, A. M., Binns, R., and Haskard, D. O. (1994) Characterisation of E-selectin expression in vivo using a radiolabeled monoclonal antibody. *Am. J. Physiol.* **266**, H279–H290.

17. Chapman, P. T., Jamar, F., Harrison, A. A., et al. (1996) Divergence between E-selectin expression, leukocyte migration and clinical sequelae in the onset and resolution of urate crystal-induced inflammation. *Br. J. Rheumatol.* **35**, 323–334.

18. Keelan, E., Harrison, A., Chapman, P., Binns, R., Peters, A. M., and Haskard, D. O. (1994) Imaging of vascular endothelial activation: a novel approach using radiolabelled monoclonal antibody against the endothelial cell adhesion molecule E-selectin. *J. Nucl. Med.* **35**, 276–281.

19. Chapman, P. T., Jamar, F., Keelan, E. T. M., Peters, A. M., and Haskard, D. O. (1996) Imaging endothelial activation in inflammation using a radiolabelled monoclonal antibody against E-selectin. *Arthr. Rheum.* **39**, 1371–1375.

20. Bhatti, M., Chapman, P., Peters, M., Haskard, D., and Hodgson, H. J. F. (1998) Visualizing E-selectin in the detection and evaluation of inflammatory bowel disease. *Gut* **43**, 40–47.

21. Jamar, F., Chapman, P. T., Harrison, A. A., Binns, R. M., Haskard, D. O., and Peters, A. M. (1995) Inflammatory arthritis: imaging of endothelial cell activation with an In-111 labeled F(ab')$_2$ fragment of anti-E-selectin monoclonal antibody. *Radiology* **194**, 843–850.

22. Harrison, A. A., Stocker, C. J., Chapman, P. T., Tsang, Y. T., Heuhns, T. Y., Gundel, R. H., Peters, A. M., Davies, K. A., George, A. J., Robinson, M. K., and Haskard, D. O. (1997) Expression of VCAM-1 by vascular endothelial cells in immune and non-immune inflammatory reactions in the skin. *J. Immunol.* **159**, 4546–4554.

23. Sasso, D. E., Gionfriddo, M. A., Thrall, R. S., Syrbu, S. I., Smilowitz, H. M., and Weiner, R. E. (1996) Bio-distribution of indium-111-labeled antibody directed against intercellular adhesion molecule-1. *J. Nucl. Med.* **37**, 656–661.

24. Ohtani, H., Strauss, H. W., Southern, J. F., et al. (1993) Imaging of intercellular adhesion molecule-1 induction in rejecting heart: a new scintigraphic approach to detect early allograft rejection. *Transplant Proc.* **25**, 867–869.

25. Danilov, S., Martynov, A., Klibanov, A., et al. (1989) Radioimmunoimaging of lung vessels: an approach using 111In-labeled monoclonal antibody to ACE. *J. Nucl. Med.* **30**, 1686–1692.

26. Muzykantov, V. R., Atochina, E. N., Gavriljuk, V., Danilov, S. M., and Fisher, A. B. (1994) Immunotargeting of streptavidin to the pulmonary endothelium. *J. Nucl. Med.* **35**, 1358–1365.

27. Jain, R. K. (1990) Physiological barriers to delivery of monoclonal antibodies and other macromolecules in tumors. *Cancer Res.* **50(Suppl.),** 814s–818s.

28. Khawli, L. A. and Epstein, A. L. (1997) Exploration of novel strategies to enhance monoclonal antibodies targeting. *Q. J. Nucl. Med.* **41,** 25–35.

29. Kalofonos, H. P., Rusckowski, M., and Siebecker, D. A. (1990) Imaging of tumor in patients with indium-111-labeled biotin and streptavidin-conjugated antibodies: preliminary communication. *J. Nucl. Med.* **31,** 1791–1796.

30. Huang, X., Molema, G., King, S., Watkins, L., Edgington, T. S., and Thorpe, P. E. (1997) Tumor infarction in mice by antibody-directed targeting of tissue factor to tumor vasculature. *Science* **275,** 547–550.

31. Maini, C. L., Tofani, A., Sciuto, R., et al. (1997) Technetium-99m-MIBI scintigraphy in the assessmnet of neoadjuvant chemotherapy in breast carcinoma. *J. Nucl. Med.* **38,** 1546–1551.

32. Cook, G. J. R. and Maisey, M. N. (1996) The current status of clinical PET imaging. *Clin. Rad.* **51,** 603–613.

33. Del Vecchio, S., Ciarmiello, A., Pace, L., et al. (1997) Fractional retention of technetium-99m-sestamibi as an index of P-glycoprotein expression in untreated breast cancer patients. *J. Nucl. Med.* **38,** 1348–1351.

34. Strauss, L. G. (1996) Fluorine 18 deoxyglucose and false positive results: a major problem in the diagnosis of oncological patients. *Eur. J. Nucl. Med.* **23,** 1409–1415.

35. Collier, B. D., Abdel-Nabi, H., and Doerr, R. J. (1993) Radioimmunoscintigraphy performed with In-111-labeled CYT-103 in the management of colorectal cancer: comparison with CT. *Radiology* **185,** 179–186.

36. Alexander, C., Villena-Heinsen, C. E., Trampert, K., et al. (1995) Radioimmunoscintigraphy of ovarian tumors with technetium-99m labeled monoclonal antibody-170; first clinical results. *J. Nucl. Med.* **22,** 645–651.

37. Biassoni, L., Granowska, M., Carroll, M. J., et al. (1998) Tc-99m labelled SM3 in the pre-operative evaluation of axillary lymph nodes in primary breast cancer with change detection statistical processing as an aid to tumour detection. *Br. J. Cancer* **77,** 131–138.

38. Chengazi, V. U., Fenley, M. R., Ellison, D., et al. (1997) Imaging prostate cancer with the monoclonal radioimmunoconjugate technetium-99m-7E11-C5.3 (CYT-351). *J. Nucl. Med.* **38,** 675–681.

39. Kaminski, M. S., Zasady, K. R., Francis, I. R., et al. (1993) Radioimmunotherapy of B cell lymphoma with 131I-anti-B1 (anti-CD20) antibody. *N. Engl. J. Med.* **329,** 459–465.

40. Siccardi, A. G., Buraggi, G. L., Natali, P. G., et al. (1990) European multicentre study on melanoma immunoscintigraphy by means of 99mTc-labelled monoclonal antibody fragments. *Eur. J. Nucl. Med.* **16,** 317–323.

41. Isobe, M. (1993) Scintigraphic imaging of MHC class II antigen induction in mouse kidney allografts: a new approach to noninvasive detection of early rejection. *Transplant Int.* **6,** 263.

42. Heelan, B. T., Thompson, M., McCormack, M., Peters, A. M., Batchelor, J. R., and George, A. J. T. (1996) The kinetics of MHC class I and class II expression in rat renal allografts: in vivo localisation with radiolabeled antibodies. *Transplantation* **61,** 1274–1277.

43. Jamar, F., Field, C., Leners, N., and Ferrant, A. (1995) Scintigraphic evaluation of the haemopoietic bone marrow using a ^{99m}Tc-anti-granulocyte antibody: a validation study with [52]Fe. *Br. J. Haematol.* **90,** 22–30.

44. Khaw, B. A., Yasuda, T., Gold, H. K., et al. (1987) Acute myocardial infarct imaging with indium-111 labeled monoclonal antimyosin Fab. *J. Nucl. Med.* **28,** 1671–1678.

45. Rubin, R. H., Young, L. S., Hansen, W. P., et al. (1988) Specific and non-specific imaging of localized Fisher immunotype 1 Pseudomonas aeroginosa infection with radiolabeled monoclonal antibody. *J. Nucl. Med.* **29,** 651–656.

46. Claessens, R. A. M. J., Koenders, E. B., Boerman, O. C., Oyen, W. J. G., Borm, G. F., van der Meer, J. W. M., and Corstens, F. H. M. (1995) Dissociation of indium from indium-111-labelled diethylene triamine penta-acetic acid conjugated non-specific polyclonal human immunoglobulin G in inflammatory foci. *Eur. J. Nucl. Med.* **22,** 212–219.

47. Jamar, F., Leners, N., Beckers, C., and Manicourt, D.-H. (1997) ^{99m}Tc-labelled immunoglobulin scintigraphy in arthritis: an analysis of synovial fluid activity. *Scand. J. Clin. Lab. Invest.* **57,** 621–628.

48. Arfors, K.-E., Rutili, G., and Svensjo, E. (1979) Microvascular transport of macromolecules in normal and inflammatory conditions. *Acta Physiol. Scand.* **463(Suppl.),** 93–103.

49. Katz, M. A. (1980) Interstitial space—the forgotten organ *Med. Hypotheses* **6,** 885–898.

50. Riva, P., Tison, V., Arista, A., et al. (1993) Radioimmunotherapy of gastrointestinal cancer and glioblastoma. *Int. J. Biol. Markers* **8,** 192–207.

51. Hird, V., Maraveyas, A., Snook, D., et al. (1993) Adjuvant therapy of ovarian cancer with radioactive monoclonal antibody. *Br. J. Cancer* **68,** 403–406.

52. George, A. J. T., Jamar, F., Tai, M.-S., Heelan, B. T., Oppermans, H., Peters, A. M., and Huston, J. S. (1995) Radiometal labeling of recombinant proteins by a genetically engineered minimal chelation site: technetium-99m coordination by single-chain Fv antibody fusion proteins through a C-terminal cysteinyl peptide. *Proc. Natl. Acad. Sci. USA* **92,** 8358–8362.

13

Animal Models for Tumor Localization

Gail Rowlinson-Busza

1. Introduction

Many factors influence the uptake of radiolabeled monoclonal antibodies (mAbs) in tumors. Some are dependent on the antibody, such as affinity, intact immunoglobulin or fragment, route of administration, choice of radio isotope, or method of labeling. Others depend on properties of the tumor, such as site, size, vasculature, and antigen density on the tumor cell surface. Animal models for studying these parameters are usually based on mice or rats bearing transplanted tumors. In this chapter, various tumor model systems will be described with some discussion of what data can be obtained using them.

2. Immunodeficient Animals

2.1. History

The idea of transplanting tumors into foreign hosts is not new, but it was not until the beginning of this century that it was realized that this was most successful if the donor animal was related to the recipient (1). This led to a proposed theory of inheritable susceptibility to tumor transplantation (2), but the nature of the process was unknown. It was initially supposed that antibodies against the tumors were responsible for their rejection. A major advance was the advent of inbred strains of mice, in which many generations of sibling matings produced animals that were all homozygous for the same genes. This allowed the allotransplantation of tumors and other tissues from one animal to another in these genetically homogeneous mice, and also to F_1 hybrids of the pure line and another strain. This led Haldane (3) to propose that there were antigenic variations on all tissues, similar to blood group antigens. Medawar (4) demonstrated, in experiments on skin-grafting in rabbits, that a second

From: *Methods in Molecular Medicine, Vol. 40: Diagnostic and Therapeutic Antibodies*
Edited by: A. J. T. George and C. E. Urch © Humana Press Inc., Totowa, NJ

allograft to the same recipient from the same donor was rejected more quickly than the first.

In 1961, Miller *(5)* elucidated the immunological function of the thymus. He demonstrated that neonatally thymectomized mice tolerated skin grafts from a different mouse strain for up to 2 mo, but that intact mice and thymectomized mice, which were then grafted with thymuses, rejected the grafts within 2 wk. Warner et al. *(6)* reported similar findings in bursectomized chickens. Therefore, if human tumors were to be transplanted successfully in experimental animals, some method of overcoming immunological rejection had to be found.

2.2. Immunologically Privileged Sites

Initially, immunologically privileged sites were found to be capable of sustaining tumor xenograft growth. Murphy *(7)* was able to grow rat sarcomas in the outer membrane of chick embryos. Successful transplants of some human tumors in the anterior chamber of the eye in rabbits and guinea pigs was reported by Greene *(8)* but most tumors regressed or did not grow at all. In a review of his attempts between 1939 and 1950 to transplant tumors into the anterior chamber of the eye, Greene *(9)* noted that metastatic tumors grew in many more cases than did primary tumors. Chesterman *(10)* implanted 20 different human tumors intracranially into the brains of mice, and observed growth of three of these tumors in some of the mice, although Greene *(11)* had a higher success rate with human tumors that had first been grown in the eye prior to transfer to the brain in experimental animals. Handler et al. *(12)* treated hamsters with cortisone and found that 26 out of 68 tested human tumors survived as viable nodules in their cheek pouches, although only 10 of the tumors actually grew. Toolan *(13)* also treated rats and hamsters with cortisone, in addition to X-irradiation, and found that human tumors could be serially transplanted as subcutaneous xenografts. Tumors grown in immunologically privileged sites, or in animals treated to make them less able to reject foreign tissue, were used for a number of studies of therapeutic agents *(14)*. However, not only did tumors fail to grow consistently in these animals, but it was also difficult to measure tumor growth in privileged sites, such as the hamster cheek pouch, although this model was used to study the localization of radiolabeled polyclonal antibody by photoscanning *(15)*. Animals treated with drugs to render them immunologically incompetent regained their immunity after a time and the resulting tumor rejection could be confused with tumor regression following experimental therapy.

2.3. Immune-Deprived Animals

More reliable hosts for human tumors were produced by neonatal thymectomy followed either by antithymocyte serum or by potentially lethal whole-body irradiation with reconstitution of the bone marrow by injection of syngeneic bone marrow cells *(16)*. This technique was refined by Steel et al. *(17)*, who eliminated the need for bone marrow reconstitution by protecting the mice with an injection of cytosine arabinoside (Ara-C) 2 d prior to irradiation. Mice prepared by this method were found to be good hosts for human tumor xenografts, which maintained the characteristics of the original tumors in terms of histology, chromosome analysis, and antigen expression *(18)*. Human colorectal tumors grown in these immune-suppressed mice were used in growth delay experiments following chemotherapy, and a correlation of the response of the xenograft with that of the original tumor in the patient was reported in cases where a comparison was possible *(19)*. However, immune-deprived mice are liable to regain their immunity after a period of time, making them unsuitable for long-term experiments.

3. Human Tumor Xenografts in Nude Mice

The hairless mutant "nude" *(nu/nu)* was first described by Flanagan *(20)*, who noted that the majority of the mice died before weaning, and that those that survived grew slowly, were poorly fertile, and eventually developed a fatal liver disease. Pantelouris *(21)* reported that the *nu/nu* homozygote (nude phenotype) was essentially athymic, although heterozygous (phenotypically normal) littermates had a normally developed thymus. In addition, blood leukocyte counts were very low both in *nu/nu* homozygotes and in heterozygotes. In 1969, Rygaard and Povlsen *(22)* were the first to grow human tumors in nude mice, using a surgical specimen of a resected colonic tumor. The same group later demonstrated that serial transplantation of human tumors was possible in nude mice *(23)*. Since that time these animals have become established as the primary host for human tumor xenografts. They have the advantage of permanent lack of immunity, although this makes animal husbandry difficult, since all food, water, and bedding must be sterile. This problem is minor, however, compared with the enormous advantage this animal has brought to cancer research.

Not all human tumors will grow in nude mice, however, with surgical specimens taken directly from the patient being less successful than established cell lines *(24)*. As found in early experiments in immunologically privileged sites *(9)*, xenografts were more easily established from metastases than from primary tumors *(25)*. Fogh et al. *(26)* reported that 127 out of 162 cultured human tumor cell lines (78%) grew as xenografts in nude mice and retained the histopathology of the original tumor. Almost all reports of the successful establishment of a xenograft line report that the histological characteristics of the original human tumor are maintained, although the degree of differentiation may change *(27)*. This change usually occurs during transfer from human to mouse, the xenograft then remaining stable in subsequent passages from mouse to mouse *(28)*. Chromosome analysis of xenografts has shown that they retain their human karyotype *(29)*. In addition, it has been reported that biochemical parameters, such as the presence of intracellular enzymes, are maintained in xenografts, for example in melanomas and pancreatic adenocarcinomas *(30)*. A comparison of tumor vasculature in human squamous cell carcinoma xeno-grafts and the original tumors revealed that the qualitative histology of the tumors was preserved in the xenografts, with proliferation of tumor cells con-centrated around blood vessels *(31)*. The median distance between interphase tumor cells and blood vessels in the xenograft was shorter than in the original tumor, as were the distances between blood vessels.

3.1. Metastasis

The incidence of metastasis is low following subcutaneous implantation of human tumors in nude mice, although intraperitoneal inoculation of tumor cells significantly increases the incidence of metastases *(32)* and intravenous injec-tion can result in lung colony formation *(33)*. Intrasplenic injection of tumor cells is a useful technique for inducing liver metastases in nude mice for the study of metastatic potential of different tumors *(33)*. Inoculation of the xeno-graft into the animal organ from which the human tumor was originally derived increases the incidence of metastatic spread. For example, human renal cell carcinoma cells were found to metastasize to lungs and all peritoneal organs following implantation into the renal subcapsule *(34)*, and growth of human bladder tumors in the bladders of nude rats resulted in metastasis to distant organs in 25% of cases *(35)*. Sharkey and Fogh *(36)* found dissemination in only 14 out of 801 mice (1.7%) bearing subcutaneous xenografts, which repre-sented 10% of 106 different primary tumors not previously cultured in vitro. This figure is similar to that usually found in such studies, but Neulat-Duga et al. *(37)* reported a much higher incidence (13.2% of mice having metastases) in a series of 831 nude mice bearing a total of 63 different malignant tumors. These authors found metastatic deposits in lungs, and to a lesser extent in lymph nodes, but these were small and therefore usually only detectable microscopi-cally. In addition, they found that metastatic human tumors exhibited higher metastatic ability in nude mice (46% of metastatic tumors compared with 13% of primary tumors). These factors could account for the discrepancy between this and other studies, as well as the fact that many mice are killed for experi-ment or die from infection before the appearance of detectable metastases.

3.2. Factors Affecting Growth of Xenografts

Several factors can affect the growth of human tumors in nude mice. The strain of mouse can influence the growth rate of xenografts *(38)*. The age of the animal at the time of tumor inoculation can affect the incidence of tumors, a higher proportion of "takes" occurring in younger animals, with a faster growth rate *(39)*. The site of tumor implantation has also been shown to affect the growth of murine tumors in mice, tumors implanted nearer the head growing two to three times more rapidly than those implanted nearer the tail *(40)*. Pimm and Morris *(41)* have demonstrated that human tumor xenografts implanted on the left flank grow significantly faster than those on the right flank. It was suggested that these differences were caused by morphogenic gradients similar to those believed to control differentiation during ontogeny.

The cancer type also affects the success rate of establishing xenografts in nude mice. For example, human lymphoid tumors have proved more difficult to grow than many other tumors. The severe combined immunodeficient (SCID) mouse lacks both B- and T-cell function owing to an autosomal mutation that greatly impairs lymphopoiesis *(42)*. These mice have been shown to be suitable hosts for several Hodgkin's lymphoma cell lines, which would not grow in nude mice *(43)*. In addition, SCID mice can be grafted with lymphoid tissue, which can reconstitute a functional immune system. This has been shown using murine bone marrow cultures *(44)* and human peripheral blood lymphocytes *(45)*. In the latter case, the mice were shown to have circulating human B- and T-cells.

In the context of comparing different targeting strategies in vivo, the nude or SCID mouse provides a convenient model, since genetically identical tumors can be induced in several animals, allowing direct comparisons to be made. However, for the reasons outlined above, when using xenograft models for cancer research, it is important to use the same strain of mouse of the same sex and of approximately the same age throughout each experiment. Tumors should be implanted at the same location in the mice. In this way, the variability between repeats of experiments is minimized.

4. Antibody Localization in Xenografts

Targeting of radiolabeled antibodies began with the work of Pressman and Keighley *(46)*, who demonstrated that radiolabeled rabbit antiserum raised against normal rat kidney could localize in the kidneys following intravenous injection into normal rats. The same group later targeted radiolabeled rabbit antisera to a rat osteogenic sarcoma *(47)*. Specific localization was confirmed by the use of the dual-label technique *(48)*. In these experiments, specific antitumor antiserum was radiolabeled with ^{131}I and coinjected with ^{133}I-labeled normal serum immunoglobulin into rats bearing syngeneic lymphosarcoma, resulting in a higher tumor uptake of the antitumor antiserum than the normal immunoglobulin.

Following the pioneering work of Pressman and Korngold *(47)* in targeting tumors with radiolabeled antitumor antiserum, the discovery of antigens that are more specific for tumors led to the development of tumor-associated antibodies. Many of these antigens are either inappropriately expressed, for example fetal proteins in adult tissues, or are aberrant forms of normal proteins, which may be truncated or incorrectly glycosylated, or may be oncogene products. For example, Gold and Freedman *(49)* identified carcinoembryonic antigen (CEA) in colonic carcinomas but not in normal adult tissues. Human tumor xenograft models were developed to study the localization of polyclonal antibodies against CEA in vivo; these demonstrated specific uptake by the tumor using both immunoscintigraphy and γ-counting of tissues *(50)*. These, and many similar studies, showed that it was feasible to target human tumors with radiolabeled antibodies against tumor-associated antigens, and that a specific antibody localized at higher levels in tumor than did an irrelevant control antibody. Sharkey et al. *(51)* compared tumor localization of a purified goat polyclonal and four mouse monoclonal anti-CEA antibodies and found that the mAbs generally showed better uptake. The advent of mAb technology has allowed the production of highly specific antibodies that have been studied extensively in human tumor xenograft systems in nude mice.

4.1. Factors Affecting Antibody Localization

Several factors have been reported to affect the localization of radiolabeled mAbs in xenografts. Tumor vascular permeability has been shown to correlate with the uptake of antibody in two different human tumors in nude mice *(52)*. Shockley et al. *(53)* have shown that variables relating to the tumor target (antigen expression levels, vascular volume and permeability) are important factors in determining antibody accumulation in tumors, whereas differences in antibody affinity for the antigen varying by 100-fold had little effect on tumor uptake. Even within the same tumor and antibody model, differences in the host animal can affect antibody uptake. Hagan *(54)* reported that tumor size was inversely proportional to uptake (in % id/g) of ^{75}Se endogenously labeled, as well as ^{125}I- and ^{111}In-labeled, specific antibody in three different xenografts. This is probably because of tumor necrosis in larger tumors and a decrease in blood flow. Eccles et al. *(55)* found that the age of the host influenced the nonspecific uptake of antibodies by normal organs and tumor in nude rats, although there was no difference in specific uptake by tumor. In very young (3 wk old) rats, the nonspecific uptake in tumor and liver was much lower than in 8 and 12 wk old animals, resulting in higher specific uptake ratios. The authors attribute these findings to Fc receptor activity. The uptake of antibody in xenografts also depends on the administered antibody dose. Pimm and

Baldwin *(56)* found a direct correlation between the radioiodinated antibody dose and the amount localized in the tumor, although tumor-bound antibody could not be displaced by a subsequent injection of a large amount of unlabeled antibody. Adams et al. *(57)* found that hepatic uptake of ^{111}In-labeled antibody depended on the antibody dose. Similar results have been reported in clinical imaging studies, in which the total dose of ^{111}In-labeled antibody correlated with the scanning sensitivity *(58)*.

4.2. Limitations and Benefits

Obviously, human tumor xenografts in nude mice have their limitations as a model of mAb uptake by human cancer. The tumor is the only human component in the mouse, so there will be no crossreactivity with human antigens, such as CEA, or nonspecific crossreacting antigen (NCA) in normal colon mucosa, as would be found in patients *(59)*. The absolute uptake of antibody by xenografts is of the order of 10% id/g, around 1000-fold higher than that found in tumors in patients *(60)*. This is probably the result of the small blood volume in the mouse in relation to the size of the tumor, and may give misleading results if experimental therapy of xenografts is attempted. Subcutaneous xenografts are discrete and clearly distinguishable from surrounding normal tissues, and therefore more favorable for γ-camera imaging than most human tumors in patients. In addition, the nude mouse has an abnormal immune system, which allows the growth of human tumors, but which also implies that immune complexes will not be formed, so that clearance of the antibody may differ from that in an immunocompetent patient. For the same reason, the nude mouse model cannot be used for vaccination studies or, for example, in strategies aimed at recruiting effector functions, such as antibody-directed cell-mediated cytotoxicity (ADCC) or T cells, for tumor cell killing.

Nevertheless, the xenograft model is valuable for comparing, within the system, various different strategies to improve antibody localization in vivo, in a physiological system that mimics the human disease. Factors affecting antibody uptake that can be studied in this model include: intact mAbs versus enzymatically generated fragments or recombinantly produced antigen-binding molecules (e.g., single-chain Fv regions), the choice of radioisotope and its stability in vivo, antibody affinity, injected protein dose, route of administration (systemic or locoregional), the use of biological response modifiers (e.g., cytokines), and two-step pretargeting approaches (e.g., the avidin/biotin system). In addition, studies can be carried out to compare different therapeutic strategies, such as ADEPT (antibody-directed enzyme prodrug therapy), drugs entrapped within liposomes compared with free drug, antibody-toxin conjugates, and so forth. Care must be taken in interpreting results of therapy experiments, because the relative uptake of mAbs is very much higher in xenografted tumors than in human tumors in clinical trials. However, as a proof of concept, xenograft models can give useful information.

5. Other Model Systems

Antigen-coated polymer beads have been implanted into normal animals as an artificial target for antibody localization, either subcutaneously, intraperitoneally, or intravenously; in the latter case the particles are sequestered in the lung capillary bed (61). This approach has the major disadvantage that there is no tumor vasculature and so it is very far removed from the human tumor situation. However, it is relatively cheap as an initial test of antigen binding in vivo or as a test of two-step targeting, for example using avidin or biotin conjugated to agarose beads (62). This model does have the advantage that the amount of antigen present is known and can be varied, and therefore it can be used in quantitative studies of antibody uptake as well as for the comparison of different antibodies and fragments in immunocompetent animals. A refinement of this technique is the implantation of a micropore diffusion chamber containing antigen-coated particles (63). The chamber walls allow free diffusion of proteins, but the pores do not allow host immune cells to enter and possibly destroy the antigen. The model has even been used with human tumor cells inside the diffusion chamber implanted into the peritoneal cavity of immunocompetent mice (64).

Other models used for cancer research include transplantation of syngeneic tumors in normal mice. Some of these murine tumors have been shown to have similar biological behavior to the equivalent human tumor (65). Although these mice have the advantage of being immunocompetent, the tumor is of murine origin and most mAbs are raised against human antigens, so they may be of limited use for localization studies. It is possible to use murine cell lines transfected with a human antigen, such as the human polymorphic epithelial mucin (PEM), associated with breast and other epithelial cancers (66). However, these cell lines are not always stable and may not be as tumorigenic in the mice, owing to their foreign component.

Spontaneous tumors most closely resemble the human cancer situation, but this is not a reliable model for cancer research, because the animals are usually too old before tumors develop. If a spontaneous tumor does develop in a rodent, it can be serially transplanted to other animals of the same strain to establish a murine tumor line. Carcinogens can be employed to generate tumors fairly rapidly and predictably (67). Surprisingly, considering the lack of immunity in nude mice and the hypothesis of immunological surveillance, the incidence of spontaneous tumors in these animals is very low (68).

6. Transgenic Mice

Transgenic mice are mice that have had a foreign gene stably inserted into their germ line. The most commonly used and successful method of achieving this is microinjection of DNA into the one-cell embryo. The first account of transgenic mice associated with the development of cancer was in 1984 *(69)*, when mouse embryos were microinjected with plasmids containing the early region of the SV40 chromosome, whose gene product has been shown to transform cells in culture *(70)*. Nearly every animal that carried the transgene developed spontaneous brain tumors of the choroid plexus. This is not the case with all transgenic mice, in which transgene expression alone is not sufficient for tumorigenesis. Transgenic mice have been produced carrying the c-*myc* oncogene under the control of a hormonally inducible mouse mammary tumor promoter *(71)*. Only multiparous females developed mammary tumors at around 4–5 mo of age. In fact, multistep tumorigenesis can be studied in similar transgenic mice *(72)*.

Transgenic mice can be made susceptible to spontaneous tumor growth by the incorporation of an oncogene *(73)* or by the mutation of the *p53* tumor-suppresser gene *(74)*. Particularly useful models for research into mAb localization are those in which a human tumor-associated antigen is expressed in transgenic mouse tissues. Peat et al. *(75)* have developed transgenic mice that express the human MUC1 gene product (PEM) in a tissue-specific manner with a very similar profile to that seen in humans. PEM is overexpressed and aberrantly glycosylated in many tumors of epithelial origin, such as breast cancer. Antibodies against the core protein of the human mucin were shown to stain the mouse tissue, although they do not react with tissues of normal mice, owing to the lack of homology between the human and mouse mucin. Thompson et al. *(76)* have taken the model one stage further by developing mice transgenic for human CEA, which is expressed by a variety of adenocarcinomas, such as those of colon. These mice were then crossed with mice genetically predisposed to tumor development, resulting in F_1 mice that developed CEA-positive tumors of the small intestine and colon. These mice are a good model for antibody-guided therapy using anti-CEA antibodies, since the damage to CEA-expressing normal tissues can be assessed. Since these mice are immunocompetent and also tolerant to human CEA, they could be used in immunotherapeutic studies, which would not be possible in nude mice.

There are several advantages of transgenic mice for cancer research, but there are also many disadvantages compared with xenograft models. A major advantage is that spontaneously occurring tumors in immunocompetent animals more closely resemble human cancers. Metastases should occur in these mice in the same manner as in patients. The main disadvantage is the inefficiency of production of tumors in transgenic mice. Only around 10% of mice born from injected embryos carry the injected DNA incorporated into the genome and there is no way of knowing from the phenotype of the mice which are transgenic; screening for the transgene is time-consuming and labor intensive. For subsequent generations, the transgenic mouse is usually mated with a normal mouse, leading to further waste. In addition, not all transgenic mice will develop tumors and in those that do, they will occur at different times and possibly at different sites. This makes the transgenic mouse a very expensive model, and unsuitable for routine screening of new tumor-targeting molecules.

For the foreseeable future, the nude mouse xenograft model is likely to remain the most widely used for tumor localization studies using mAbs; most radiolabeled antibodies undergoing clinical trials will have been tested initially in this preclinical model for stability and their ability to localize to their respective antigens in vivo.

References

1. Tyzzer, E. E. (1909) A study of inheritance in mice with reference to their susceptibility to transplantable tumors. *J. Med. Res.* **21,** 519–573.
2. Little, C. C. and Tyzzer, E. E. (1916) Further experimental studies on the inheritance of susceptibility to a transplantable tumor, carcinoma (J.w.A.) of the Japanese waltzing mouse. *J. Med. Res.* **33,** 393–453.
3. Haldane, J. B. S. (1933) The genetics of cancer. *Nature* **132,** 265–267.
4. Medawar, P. B. (1944) The behaviour and fate of skin autografts and skin homografts in rabbits. *J. Anat.* **78,** 176–199.
5. Miller, J. F. A. P. (1961) Immunological function of the thymus. *Lancet* **2,** 748,749.
6. Warner, N. L., Szenberg, A., and Burnet, F. M. (1962) The immunological role of different lymphoid organs in the chicken. I. Dissociation of immunological responsiveness. *Aust. J. Exp. Biol.* **40,** 373–388.
7. Murphy, J. B. (1912) Transplantability of malignant tumors to the embryos of a foreign species. *JAMA* **59,** 874–875.
8. Greene, H. S. N. (1941) Heterologous transplantation of mammalian tumors. II. The transfer of human tumors to alien species. *J. Exp. Med.* **73,** 475–486.
9. Greene, H. S. N. (1952) The significance of the heterologous transplantability of human cancer. *Cancer* **5,** 24–44.
10. Chesterman, F. C. (1955) Intracranial heterotransplantation of human tumors. *Br. J. Cancer* **9,** 541–561.
11. Greene, H. S. N. (1951) The transplantation of tumors to the brains of heterologous species. *Cancer Res.* **11,** 529–534.
12. Handler, A. H., Davis, S., and Sommers, S. C. (1956) Heterotransplantation experiments with human cancers. *Cancer Res.* **16,** 32–36.

13. Toolan, H. W. (1954) Transplantable human neoplasms maintained in cortisone-treated laboratory animals: H.S.#1; H.Ep.#1; H.Ep.#2; H.Ep.#3; and H.Emb.Rh.#1. *Cancer Res.* **14,** 660–666.
14. Teller, M. N., Merker, P. C., Palm, J. E., and Woolley, G. W. (1958) The human tumor in cancer chemotherapy in the conditioned rat. *Ann. NY Acad. Sci.* **76,** 742–751.
15. Goldenberg, D. M., Preston, D. F., Primus, F. J., and Hansen, H. J. (1974) Photoscan localization of GW-39 tumors in hamsters using radiolabeled anticarcinoembryonic antigen immunoglobulin G. *Cancer Res.* **34,** 1–9.
16. Stanbridge, E. J., Boulger, L. R., Franks, C. R., Garrett, J. A., Reeson, D. E., Bishop, D., and Perkins, F. T. (1975) Optimal conditions for the growth of malignant human and animal cell populations in immunosuppressed mice. *Cancer Res.* **35,** 2203–2212.
17. Steel, G. G., Courtenay, V. D., and Rostom, A. Y. (1978) Improved immune-suppression techniques for the xenografting of human tumors. *Br. J. Cancer* **37,** 224–230.
18. Selby, P. J., Thomas, J. M., Monaghan, P., Sloane, J., and Peckham, M. J. (1980) Human tumor xenografts established and serially transplanted in mice immunologically deprived by thymectomy, cytosine arabinoside and whole body irradiation. *Br. J. Cancer* **41,** 52–61.
19. Nowak, K., Peckham, M. J., and Steel, G. G. (1978) Variation in response of xenografts of colo-rectal carcinoma to chemotherapy. *Br. J. Cancer* **37,** 576–584.
20. Flanagan, S. P. (1966) 'Nude', a new hairless gene with pleiotropic effects in the mouse. *Genet. Res.* **8,** 295–309.
21. Pantelouris, E. M. (1968) Absence of thymus in a mouse mutant. *Nature* **217,** 370,371.
22. Rygaard, J. and Povlsen, C. O. (1969) Heterotransplantation of a human malignant tumor to "nude" mice. *Acta Pathol. Microbiol. Scand.* **77,** 758–760.
23. Povlsen, C. O. and Rygaard, J. (1971) Heterotransplantation of human adenocarcinomas of the colon and rectum to the mouse mutant nude. A study of nine consecutive transplantations. *Acta Pathol. Microbiol. Scand.* **79,** 159–169.
24. Schmidt, M., Deschner, E. E., Thaler, T., Clements, L., and Good, R. A. (1977) Gastrointestinal cancer studies in the human to nude mouse heterotransplant system. *Gastroenterology* **72,** 829–837.
25. Fogh, J., Orfeo, T., Tiso, J., and Sharkey, F. E. (1979) Establishment of human colon carcinoma lines in nude mice. *Exp. Cell Biol.* **47,** 136 144.
26. Fogh, J., Fogh, J. M., and Orfeo, T. (1977) One hundred and twenty-seven cultured human tumor cell lines producing tumors in nude mice. *J. Natl. Cancer Inst.* **59,** 221–226.
27. Hajdu, S. I., Lemos, L. B., Kozakewich, H., Helson, L., and Beattie, E. J. (1981) Growth pattern and differentiation of human soft tissue sarcomas in nude mice. *Cancer* **47,** 90–98.
28. Sharkey, F. E., Fogh, J. M., Hadju, S. I., and Fitzgerald, P. J. (1978) Experience in surgical pathology with human tumor growth in the nude mouse, in *The Nude*

Mouse in Experimental and Clinical Research (Fogh, J. and Giovanella, B. C., eds.), Academic, New York, pp. 187–214.

29. Giovanella, B. C., Yim, S. O., Stehlin, J. S., and Williams, L. J., Jr. (1972) Development of invasive tumors in the "nude" mouse after injection of cultured human melanoma cells. *J. Natl. Cancer Inst.* **48,** 1531–1533.

30. Grant, A. G., Duke, D., and Hermon-Taylor, J. (1979) Establishment and characterization of primary human pancreatic carcinoma in continuous cell culture and in nude mice. *Br. J. Cancer* **39,** 143–151.

31. Lauk, S., Zietman, A., Skates, A., Fabian, R., and Suit, H. D. (1989) Comparative morphometric study of tumor vasculature in human squamous cell carcinomas and their xenotransplants in athymic nude mice. *Cancer Res.* **49,** 4557–4561.

32. Kyriazis, A. P., DiPersio, L., Michael, G. J., Pesce, A. J., and Stinnett, J. D. (1978) Growth patterns and metastatic behavior of human tumors growing in athymic mice. *Cancer Res.* **38,** 3186–3190.

33. Giavazzi, R., Campbell, D. E., Jessup, J. M., Cleary, K., and Fidler, I. J. (1986) Metastatic behavior of tumor cells isolated from primary and metastatic human colorectal carcinomas implanted into different sites in nude mice. *Cancer Res.* **46,** 1928–1933.

34. Naito, S., von Eschenbach, A. C., Giavazzi, R., and Fidler, I. J. (1986) Growth and metastasis of tumor cells isolated from a human renal cell carcinoma implanted into different organs of nude mice. *Cancer Res.* **46,** 4109–4115.

35. Russell, P. J., Ho Shon, I., Boniface, G. R., Izard, M. E., Philips, J., Raghavan, D., and Walker, K. Z. (1991) Growth and metastasis of human bladder cancer xenografts in the bladder of nude rats. A model for intravesical radio-immunotherapy. *Urol. Res.* **19,** 207–213.

36. Sharkey, F. E. and Fogh, J. (1979) Metastasis of human tumors in athymic nude mice. *Int. J. Cancer* **24,** 733–738.

37. Neulat-Duga, I., Sheppel, A., Marty, C., Lacroux, F., Pourrat, J., Cavervière, P., and Delsol, G. (1984) Metastases of human tumor xenografts in nude mice. *Invasion Metastasis* **4,** 209–224.

38. Maruo, K., Ueyama, Y., Hoiki, K., Saito, M., Nomura, T., and Tamaoki, N. (1982) Strain-dependent growth of a human carcinoma in nude mice with different genetic backgrounds. Selection of nude mouse strains useful for anticancer agent screening system. *Exp. Cell Biol.* **50,** 115–119.

39. Maruo, K., Ueyama, Y., Kuwahara, Y., Hioki, K., Saito, M., Nomura, T., and Tamaoki, N. (1982) Human tumor xenografts in nude rats and their age dependence. *Br. J. Cancer* **45,** 786–789.

40. Auerbach, R., Morrissey, L. W., and Sidky, Y. A. (1978) Regional differences in the incidence and growth of mouse tumors following intradermal or subcutaneous inoculation. *Cancer Res.* **38,** 1739–1744.

41. Pimm, M. V. and Morris, T. M. (1990) Growth rates of human tumors in nude mice. *Eur. J. Cancer* **26,** 764–765.

42. Bosma, G. C., Custer, R. P., and Bosma, M. J. (1983) A severe combined immunodeficiency mutation in the mouse. *Nature* **301,** 527–530.

43. von Kalle, C., Wolf, J., Becker, A., Sckaer, A., Munck, M., Engert, A., Kapp, U., Fonatsch, C., Komitowski, D., Féaux de Lacroix, W., and Diehl, V. (1992) Growth of Hodgkin cell lines in severely combined immunodeficient mice. *Int. J. Cancer* **52,** 887–891.

44. Dorshkind, K., Denis, K. A., and Witte, O. N. (1986) Lymphoid bone marrow cultures can reconstitute heterogeneous B and T cell-dependent responses in severe combined immunodeficient mice. *J. Immunol.* **137,** 3457–3463.

45. Mosier, D. E., Gulizia, R. J., Baird, S. M., and Wilson, D. B. (1988) Transfer of a functional human immune system to mice with severe combined immunodeficiency. *Nature* **335,** 256–259.

46. Pressman, D. and Keighley, G. (1948) The zone of activity of antibodies as determined by the use of radioactive tracers: the zone of activity of nephritoxic antikidney serum. *J. Immunol.* **59,** 141–146.

47. Pressman, D. and Korngold, L. (1953) The in vivo localization of anti-Wagner-osteogenic-sarcoma antibodies. *Cancer* **6,** 619–623.

48. Pressman, D., Day, E. D., and Blau, M. (1957) The use of paired labeling in the determination of tumor-localizing antibodies. *Cancer Res.* **17,** 845–850.

49. Gold, P. and Freedman, S. O. (1965) Specific carcinoembryonic antigens of the human digestive system. *J. Exp. Med.* **122,** 467–481

50. Mach, J.-P., Carrel, S., Merenda, C., Sordat, B., and Cerottini, J.-C. (1974) *In vivo* localisation of radiolabelled antibodies to carcinoembryonic antigen in human colon carcinoma grafted into nude mice. *Nature* **248,** 704–706.

51. Sharkey, R. M., Primus, F. J., Shochat, D., and Goldenberg, D. M. (1988) Comparison of tumor targeting of mouse monoclonal and goat polyclonal antibodies to carcinoembryonic antigen in the GW-39 human tumor-hamster host model. *Cancer Res.* **48,** 1823–1828.

52. Sands, H., Jones, P. L., Shah, S. A., Palme, D., Vessella, R. L., and Gallagher, B. M. (1988) Correlation of vascular permeability and blood flow with monoclonal antibody uptake by human Clouser and renal cell xenografts. *Cancer Res.* **48,** 188–193.

53. Shockley, T. R., Lin, K., Sung, C., Nagy, J. A., Tompkins, R. G., Dedrick, R. L., Dvorak, H. F., and Yarmush, M. L. (1992) A quantitative analysis of tumor specific monoclonal antibody uptake by human melanoma xenografts: effects of antibody immunological properties and tumor antigen expression levels. *Cancer Res.* **52,** 357–366.

54. Hagan, P. L., Halpern, S. E., Dillman, R. O., Shawler, D. L., Johnson, D. E., Chen, A., Krishnan, L., Frincke, J., Bartholomew, R. M., David, G. S., and Carlo, D. (1986) Tumor size: effect on monoclonal antibody uptake in tumor models. *J. Nucl. Med.* **27,** 422–427.

55. Eccles, S. A., Pervies, H. P., Styles, J. M., Hobbs, S. M., and Dean, C. J. (1989) Pharmacokinetic studies of radiolabelled rat monoclonal antibodies recognising syngeneic sarcoma antigens. II. Effect of host age and immune status. *Cancer Immunol. Immunother.* **30,** 13–20.

56. Pimm, M. V. and Baldwin, R. W. (1984) Quantitative evaluation of the localization of a monoclonal antibody (791T/36) in human osteogenic sarcoma xenografts. *Eur. J. Cancer Clin. Oncol.* **20,** 515–524.

57. Adams, G. P., DeNardo, S. J., Deshpande, S. V., DeNardo, G. L., Meares, C. F., McCall, M. J., and Epstein, A. L. (1989) Effect of mass of ^{111}In-benzyl-EDTA monoclonal antibody on hepatic uptake and processing in mice. *Cancer Res.* **49,** 1707–1711.
58. Patt, Y. Z., Lamki, L. M., Haynie, T. P., Unger, M. W., Rosenblum, M. G., Shirkhoda, A., and Murray, J. L. (1988) Improved tumor localization with increasing dose of indium-111-labeled anti-carcinoembryonic antigen monoclonal antibody ZCE-025 in metastatic colorectal cancer. *J. Clin. Oncol.* **6,** 1220–1230.
59. Kodera, Y., Isobe, K., Yamauchi, M., Satta, T., Hasegawa, T., Oikawa, S., Kondoh, K., Akiyama, S., Itoh, K., Nakashima, I., and Takagi, H. (1993) Expression of carcinoembryonic antigen (CEA) and nonspecific crossreacting antigen (NCA) in gastrointestinal cancer; the correlation with degree of differentiation. *Br. J. Cancer* **68,** 130–136.
60. Epenetos, A. A., Snook, D., Durbin, H., Johnson, P. M., and Taylor-Papadimitriou, J. (1986) Limitations of radiolabeled monoclonal antibodies for localization of human neoplasms. *Cancer Res.* **46,** 3183–3191.
61. Otsuka, F. L., Welch, M. J., McElvany, K. D., Nicolotti, R. A., and Fleischman, J. B. (1984) Development of a model system to evaluate methods of radiolabeling monoclonal antibodies. *J. Nucl. Med.* **25,** 1343–1349.
62. Hnatowich, D. J., Virzi, F., and Rusckowski, M. (1987) Investigations of avidin and biotin for imaging applications. *J. Nucl. Med.* **28,** 1294–1302.
63. Fjeld, J. G., Benestad, H. B., Stigbrand, T., and Nustad, K. (1988) In vivo evaluation of radiolabelled antibodies with antigen-coated polymer particles in diffusion chambers. *J. Immunol. Methods* **109,** 1–7.
64. Fjeld, J. G., Bruland, Ø. S., Benestad, H. B., Schjerven, L., Stigbrand, T., and Nustad, K. (1990) Radiotargeting of human tumuor cells in immunocompetent animals. *Br. J. Cancer* **62,** 573–578.
65. Ziegler, M. M., Ishizu, H., Nagabuchi, E., Takada, N., and Arya, G. (1997) A comparative review of the immunobiology of murine neuroblastoma and human neuroblastoma. *Cancer* **79,** 1757–1766.
66. Lalani, E.-N., Berdichevsky, F., Boshell, M., Shearer, M., Wilson, D., Stauss, H., Gendler, S. J., and Taylor-Papadimitriou, J. (1991) Expression of the gene coding for a human mucin in mouse mammary tumor cells can affect their tumorigenicity. *J. Biol. Chem.* **266,** 15,420–15,426.
67. Taguchi, O., Michael, S. D., and Nishizuka, Y. (1988) Rapid induction of ovarian granulosa cell tumors by 7,12-dimethylbenz(a)anthracene in neonatally estrogenized mice. *Cancer Res.* **48,** 425–429.
68. Rygaard, J. and Povlsen, C. O. (1976) The nude mouse vs. the hypothesis of immunological surveillance. *Transplant. Rev.* **28,** 43–61.
69. Brinster, R. L., Chen, H. Y., Messing, A., van Dyke, T., Levine, A. J., and Palmiter, R. D. (1984) Transgenic mice harboring SV40 T-antigen genes develop characteristic brain tumors. *Cell* **37,** 367–379.
70. Tegtmeyer, P. (1975) Function of simian virus 40 gene A in transforming infection. *J. Virol.* **15,** 613–618.

71. Stewart, T. A., Pattengale, P. K., and Leder, P. (1984) Spontaneous mammary adenocarcinomas in transgenic mice that carry and express MTV/*myc* fusion genes. *Cell* **38,** 627–637.
72. Hanahan, D. (1988) Dissecting multistep tumorigenesis in transgenic mice. *Annu. Rev. Genet.* **22,** 479–519.
73. Thomas, H. and Balkwill, F. R. (1994) Oncogene transgenic mice as therapeutic models in cancer research. *Eur. J. Cancer* **30A,** 533–537.
74. Donehower, L. A., Harvey, M., Slagle, B. L., McArthur, M. J., Montgomery, C. A., Jr., Butel, J. S., and Bradley, A. (1992) Mice deficient for p53 are developmentally normal but susceptible to spontaneous tumors. *Nature* **356,** 215–221.
75. Peat, N., Gendler, S., Lalani, E.-N., and Taylor-Papadimitriou, J. (1992) Tissue-specific expression of a human polymorphic epithelial mucin (MUC1) in transgenic mice. *Cancer Res.* **52,** 1954–1960.
76. Thompson, J. A., Eades-Perner, A.-M., Ditter, M., Muller, W. J., and Zimmermann, W. (1997) Expression of transgenic carcinoembryonic antigen (CEA) in tumor-prone mice: an animal model for CEA-directed tumor immunotherapy. *Int. J. Cancer* **72,** 197–202.

14

Antibodies for Immunoassays

David J. Newman

1. Introduction
1.1. What Can Antibodies Do for Us in Immunoassays?

What is an immunoassay without an antibody? Clearly the name provides the answer to this question; without antibodies there would be no immunoassays. An immunoassay is an analytical technique, quantitative or qualitative, that relies absolutely on the specificity and affinity of the interaction between epitope and paratope for generation of a detectable response. The actual detection of this binding interaction can be via one of literally hundreds of different signal transduction mechanisms, e.g., fluorimetry, chemiluminescence, agglutination (turbidimetry or nephelometry) enzyme reactions, and so forth (1–4), but these are simply transducing systems for the primary binding interaction. Antibodies thus provide us with an exquisitely sensitive and specific analytical technology for detecting and quantifying epitopic structures. These structures include amino-acid derivatives, e.g., thyroid hormones, peptides, e.g., vasopressin, proteins, e.g., cytokines, as well as carbohydrate structures, e.g., CA-125. Immunoassay technology has developed to such an extent that it is probably the most versatile analytical tool available able to identify and quantify epitopic structures across the milli- to zeptomolar concentration ranges (2).

The structure of the epitope can be sequence-specific or conformational, and it can be closely related to the biological function of the complete molecule or completely unrelated. It is particularly important to discover which of the first is the case when selecting the format for an assay. For instance, if it is a conformational epitope that is recognized by an antibody then subtle differences in purification technique or method of conjugation to detection transducers or solid phases may alter the conformation of the epitope in such a way that it is no longer bound with the same affinity as the native molecule. This can

From: *Methods in Molecular Medicine, Vol. 40: Diagnostic and Therapeutic Antibodies*
Edited by: A. J. T. George and C. E. Urch © Humana Press Inc., Totowa, NJ

Table 1
Advantages of Immunoassays vs PCR

Immunoassay	PCR
Fully quantitative	Semiquantitative
Provides proof of protein synthesis	Provides proof of existence of mRNA
Provides evidence of posttranslational modifications	Provides evidence of genetic differences
Detects conformation as well as sequence	Detects sequences only
Can be used for nonprotein structures, e.g., carbohydrates	Not applicable
Can be used for haptenic molecules, e.g., steroid and thyroid hormones	Not applicable
Virtually infinite assay formats and detection systems	Restricted formats currently but potential for many more

significantly alter the specificity of any immunoassay developed using such an antibody. Regarding the biological activity of the structure of interest, because an antibody recognizes a structural determinant the only means of evaluating whether an antibody recognizes a determinant closely related to biological function is to perform comparison experiments with an appropriate bioassay. However, surprisingly often this is not attempted. One comparitively straight-forward way of evaluating this would be to see whether the antibody inhibits the biological activity of the molecule in an in vitro model system.

1.2. Why Are They Useful?

Immunoassays, and by association antibodies, are still essential scientific tools in biological research because they offer something completely different from the polymerase chain reaction (PCR). Both depend on the affinity of an interaction between two complimentary sequences linked to signal generation. Both can involve an amplification step, and both can be qualitative and quanti-tative in nature. However, as shown in **Table 1** comparing antibody and DNA/RNA technologies, the distinct features of antibody technology give it a safe future in the fields of both research and diagnosis. Both technologies require careful optimization and validation and provide complementary information. Also, when investigating for the first time whether a cell line synthesis is a cytokine or growth factor in response to an insult it may even be better to use an immunoassay rather than RT-PCR because the immunoassays may well be the more sensitive tool. Furthermore, as mentioned previously, immunoassays and antibodies have a much broader potential applicability as analytical tools than does DNA technology.

1.3. What Are We Aiming to Do Here?

Within the format of a chapter such as this, where practical information is required, it is difficult to select examples because methods vary enormously with regard to the buffers used, concentrations of antibody, solid-phases, detection systems, and so forth. I have assumed that the reader is working in a general research laboratory with a microtiter plate reader, electrophoresis equipment, and possibly an automated spectrophotometer. I have asked myself the question "How would I set out measure a new protein antigen and a new hapten for neither of which have immunoassays been previously developed?" I assume that a source of purified antigen is available but no reference analytical procedure is available.

A wide range of immunoassays is available on the market, with assays for novel antigens soon appearing in catalogs, albeit at a price. It is always worth bearing in mind that it is not reagent costs that are expensive, but salaries, and that developing "in-house" assays can be a false economy. It can even be worthwhile contracting out the production of the antiserum for your novel antigens because a wide variety of companies offer this service at reasonable cost.

2. Materials

2.1. Immunogen/Calibrant

To generate an antibody a purified source of the antigen is required. The less contaminating material present the easier it is going to be to generate a specific antibody to the epitopic structure of interest. To develop any quantitative assay a calibrant will also be required, and for a novel antigen this will be the purified or synthesized molecule that was used to generate the antibody. For calibration purposes the molecule should be homogeneous, as assessed by electrophoresis/chromatography, and so forth. Some idea of its lability in storage is required, but a safe option is to store aliquots at a reasonably high concentration and at −70°C. Once an antibody is available immunoblotting is required to look at antigen purity and suitability as a calibrant. Immunoblotting can also be used to assess whether purified or synthetic anitgens are recognized to the same extent as the antigen found in the fluid to be analyzed. However, electrophoresis can itself be a denaturing process.

2.2. Antibody Generation

Generation of antibodies is covered in other chapters in this volume. Antibody quantity, affinity, and specificity are the key requirements for their use in an immunoassay (*see* **Table 2**). Immunoglobulins from an enormous range of animal species have been used in immunoassays; rabbit, sheep, goat, mouse, rat, horse, pig, and chicken are probably the most commonly used, each offer-

**Table 2
Desirable Characters of an Antibody for Use in an Immunoassay**

In general select IgG in favor of IgM: Affinity is more important than avidity.
Decide whether the system is to be quantitative or qualitative
    Quantitative systems require higher affinity antibodies.
    Fast assays require higher affinity antibodies.
Decide whether the system is to be single or multiple use
    Stability of antibody is vital if multiple use is required.
Decide whether the system is to use multiple wash steps
    Dissociation constant will need to be slow.
What is the molar concentration of the ligand?
    Equilibrium constant of antibody should be of some magnitude.
    Higher affinity antibodies will in general give greater sensitivity and speed.

---

ing something slightly different in terms of quantity, ease of purification, affinity, and stability. For instance, chicken antibodies can be harvested from the eggs whence the unusual chicken immunoglobulin IgY can be easily purified *(5)*. In general, when developing an immunoassay for a novel antigen it is best to go for polyclonal antibody first and to leave monoclonal antibody (mAb) development until the polyclonal specificity has been shown to be insufficient or a large-scale continuous supply is needed. However, if considerable experience in monoclonal technology is available then an advantage of a mAb first approach for proteins is that panels of antibodies can be relatively easily developed, so matching pairs will be readily available for two-site assays (*see* Chapter 30).

For conjugation of antibodies to solid phases or to label molecules further purification is required. Preparation of an immunoglobulin fraction using ammonium sulfate precipitation or protein A/G (*see* **Table 3** and later chapters for more detail) increases the specific immunoglobulin concentration. If affinity purification against immobilized antigen is performed enhanced affinity populations can be prepared as well *(6)*, although exposure of immunoglobulins to the low pH used to elute them from antigen columns can cause an increased sensitivity to protease digestion (*see* Chapter 18).

Interference from rheumatoid factors in human serum-based immunoassays previously required the use of antibody fragments with the Fc region removed by enzyme digestion. The production of Fab fragments requires some degree of optimization for each successive antibody and yields of active antibody are rarely in excess of 60% *(7)*. Thus, this is an expensive step to take and it is perhaps better to first establish whether there is a problem in the first place. In my experience with latex particle-based assays, which were thought to be par-

Table 3
Purification of Immunoglobulins in Order of Increasing Purity[a]

Fractional precipitation: ammonium sulfate (commonly 20%)
DEAE ion-exchange (now available attached to magnetic particles removing
    albumin in one step)
Protein A/G (depending on species and immunoglobulin isotype) affinity
    chromatography
Affinity chromatography on an antigen column.

[a]Costs: Ab fragments > monoclonal = affinity purified > IgG Fraction > antiserum

ticularly prone to this type of interference, the conjugation to a solid phase can
significantly ameliorate this effect and Fab fragments were not found to be
essential at all. Other potential interferences that can influence the choice of
final immunoreagent are HAMA (human antimouse antibodies) and other
antispecies antibodies. However, the best means of reducing this type of interference appears to be the inclusion of excess immunoglobulin of the same species in the assay buffer.

When working toward an assay for a novel antigen I would start with the
simplest reagent, an immunoglobulin fraction of a polyclonal antibody, and
include blocking immunoglobulin of the same species in the assay buffer.

2.3. Factors Influencing Immunoassay Performance

Which antibody or antiserum to choose is clearly of vital importance. The
specificity required will depend on the purposes to which the assay is to put to
use. For instance, early immunoassays for follicle-stimulating hormone (FSH)
were evaluated in such way that it ensured that there was limited crossreaction
with luteinizing hormone (LH). However, now that we know that different
isoforms of FSH, differing mainly in their attached carbohydrate chains, have
different biological activities, it is important to know which of the isoforms are
recognized by an antibody. Alternatively, when measuring a drug in a patient's
serum that is metabolized into a variety of active and inactive metabolites it
may be useful to have an antibody that can measure only the active metabolites. This has now led to some authors suggesting that receptor-based assays,
possibly using recombinant receptor molecules (8), might be more useful than
antibodies for this purpose.

2.4. Assay Format

In general, the solid-phase, two-site assay is the best choice for proteins,
with a matched pair of antibodies selected by some form of epitope mapping or
competition experiments. For haptens the chemical structure of the hapten will

determine how it can be linked either to a solid phase or to a transducer system. To develop a viable assay a different protein:hapten conjugate will be required from that used as an immunogen; however, this will have also been required for screening the different antisera. When designing a screening test for antisera or monoclonals it will always be preferable to screen in a format as close as possible to the final assay format to avoid unforeseen complications. Thus, for haptens in particular if a fluorescence-labeled system is to be used then a fluorescence conjugate should be used for screening purposes. Thus, in order to screen suitable antibodies a choice will already have been made about the assay format, probably based on the available resources; microtiter plate "sandwich" assays for proteins and probably microtiter-based immobilized antigen-based competitive assays for haptens. In commercial assay development different choices will be made depending on the instrumentation onto which the assay is to be placed.

2.5. Solid Phase

The most common solid phase will probably be microtiter plates, as mentioned previously, but several choices must be made even here *(9,10)*. Different shaped wells and surfaces are available, with some advantages to "treated" ones for enhancement of protein adsorption or coupling. Microtiter plates have slow assay kinetics, mainly because of the small surface areas for antibody/protein immobilization. Microparticulate solid-phases, e.g., latex particles or magnetic particles, offer more reproducible immobilization and provide better assay kinetic characteristics, and can also be used in microtiter plates *(2,11)*.

Although adsorption of antibodies to solid phases produces quite a stable reagent, it is a random process that can result in significant proportions of the immunoglobulins attaching in a manner rendering them unable to recognize the antigen *(12–14)*. Covalent coupling of protein provides an opportunity for improved orientation of antibodies and a detergent-resistant conjugation, which enables more stringent washing conditions to be used *(15–17)*. For in-house procedures development, with adsorption is probably the best first option, moving to covalent attachment if necessary. As experience with this approach develops, move toward covalent attachment as the first option. For measurement of analytes in difficult matrixes, e.g., health and safety or environmental work where stringent washing may be essential, covalent linkage is probably best. When choosing which covalent coupling method to use the mildest reaction conditions are preferred in order to retain as much functional activity as possible *(18)*. Glutaraldehyde is simple to use but crude and relatively aggressive; carbodiimide less so, but if available the use of activated surfaces, such as chloromethylstyrene or aldehyde, are preferred because they are much more gentle chemistries. A good compromise is to buy pre-prepared streptavidin-coated solid phases and to prepare biotinylated antibodies/conjugates for capture. Biotinylation is extremely straightforward. Clearly this latter approach cannot be used if a biotin:strepatavidin detection system is planned!

In practice, different antibodies/conjugates can vary in their resistance to damage induced by adsorption and covalent coupling techniques. Experimental optimization of protein loading and the pH/ionic strength conditions used will be required. It is possible that the ability of an antibody/conjugate to function after conjugation is part of the selection procedure of which one to use. It should be remembered that differences in titer/active antibody concentration will be important in determining the success of a conjugation. Optimization of the amount of antibody/conjugate to put on the surface of a solid phase is an important prerequisite of developing a good reagent; more is definitely not always better. Steric hindrance and increased nonspecific interactions with sample matrix components can result from too high a protein loading *(12)*.

2.6. Detection System

It is best to go for as simple as possible a system to start. Assuming most laboratories will have a microtiter plate reader it would be best to go for biotinylating the detection antibody and buying streptavidin, conjugated to either alkaline phosphatase or horse radish peroxidase (probably the former), from a reputable supplier, of which there are many. Preparation of enzyme–labeled antibodies is a complex process requiring careful optimization and purification probably best left to those with significant experience *(19)*. A wide range of substrates is available for either enzyme, in the Sigma (St. Louis, MO) catalog for instance. There is the possibility of starting off with a colorimetric detection system and then extending the sensitivity of the assay by using a fluorimetric or chemiluminometric substrate at a later stage if the detection technology is available and the improved performance is needed (*see* Chapter 30).

2.7. Assay Matrix: Buffers

Most immunoassay buffers tend to be based on phosphate salts because they provide good buffering capacity in the most common pH range used, 7.0–7.4. At around 100 mM and preferably containing some NaCl (50–100 mM) this provides a suitable buffer ionic strength for most analytical purposes; however, if particular matrices incompatible with phosphate are to be used then alternatives need to be sought. Tris-HCl and borate buffers have been used. More extreme buffer conditions have also been used by some authors to reduce nonspecific binding for particular circumstances, e.g., pH 10.0, but the need for this can be removed by careful addition of detergents, for instance. *(20)*.

The development of an immunoassay requires the potentiation of the intermolecular forces that drive the antibody:antigen reaction while reducing the forces that cause nonspecific binding and agglutination *(21)*. This balancing act is performed by selecting a suitable assay buffer and requires careful optimization and assay validation to ensure that the buffer is appropriate for use with different analytical matrices. For instance, an assay that is valid for analyzing chromatography fractions or tissue culture fluid is not necessarily going to provide an accurate answer in animal or human patient serum. As the protein concentration in the analytical matrix increases the further protein should be added to the buffer, e.g., bovine or human serum albumin. This will increase the viscosity, which alone can cause methodological problems and matrix effects *(22)*, but also helps block nonspecific binding from serum components. Analysis of water samples for environmental monitoring may require the use of a higher ionic strength buffer to compensate for the lack of ions in the water matrix, since changes in ionic strength can greatly influence the kinetics of the antibody:antigen reaction, particularly when haptens are being assayed *(21)*.

Detergents can play a very important role in minimizing nonspecific binding, and although more commonly used in enzyme-linked immunosorbent assays (ELISA) formats in the wash buffers, have proved invaluable in assay buffers. Nonionic detergents, e.g., Tween-20, are more commonly used than ionic detergents, such as sodium dodecyl sulfate (SDS). Concentrations range from 0.05 up to 0.5% in some assay systems *(10,15)*. A further addition that is often required is that of a bateriostat. Although almost ubiquitous a few years ago, use of sodium azide is declining and is being replaced with selective antibiotics, at least in commercial applications.

Any assay using a solid-phase format will require suitable washing of the solid-phase prior to the final signal generation. It is thus important that the antibody selected has a low dissociation rate constant. Otherwise, significant dissociation can occur during the wash step. Wash buffers need also have similar pH, ionic strength, detergent, and protein concentrations to that used in the assay buffer, but may need to use a different buffer salt, e.g., not phosphate if an alkaline phosphatase detection system is to be used. Tris-based buffers offer a good alternative.

3. Methods

In **Fig. 1** I have shown a suggested development pathway or decision tree for the selection of antibodies for both a novel hapten and a novel protein antigen. This is based around the premises already mentioned in the earlier parts of this chapter and delineates the decisions to be made. The first is not exactly a

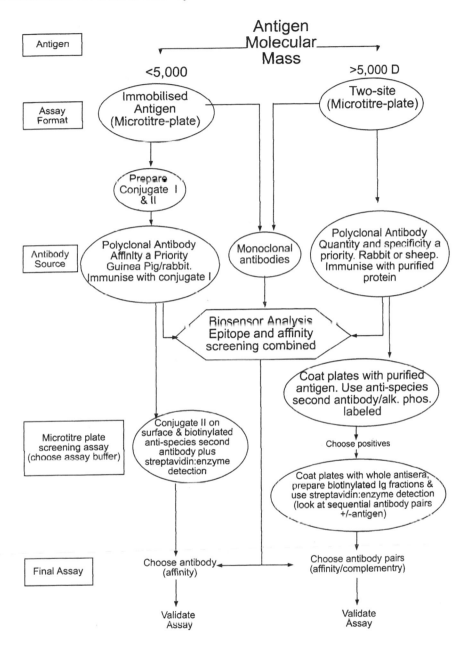

Fig. 1. Possible development pathways for immunoassays for a protein and hapten.

choice, but the molecular weight of the antigen will determine which arm of the tree to follow. Regarding the assay format, a solid-phase system, essentially a microtiter plate is assumed. The primary source of antibody is likely to be that of a polyclonal antibody, but mAbs do offer certain advantages if the technology and experience are available. The initial primary screening of the available test bleeds from the animals used or the positive clones of mAbs is likely, in most laboratories, to be using a microtiter-based assay system. However, also included is what is becoming increasingly important, if not the most widely recommended, technique for screening antibodies, i.e., the use of optical biosensor analysis, which is described elsewhere in this book. The advantages of biosensor analysis are that both epitopic mapping and affinity determination can be combined using the very low amounts of material available in test bleeds and the initial phase of mAb development using a microtiter-based approach relative to titer, affinity, and specificity can be determined after "any binding at all" has been discovered. Essentially dilutions of antisera/hybridoma supernatants (in assay buffer) are reacted with immobilized antigen and binding determined using a labeled antispecies antibody detection system. Positives can be retested looking at competition with free antigens to inhibit binding from which relative affinities can be determined. If there is a particularly important molecule that must not be recognized by the selected antibody, an excess of this molecule should be included in the initial experiments. The use of the microtiter-based screening assay requires essentially a final assay format to have been selected prior to any evaluation of the antibody. As indicated earlier, one contraindication for using the biosensor is if a microtiter-based format is used for the final assay with an enzyme labeled system. In this case screening using this format is the nearest possible environment to the final assay and is likely to give more representative performance of the selected antibody reagents in the final assay.

3.1. Generation of Antibodies

As indicated in **Subheading 2.1.**, in order to generate an antibody, a purified source of the antigen is required. Whereas for a high-mol-wt protein antigen one fully characterized source of this material is all that is essential, for a hapten one will need to develop at least two different conjugates of the hapten: conjugate 1, to be used during the immunization, for instance conjugating the hapten to keyhole limpet hemocyanin; and then conjugate 2, to be used in the antibody screening, in which the carrier protein to which the hapten is linked must be of a different type. Preferably the conjugation reaction used or the bridging molecule should also be of a different type. This prevents selection of antibodies that recognize the carrier protein used during the immunization stage. Guidelines are given elsewhere in this book and in a variety of references, for instance **ref.** *32*, that mention the importance of optimizing the molar ratio of hapten to carrier protein for both the conjugate used for immunization and that used for screening. In particular with the conjugate used for screening, too high a molar ratio of hapten to conjugate will provide too high a concentration of hapten on the surface, capturing too much of the free solution antibody, thus preventing effective competition during assay development by the soluble ligand. It would be fair to say that in general, for the development of specific immunoassay, the purity of the conjugate or protein should be as high as possible for the screening step. Some degree of minor contamination can be allowed for the preparation used during the immunization but it is clearly most important to select only for the desired characteristics.

3.2. Selection of an Antibody for Immunoassay

Selection of an antibody for immunoassay requires an appreciation of both specificity and affinity. As indicated earlier, this is best achieved by means of biosensor analysis; however, relative affinity constants can be easily determined using microtiter-based assay systems by looking at the competition of decreasing concentrations of free ligand with fixed amounts of antibody.

For molecules that have not had assays previously developed for them, an alternative reference procedure is required to evaluate whether the assay developed using the screening format is indeed specific. The simplest means to evaluate the antibody specificity is using Western blots (Chapter 32) to see if in the biological matrix of interest the antibody binds to an appropriate molecular weight or p.I. The problem with this approach is that, particularly if SDS polyacrylamide gels are used, there can be significant conformational change in the antigen, which may mean that the antibody will no longer recognize it even though it might recognize the native material in the biological fluid. Alternatively, early verification of specificity can be determined by evaluating, for instance, chromatographic profiles of the biological fluid of interest, demonstrating that the antibody only recognises that peak in which the desired molecule is present.

After affinity and specificity one further characteristic may be important if the antibody is to be used in a multiple use format, particularly in some of the new immunosensors (*17*). If this is the case, some evidence of the stability of that antibody to the regeneration conditions likely to be used during the operation of the immunosensor is required. This can be best performed on biosensor systems but also can be performed on microtiter-based formats. Recovery of antigen binding is the most appropriate control for this format.

3.3. Summary of Design Criteria

Although selection of the appropriate assay design is a prerequisite for designing an appropriate screening format, it is worthwhile reiterating some of the important criteria. As indicated in **Table 2**, if a qualitative or semi-quantitative system is the final format in which the antibodies are to be used, less stringent requirements on the affinity of the antibody are necessary. For a quantitative assay the affinity constant becomes more important and it should be of the same order of magnitude as the molar concentration of the ligand to be measured. The fundamental criteria associated with the optimization of immunoassays and the rules to be followed have been well described by numerous articles by Prof. Roger Ekins (e.g., **ref. 24**). In summary, if an assay format using an immobilized hapten is to be used then the affinity constant of the antibody is going to be of primary importance. In the development of a two-site assay, e.g., an ELISA for a protein using a matched pair of complementary antibodies recognizing different or at least multiple epitopes on the molecule of interest, affinity constants are less important. The relative concentration of immunoreagents used tends to be higher, and what becomes most important is minimizing the nonspecific binding that occurs in the reaction matrix. These general rules are important when selecting the appropriate antibodies for a hapten versus a higher molecular weight analyte.

To effectively identify the appropriate antibodies for use in a two-site assay (after initial screening) if a biosensor is unavailable, it is preferable to prepare at least an IgG for action of all the available antibodies and to biotinylate 50% of the available immunoglobulin. Then the nonbiotinylated fraction can be used to coat microtiter plates and a biotinylated fraction can be used in conjunction with a streptavidin-linked enzyme as a labeled antibody system. Different combinations of coated plates and biotinylated antibodies can be used to select complementary pairs. Because initial "yes/no" screening often uses immobilized antigen, which is often denatured antigen, if a denatured antigen is not to be present in the final assay it is possible that inappropriate antibodies may be selected in this primary screen. Thus, whereas all positively screening hybridomas clearly need to be re-evaluated, some of the negative but high immunoglobulin-producing hybridomas may be worthwhile screening in a sandwich format.

3.4. Reaction Conditions

A preliminary selection of reaction conditions, particularly buffer, ionic strength, pH, and so forth, will have been taken to develop an appropriate screening assay. However, once antibodies have been selected more complete assay optimization is necessary. This will include the selection of the appropriate calibration matrix for use in the final assay format. A general rule that cannot be escaped is that the calibration matrix used should be as near as possible identical with the matrix in which the analyte of interest is to be measured. If there are significant differences between these two matrices it is unlikely that a valid assay will be developed. For instance, if a serum-based assay is required serum-based or high-protein concentration synthetic matrices are essential. If extraction steps are necessary, for instance, with particular haptens in certain nonaqueous matrices, the final buffer in which the extracted material is dissolved needs to be the same as that in which the calibrant is dissolved.

3.5. Detection System

I would always recommend in the first instance that an enzyme-based assay is probably the most appropriate, generally applicable, detection system. If, for instance, alkaline phosphatase is selected as the enzyme label it is preferably bought from a commercial supplier conjugated to streptavadin. This can be used in combination with a biotinylated antibody, and biotinylation of immunoglobulin fractions is extremely straightforward, with a number of protocols available in the literature. Conjugation of enzymes to immunoglobulins is fraught with difficulties requiring careful attention to the molar ratio of the two components and considerable experience of protein purification subsequent to that. The advantage of selecting an enzyme, such as alkaline phosphatase, is that a colometric substrate can be used initially for simple optimization. However, if the resultant assay does not obtain the detection limits necessary for the quantification of the molecule of interest, higher sensitivity can be gained by using either fluorescent, for instance, methyl umbelliferone phosphate, or chemiluminescence substrates if the appropriate detectors are available. Increasing the sample volume used in an assay is not something to be undertaken lightly simply to improve the detection limit of the assay. Major alterations in the reaction conditions can be induced by such alterations and complete revalidation of the assay is essential before these changes can be taken as acceptable.

3.6. Validation of the Assay/Antibodies Finally Selected

Even assuming that an appropriate pair of antibodies or individual antibody with high enough affinity have been selected, there still remains doubt that the assay formulation will provide a valid assay. Recovery experiments using added analyte and experiments using serial dilutions of a high concentration containing sample in the calibration matrix need to be performed. Simple estimations of within- and between-assay precision are also necessary. These simple steps can indicate that an inappropriate selection of either reaction conditions or immunoreagent has been reached. This may require revisiting the original stocks of antibody that were discarded initially. It is worth emphasizing that all immunoreagents should be stored appropriately for subsequent re-evaluation in light of discoveries to be made during the validation step. The complete validation of an assay requires determination of sensitivity and preferably precision profiles, as indicated in articles by Prof. Ekins, alluded to earlier *(24)*. However, with a new novel analyte there remains the lack of a reference procedure to ultimately confirm the accuracy of the method or the specificity of the antibodies, which at this stage can be almost synonymous. Normally with novel antigens there will have been a biological response observed. This can be used to assess the measure of agreement between the structure measured in the assay and the function represented by the biological activity. An example from my own experience was the development of novel assays for a protein called cystatin C, which had been suggested as a marker for glomerular filtration rate. To validate this assay, I and my coworkers compared the preliminary optimized immunoassay with an enzyme-enhanced radial immunodiffusion (RID) assay using the same antibody. The advantage of the RID approach was that it placed fewer constraints on the antibody and required, in principle at least, less optimization because the conditions were much simpler. However, the fundamental verification of the assay was to compare the serum concentration of cystatin C measured by the new assay against glomerular filtration rate measured by an alternative technique. The demonstration of a good agreement confirmed that the molecule we were measuring, or rather the structure that we were measuring, agreed well with the biological function we wished to use it to determine. If other assays do exist then clearly a direct comparison can be made with those and the measure of agreement assessed.

For low-molecular haptens, high-performance liquid chromatography (HPLC) or other chromatographic means of isolating the molecule of interest can be used to quantify the amount of analyte present using an entirely different analytical technique. Correlation between these two parameters, that is, chromatographic retention time and immunological activity, can give an indication of the specificity of the immunological assay. However, it should always be remembered that these are different analytical techniques, measuring different aspects, and comparison of the two methodologies may not give the same answer. If this is the case, a third technique needs to be used to discover which of the analytical tools is giving the more desirable information.

4. Conclusion

In summary, the main points for selection of an antibody for use in an immunoassay have been described in **Fig. 1** and **Tables 1–3**. The direction to take depends on the molecular weight of the molecule to be measured. A decision is required based on whether structure or function is likely to be the most important characteristic, and indeed this may not be possible until after the assay has been developed. It is always better to use commercial sources of detection systems because this will save time and money and may well improve the robustness of both the screening test and final assay. It is often worth writing to authors of published works if they indicate that antibodies or purified antigens have been previously discovered or generated.

Removal of matrix effect and complete validation of assays are essential. Do not assume that an assay developed for chromatography fractions or tissue culture medium will give the appropriate result in serum or urine; it will not. Reoptimization is essential.

In summary, the conditions in which you use your immunoreagents can be extremely varied in immunoassays. When selecting the antibodies for use in an immunoassay the final assay conditions need to be mimicked as closely as possible. Finally, remember that when using an immunoassay in an in vitro experiment, for instance, to measure the amount of cytokine released into the supernatant it is not nooooory that you see the same proportional increase in the supernatant, as RT-PCR shows in the cell extract. PCR and immunoassay are complementary techniques that measure different factors and will give different information.

Reagent Supplies: Useful Directories

Linscott's Directory of Immunological and Biological Reagents. Linscott's Directory, Falun, Sweden.
Web Sites: Antibody Resources http://www.antibodyresource.com

References

1. Edwards, R. (1985) *Immunoassay: An Introduction*, William Heinemann Medical Books, London, UK.
2. Price, C. P. and Newman, D. J. (eds.) (1997) *Principles and Practice of Immunoassay*, Stockton, London, UK.
3. Edwards, R. (ed.) (1998) *Practical Approaches to Immunoassay*. Oxford University Press, Oxford, UK.
4. Tijssen, P. (1985) *Practice and Theory of Enzyme Immunoassays*. Elsevier, Amsterdam, The Netherlands.
5. Polson, A. (1990) Isolation of IgY from the yolk of eggs by a chloroform polyethylene glycol procedure. *Immun. Invest.* **19**, 253–258.
6. Hodgkinson, S. C. and Lowry, P. J. (1982) Selective elution of immunoadsorbed anti-(human prolactin) immunoglobulins with enhanced immunochemical properties. *Biochem. J.* **205**, 535–541.

7. Rousseaux, J., Rousseaux-Provost, R., and Bazin, H. (1983) Optimal conditions for the preparation of Fab and F(ab')$_2$ fragments from monoclonal IgG of different rat IgG subclasses. *J. Immunol. Methods* **64,** 141–146.
8. Soldin, S. J. (1995) Receptor (immunophilin-binding) assay for immunosuppressive drugs. *Therap. Drug Monit.* **17,** 574–576.
9. Butler, J. E. (1993) The behaviour of antigens and antibodies immobilised on a solid phase, in *Structure of Antigens,* vol. 1 (Van Regenmortel, M. H. V., ed.), CRC, New York, pp. 209–260.
9a. Multiple authors. (1993) Antibodies, in *Methods of Immunological Analysis,* vol. 2 (Albert, W. H. and Staines, N. A., eds.), VCH, Basel, Switzerland, pp. 147–427.
10. Newman, D. J. and Price, C. P. (1997) Separation techniques, in *Principles and Practice of Immunoassay* (Price, C. P. and Newman, D.J., eds.), Stockton, London, UK, pp. 155–172.
11. Griffin, C., Sutor, J., and Schull, B. (1994) *Microparticle Reagent Optimisation,* Seradyn Inc, Indianapolis, IN.
12. Spitznagel, T. M. and Clark, D. S. (1993) Surface density and orientation effects on immobilised antibodies and antibody fragments. *Biotechnology* **11,** 825–829.
13. Veilleux, J. K. and Duran, L. W. (1996) Covalent immobilisation of biomolecules to preactivated surfaces. *IVD Tech.* **2,** 26–31.
14. Davies, J., Dawkes, A. C., Haymes, A. G., et al. (1995) Scanning tunnelling microscopy and dynamic angle studies of the effects of partial denaturation on immunoassay solid phase antibody. *J. Immunol. Methods* **186,** 111–123.
15. Self, C. H., Dessi, J. L., and Winger, L. A. (1996) Ultraspecific immunoassays for small molecules: role of wash steps and multiple binding formats. *Clin. Chem.* **42,** 1527–1531.
16. Thakkar, H., Davey, C. L., Medcalf, E. A., et al. (1991) Stabilisation of turbidimetric immunoassay by covalent coupling of antibody to latex particles. *Clin. Chem.* **37,** 1248–1251.
17. Newman, D. J., Olabiran, Y., and Price, C. P. (1997) Bioaffinity agents for sensing systems, in *Handbook of Biosensors and Electronic Noses: Medicine, Food and the Environment* (Kress-Rogers, E., ed.), CRC, London, UK, pp. 59–90.
18. Douglas, A. S. and Monteith, C. A. (1994) Improvements to immunoassays by use of covalent binding assay plates. *Clin. Chem.* **40,** 1833–1837.
19. Gosling, J. P. (1997) Enzyme immunoassay: with and without separation, in *Principles and Practice of Immunoassay* (Price, C. P. and Newman, D. J., eds.), Stockton, London, UK, pp. 351–388.
20. Newman, D. J., Kassai, M., Craig, A. R., et al. (1996) Validation of a particle enhanced immunoturbidimetric assay for serum β2-microglobulin on the Dade International ACA. *Eur. J. Clin. Chem. Clin. Biochem.* **34,** 861–865.
21. Newman, D. J. and Price, C. P. (1996) Molecular mechanisms in immunoassays for drugs. *Ther. Drug Monit.* **18,** 493–497.
22. Morgan, C. L., Burrin, J. M., Newman, D. J., and Price, C. P. (1998) The matrix effects on kinetic rate constants of antibody–antigen interactions are caused by viscosity. *J. Immunol. Methods* **217,** 51–60.

23. Knott, C. L., Kuss-Reichel, K., Liu, R.-S., and Wolfert, R. L. (1997) Development of antibodies for diagnostic assays, in *Principles and Practice of Immunoassay* (Price, C. P. and Newman, D. J., eds.), Stockton, London, UK, pp. 65–98.
24. Ekins, R. P. (1997) Immunoassay design and optimisation, in *Principles and Practice of Immunoassay* (Price, C. P. and Newman, D. J., eds.), Stockton, London, UK, pp. 175–207.

III

Eᴛʜɪᴄs ᴀɴᴅ Iɴᴅᴜsᴛʀʏ

15

Intellectual Property

William M. Brown

1. Introduction

"Intellectual property" (IP) is a generic legal term for patents, copyrights, and trademarks, all of which provide legal rights to protect ideas, the expression of ideas, and the inventors of such ideas *(1)*. Intellectual property has many of the characteristics of real property (houses, buildings, and so forth); intellectual property can be bought, sold, assigned, and licensed. Additionally, the owner of IP can prevent "trespass" on his property by others, though in IP this is referred to as infringement. A patent provides legal protection for a new invention, that is, an application of a new idea, discovery, or concept that is useful. Copyright provides legal protection from copying for any creative work (e.g., works of art, literature [fiction or nonfiction], music, lyrics, photographs), as well as business and scientific publications, computer software, and compilations of information. A trademark provides rights to use symbols, particular words, logos, or other markings that indicate the source of a product or service. A further method of benefitting from an invention is simply to keep it secret, rather than to disclose it; the most famous trade secret of all time is the formula for Coca-Cola, still a closely guarded secret to this day *(2,3)*. Trade secrets have the advantage that they never expire, but special measures are required to ensure the continued secrecy, and should it be violated, there is little legal protection for the owner *(2,3)*.

Intellectual property may seem like a strange topic for a chapter in a science book intended for practicing scientists, but intellectual property impinges on almost everything scientists do, as the reader will realize by the end of this chapter. Furthermore, as scientists are paid to come up with ideas and aspire to publish their work, the protection of ideas and of written works especially should be of interest and concern to all.

From: *Methods in Molecular Medicine, Vol. 40: Diagnostic and Therapeutic Antibodies*
Edited by: A. J. T. George and C. E. Urch © Humana Press Inc., Totowa, NJ

As a scientist, it is difficult to avoid intellectual property. Write a paper or review (copyright is "created" automatically once your ideas are fixed in a permanent medium; it is not even necessary [though it is advisable] to add the copyright sign [©] and the author's name), sign a copyright transfer form when submitting a paper or review to a journal, go to the library to copy a paper from a journal (read the copyright notice in the next journal you copy from, or perhaps the copyright notice attached to the photocopier in the library), open and use a software package (software is protectable under copyright law, and a copyright agreement was probably printed on the envelope from which you removed the disk), or use the polymerase chain reaction (PCR) process (PCR is covered by two US patents *[4,5]*, now assigned to Roche *[6–9]*) and you have entered the lawyer's realm of intellectual property.

A further area in which scientists may encounter the subject of intellectual property law is in employment contracts. When starting a new position at a pharmaceutical or biotech company, scientists will likely be required to assign all inventions made during their employment to their employer. That is not so unreasonable, because, of course, scientists were hired to come up with ideas, and to do so, scientists will be using the employer's resources and facilities. Under US law, the Court of Appeals for the Federal Circuit has ruled that inventions belong to the employer even without the employee formally assigning them *(10)*.

Additionally, the subject of intellectual property has hardly been out of the scientific (or lay) press in the last 20 years *(11–13)*. From the landmark case of *Chakrabarty*, in which the US Supreme Court held that genetically altered bacteria could be patented under US law *(14–17)*, the original Cohen-Boyer patent covering many of the basic recombinant DNA techniques *(18–20)*, Genentech's patent *(21)*, also covering many basic recombinant DNA methods *(22)*, the Pasteur Institute's battle with the National Institutes of Health (NIH) over the patent for the antibody test for HIV *(23,24)*, Wellcome and Genentech's patent battles over tissue plasminogen activator (t-Pa) *(25–30)*, Hybritech's battle with Monoclonal Antibodies, Inc. *(31–33)*, the patent for microinjection (to create transgenic animals *[34–36]*), Amgen's patent dispute with Genetics Institute over recombinant erythropoietin *(37–43)*, Centocor and Xoma's long-running patent battle over their monoclonal antibody (mAb) products to treat sepsis *(44–49)*, the battle between Wellcome and the NIH over the AZT patent *(50–55)*, the battle between DuPont and Cetus over the rights to PCR *(56–59)*, the European Patent Office's battle with Harvard University over patenting the Oncomouse *(60–64)*, Craig Venter and NIH's attempt to patent partial cDNA sequences (EST's, expressed sequence tags) *(65–77)*, Promega's challenge to the patents on Taq polymerase *(78–80)*, Chiron's dispute over a patent for a Hepatitis C test *(81)*, Genentech's dispute with Chiron over IGF-I *(82)*, Genentech and Novo Nordisk's still ongoing war over human growth hormone

(83–85), to the dispute between Oncormed and Myriad Genetics concerning the breast cancer susceptibility gene *BRCA1/2 (86,87)*, the scientific press has been loaded with intellectual property news. It is now rare that an edition of *Science* or *Nature* contains nothing on the subject.

It is not much of an exaggeration to claim that the world biotechnology industry hangs on two broad techniques, recombinant DNA and mAbs. The two technologies have very different and illustrative histories in terms of intellectual property.

It is somewhat ironic to be writing a chapter on intellectual property in a book concerning—of all things—antibodies; it is now part of scientific and legal folklore that neither Köhler and Milstein, nor their employer—the British Medical Research Council—recognized the commercial significance of their discovery and patented their invention. As a result, neither the inventors nor the MRC made much money out of their seminal work *(88–90)*. Since then, there have been many patents (and disputes about patents) on specific mAbs and their uses (e.g., **refs.** *31–33,44–46,48*), but the original Köhler and Milstein technique was never patented.

Contrast this with the now famous Cohen-Boyer patent *(18)* on the basic techniques of recombinant DNA *(91)* from which Stanford University (Cohen's employer) and University of California, San Francisco (Boyer's employer), made tens of millions of dollars before the patent expired in 1997 *(92)* by selling licenses to the then fledgling biotechnology industry *(20,92,93)*. Also covering basic recombinant DNA techniques were Genentech's patent (including fusion proteins, the Riggs patent *[21,22]*) and the Itakura patent (covering plasmid technology *[94]*), both of which were also widely licensed *(12)*.

2. Patents

2.1. Innovation and Invention

As a society, we greatly value innovation; it is no longer possible—except with regard to the simplest products—to succeed for very long selling a product solely because it is cheaper. We constantly demand new and more advanced products. No company making a cheap 1970-level car is going to succeed today; we want a 2000 model with airbags, antilock brakes, traction control, CD hifi stereo system, and so forth. Likewise, there is no longer a market for 8086 (or even 80386) computers, at any price. Such new and more advanced products are the result of research and development. Society has long recognized the need to encourage and stimulate inventors to bring new and useful products to the marketplace for the benefit of all and to protect and reward the innovator by protecting him or her from cheap copies made by competitors piggybacking off the innovator's expensive and time-consuming research and development efforts.

2.2. What Is a Patent?

A patent is a government-given, time-limited monopoly on an invention; that is, armed with a patent an inventor—using the power of the government—can prevent anybody else using his or her technique or making, selling, or importing the product. In return for this limited monopoly, the inventor is required to describe fully the invention for the benefit of the public and others working in the field. When the patent expires, anyone can use the invention, and during the life or term of the patent, the information in the patent is freely available to all to stimulate related work. Indeed, to make a full survey of the scientific literature, it is now essential to search the patent databases too.

Because patents are government-given, an inventor must apply for a patent separately in each country in which he or she wants protection. Furthermore, because each nation has its own patent system, there are many variations on the basic theme. There are agreements between nations such that they recognize patent filings in other countries, but there is no "world patent" and it is basically necessary to apply for a patent separately in each country. Whether it is worth doing so in every country depends on the resources of the inventor and the significance and likely commercial value of the patent and the resulting product(s).

Under US law, currently there are three types of patents: utility patents, design patents, and plant patents. A utility patents can cover any invention or discovery of a new and useful (or a new and useful improvement of any) composition of matter (e.g., a new chemical compound or mixture of compounds), process (e.g., an industrial or technical procedure or method), product, or machine. Design patents protect the appearance of an article. Plant patents cover the "invention" (by crossbreeding) or discovery of new plants, including cultivated mutants, hybrids, and seedlings.

2.3. Requirements for Patentability

To be patentable, an invention must be novel, nonobvious, and useful. That may sound simple enough, but it is far from always so.

"Novel" or new means simply that the invention must be different from what was previously known. Novel does not mean revolutionary; indeed, most patented inventions are far from revolutionary. Improvements on existing machines, devices, and processes are often sufficiently different to be patentable in their own right. "Novel" in the patentability sense includes new uses for a known invention. A good example of this is the compound minoxidil, which was invented, patented, and marketed as an antihypertensive drug before its hair growth-promoting properties were discovered. Although the molecule could not be "repatented," its new use in treating baldness could be, and minoxidil is now the active ingredient in Rogaine. Similarly, although it is not possible to repatent a previously patented mAb, it is perfectly acceptable to patent a new use for such an antibody; detecting a disease-associated protein, for example. Additionally, any new method of producing mAbs would be patentable, as would improvements on the original method of Köhler and Milstein.

"Nonobvious" means that the invention must be sufficiently novel or different from previously published work (the so-called "prior art") that it is not an obvious next step to one "skilled in the art," that is, in the scientific or technical discipline to which the invention relates. The hypothetical person "skilled in the art" is not a genius and is not the inventor; the test is not nonobvious to the inventor, but to the hypothetical person. The level of skill required varies depending on the field, but is typically someone with postgraduate education (not necessarily a PhD) and several years experience in the area.

"Useful" means simply that the invention has some known use. There is a very low threshold for usefulness; almost any use will do, so long as it is functional and not solely aesthetic. However, even such a low threshold prevents the patenting of new chemical compounds where no use or function is known.

2.4. Obtaining a Patent: "Patent Prosecution"

Obtaining a patent is, in concept anyway, fairly straightforward; the whole process is frequently referred to as "patent prosecution." The inventor invents and carefully documents everything about his or her invention and all its possible uses. The inventor takes this material to a patent agent or patent attorney who conducts a search of the prior art, that is, all the published literature and all previously granted patents (now greatly facilitated with computer databases). This search enables the inventor and attorney to learn about other related inventions and to begin to analyze whether the invention is patentable over the prior art, that is, whether it is novel and/or a sufficient advance over existing technology. At this stage, it is also advisable to assess the likely utility—commercial and otherwise—of the invention. The inventor then has to "reduce to practice" the invention, if this has not already been done; this means creating a prototype of the invention or showing how it can be carried out in a practical (as opposed to theoretical) way. A patent application is then submitted, detailing the invention and how it can be carried out.

The patent office examines the patent application both for form and substance. Typically, a patent is not granted immediately, but the application is challenged by the patent office for being insufficient or inadequate in some manner; the inventor responds to this and clarifies or narrows the application and eventually the patent application is rejected or granted.

Once a patent application has been filed, the inventor may disclose the invention publicly without jeopardizing the patent, and can seek licensees or assignees of the patent or can seek to commercialize or otherwise exploit the patent.

Scientists typically live by the mantra "publish or perish;" however, in the world of patents, if work is published before the application is filed, it is the application that may perish. As has been discussed in the medical literature recently *(95,96)*, scientists, especially those working for corporations or conducting research funded by corporations, have had publications delayed while patent protection for the work was sought. This is not just a precaution, but a requirement.

Under US patent law, an inventor has a one-year grace period after the first public disclosure or publication to file a patent application; however, in most other countries there is no such grace period. Thus, if an invention is published or disclosed publicly (e.g., by speaking about it at a conference), then the right to a patent for that invention in those countries will be forfeited. Despite this, an inventor may safely disclose an invention to, for example, an outside consultant or even a company that might be interested in licensing or assigning the invention, under a confidentiality agreement. Such a disclosure would not constitute publication or public disclosure.

2.5. First-to-File or First-to-Invent

In every nation except the United States and the Philippines, if more than one inventor comes up with the same discovery, the patent goes to the first to file a patent application (the first-to-file system). In the United States and Philippines, it is the first to invent who gets the patent; that is, if two or more inventors come up with the same invention and submit patent applications claiming that invention, they get to prove through their laboratory notebooks and other documentation who first conceived the idea and reduced it to practice.

Clearly, there are arguments for and against each system. The first-to-invent seems more just, but of course causes litigation to settle the issue, whereas the first-to-file system is clean, simple, and efficient, and it is surely not too great an imposition on an inventor to insist that the patent application be filed quickly after the invention.

2.6. The Rights of a Patent Owner

A patent owner has the right to exclude others from making, using, selling, or importing the invention for the duration of the patent. It is important to remember that a patent does not necessarily give the patent owner the right to practice his or her invention, because by doing so, the inventor may infringe someone else's patent or violate some other law or regulation. As a simple example, a perfectly valid patent on a new drug does not permit the inventor to sell the drug; the drug, patented or not, is still subject to the normal drug approval process.

The key point is that nobody else can use the invention without the patent owner's permission. The patentee (patent owner) may assign (sell, transfer) the patent rights to another (e.g., the PCR patents *[4,5]*, now assigned to Roche *[6–9]*), or may retain the rights and license them to others so that they can use the invention (e.g., the Cohen-Boyer patent *[18,20,92]*).

Once a patent has died anyone can make, use, sell, or import the invention without the patentee's authorization; the invention is said to be in the "public domain" at that point, and the patent owner has no rights once the patent term has expired (e.g., the Cohen-Boyer patent *[18]*), which expired in 1997 *[92]*).

2.7. Patenting Animals

An issue that biotechnology has brought to the fore in recent years is the patents of life forms, from microorganisms to higher animals. The patenting of living microorganisms is now generally accepted throughout the world, but the patenting of higher animals has caused great controversy.

The United States led the way in this area, from the first grant of a patent for a bacterium in 1980, following the Supreme Court's ruling in *Diamond v. Chakrabarty (14,17)*. Chakrabarty, a microbiologist, had in the early 1970s genetically engineered a *Pseudomonas* bacterium capable of breaking down oil, and it was hoped that the bacterium could be used in cleaning up oil spills. The Supreme Court held that under US patent law, a modified bacterium qualified because it was not a product of nature but was "man made" and was patentable.

Again taking the lead, in 1988 the US patent office granted a patent on the "Harvard Oncomouse" *(97–99)*, despite opposition (*see* **refs. *64,100,101***). The Oncomouse is a transgenic mouse carrying an activated mouse oncogene (*myc* plus DNA from the mouse mammary tumor virus) *(102,103)* and has a greatly increased susceptibility to malignant breast tumors during pregnancy *(99)*. It obviously has potential utility as a cancer model and testing system for anti-cancer drugs. Since then, although not quite routine, US patents have been issued on several other transgenic animals *(104)*. In Europe there has been much more opposition, both by animal rights activists *(63,105)* and the European Patent Office *(64,106)*.

3. Copyright

3.1. Protection for Creative Works

Copyright is created automatically in any creative work (e.g., fiction, non-fiction, photographs, figures, paintings, designs, patterns, sculptures) as soon as it is fixed in a tangible medium (e.g., on paper, film, canvas, or on a hard or floppy disk) and is essentially a legal right of the author to control copying of the work once it leaves the author's possession. Copyright does not protect the author's idea(s), only the form of words used to express the idea(s). Thus, someone can take an author's idea, and rewrite it, and there is no copyright violation.

Copyright law goes back to 1710 with the Statute of Anne in England and to 1790 in the United States (and there is a copyright clause in the US Constitution [Article I, Section 8], though the concept that a writer "owned" his work goes back much further than that [*see* **refs.** *107–111*). Because all scientists get to be authors at some stage, this is another important issue. Additionally, we constantly rely on the published work of others, in the form of laboratory manuals and journal articles.

A copyright does not need to be registered, unlike a patent, although it is advisable to do so to gain the fullest protection of the law. However, the protection afforded is much shallower. Independent creation is a perfect defense to a charge of copyright infringement, whereas in patent law, the first-to-invent (in the United States or the Philippines) or the first-to-file will get the patent—and the right to exclude others from practicing the invention—*even if* other inventors independently conceived the same invention.

3.2. Scientific Journals and Books

Journals and book publishers usually ask for the transfer of copyright from the author to the journal or publisher because by having all the copyrights, monitoring and enforcement of rights becomes sensible. Alternatively, publishers can—by contract—hire writers to write specific works; any such work is a "work made for hire" and the copyright belongs to the publisher. The chapters in this book were works made for hire, and so the copyright is owned by Humana Press.

Very few authors are ever going to scan the world literature constantly looking for copyright infringements, whereas publishers to which copyrights have been assigned and groups of such publishers can sensibly do so. Likewise, it made sense for journal publishers to band together to form the Copyright Clearance Center (CCC), whereas individual authors could not sensibly do so. The CCC is a centralized clearing house set up in the United States in 1977 by publishers to sell licenses to institutions and to collect copyright fees from libraries and document services for copies made of member publishers' works. Canada has introduced a similar scheme, Cancopy *(112)*.

3.3. The Texaco Case

The now famous *Texaco* case *(113,114)* cannot go unmentioned; in *Texaco*, the US Court of Appeals for the Second Circuit held that a Texaco researcher violated US copyright law by copying several articles from a journal and distributing them to colleagues at Texaco *(113)*. The Court's ruling was not quite as simple or as massively broad as it sounds, and the Court specifically refused to address the situation in which an individual copied articles for his or her own use; academics and researchers should not necessarily be quaking in their boots!

The ruling was confined to its facts, where Texaco (a large, wealthy corporation) had purchased a single copy of the journal from the publisher for its library and then systematically made multiple copies of articles for its employees, instead of paying for multiple subscriptions to the journal *(113)*. Additionally, Texaco had not purchased a license from the CCC, as many corporations and institutions had. The case was actually settled before the final decision was issued *(115)*; Texaco, without admitting fault, paid a large settlement, including retroactive license fees to the CCC *(115)*.

4. Trademarks

4.1. Introduction

A trademark is any symbol, word or series of words, logo, or other marking that indicates the source of a product or service. In the laboratory there are many examples; take your New England Biolabs® restriction enzymes from your StrataCooler® II, purify RNA with the RNeasy® kit, use your Nikon® microscope to inspect your cells, which you obtained from ATCC®, take your references from Reference Manager®, check Current Contents® each week, and it apparent that trademarks are everywhere. Outside the laboratory, the ubiquitous McDonald's golden arches, Prudential's rock, and Coca Cola's name, stylized font, and the shape of their glass bottles are obvious examples.

4.2. Trademarks and Service Marks

Strictly, trademarks apply only to products; service marks indicate services. However, "trademark" is used generically to cover both. If you open a recent edition of *Science* and look at the advertisements, you will see, for example, Stratagene®'s PathDetect™ in vivo signal transduction system. If you open a recent edition of *Business Week*, you will see Transamerica's pyramid logo (the shape of the top of their landmark office building in San Francisco), itself a registered trademark, and their slogan "The People in the Pyramid are Working for You.℠" Stratagene® indicates that Stratagene is a registered trademark, as is the Transamerica pyramid logo and PathDetect™ indicates that PathDetect is considered a trademark by Stratagene, but that it has not (yet) been registered (with the US Patent and Trademark Office) or that its registration has not (yet) been approved. Transamerica's slogan is a service mark; their service is providing insurance.

Unlike patents and copyrights, which are both based on creative products, a trademark is based on use. Unlike patents or copyrights, a trademark can be lost by not using it; there is no such obligation on a patentee who can simply sit back and prevent anyone from using his or her invention. Also, unlike trademarks and patents, trademarks can have an indefinite lifespan. Trademarks do not have to be registered; however if they are it simplifies some issues should litigation ever arise.

4.3. Trademark Litigation

It is fair to say that trademark litigation has attracted much less attention than patent disputes in recent years, but there have been several examples relating to drugs and medical services and the misuse or misappropriation of trademarks or service marks. On several occasions the renowned Mayo Clinic of Rochester, MN, has had to defend its name, literally *(116)*. The Mayo Foundation holds three trademarks: "Mayo," "Mayo Clinic," and the familiar tripleshield logo *(116)*. The Supreme Court of Minnesota held that a man whose first name was Mayo could not sell drugs through his company, "Mayo's Drug and Cosmetic Company," because there was a reasonable likelihood of confusion on the part of the public (presumably *exactly* what Mr. Mayo L. Priebe, Sr. intended!) between Mayo's Drug and the Mayo Clinic and Hospital, with the obvious inference that products sold by Mayo's Drug came with some stamp of approval from the institution *(117)*.

4.4. Scientific Trademark Examples

4.4.1. Bristol-Myers Squibb and Taxol®

A trademark issue that has been discussed in the scientific press of late is Bristol-Myers Squibb's claim to the word "Taxol" as the name of its anticancer drug *(118–120)*. The compound in question is the antileukemia drug extracted from the bark of the Pacific yew *(121)*, for which in a blaze of publicity, a total synthesis was reported several years ago *(122)*. Bristol-Myers Squibb does now own the trademark Taxol®, and the compound in question should now be referred to as paclitaxel *(118)*.

4.4.2. Bayer and Aspirin

Another example of a trademark recently in the news concerns Bayer and aspirin *(123,124)*. Aspirin was synthesized by Felix Hoffmann at Bayer in 1897. Following the expiration of the US patent in 1917, the company sought to protect its drug's name with the trademark Aspirin. The US Patent & Trademark Office canceled Bayer's trademark on aspirin in 1918 *(124)*, though the company maintained the name as a trademark in many other countries. Sterling Drug, Inc. purchased the right to use the name in the US in the 1920s, and in 1994, Bayer's US affiliate, Miles, Inc., bought Sterling Winthrop's over-the-counter drug business, including the name *(123,125)*, returning the name to Bayer.

5. Summary

Intellectual property, and the protection of ideas and the written expression of ideas, should be of concern to all scientists. We constantly use copyrighted journals and laboratory manuals, trademarked products, and patented processes. Additionally as authors, we acquire and then typically transfer copyright in our work to journals and book publishers. Scientists working outside academia are generally required to transfer all inventions made in the course of their employment to their employer. Hopefully, this brief introduction to intellectual property will heighten awareness and stimulate the reader to delve deeper into the subject.

References

1. Marshall, P. (1997) Guarding the wealth of nations. Intellectual property, copyright, and international trade and relations. *Wilson Quart.* **21,** 64–100.
2. *Coca-Cola Bottling Co. of Shreveport, Inc. v. The Coca-Cola Co.*, 563 F.Supp. 1122 (D.Del. 1983).
3. *Coca-Cola Bottling Co. of Shreveport, Inc. v. The Coca-Cola Co.*, 107 F.Supp. 288 (D.Del. 1985).
4. US Patent No. 4,683,195. Process for amplifying, detecting, and/or cloning nucleic acid sequences.
5. US Patent No. 4,683,202. Process for amplifying nucleic acid sequences.
6. Hoffman, M. (1992) Roche eases PCR restrictions. *Science* **255,** 528.
7. Dickson, D. (1993) Licenses sought from PCR users in Britain. *Nature* **361,** 291.
8. Barinaga, M. (1995) Scientists named in PCR suit. *Science* **268,** 1273,1274.
9. Cohen, J. (1997) May I see your license, please? PCR patent tangle slows quick assay of HIV levels. *Science* **276,** 1488–1491.
10. *Teets v. Chromalloy Gas Turbine Corp.*, 83 F.3d 403 (Fed. Cir. 1996).
11. Fox, J. L. (1984) Gene splicers square off in patent courts. *Science* **234,** 584–586.
12. Blecher, M. (1988) Dominating patents: a view from the bridge. *Clin. Chem.* **34,** 1705–1709.
13. Sugawara, S. (1991) Drug patent race heads to the bench. *Washington Post*, Sept. 15, p. H1.
14. Wade, N. (1980) Supreme Court hears argument on patenting life forms. *Science* **208,** 31,32.
15. Wade, N. (1980) Court says lab-made life can be patented. *Science* **208,** 1445.
16. Greenhouse, L. (1980) Science may patent new forms of life, justices rule, 5 to 4: dispute on bacteria; decision assists industry in bioengineering in a variety of projects. *The New York Times*, June 16, p. A1.
17. *Diamond v. Chakrabarty*, 447 U.S. 303 (1980).
18. US Patent No. 4,237,224. Process for producing biologically functional molecular chimeras.
19. Dickson, D. (1980) Stanford and UCLA [sic; UCSF] plasmid patent. *Nature* **288,** 527,528.

20. Beardsley, T. (1984) Cohen-Boyer patent finally confirmed. *Nature* **311**, 3.
21. US Patent No. 4,366,246. Method for microbial polypeptide expression.
22. Ezzell, C. (1987) Patent Office decision puts Genentech out in front. *Nature* **330**, 97.
23. Norman, C. (1985) Patent dispute divides AIDS researchers. *Science* **230**, 640–642.
24. Barnes, D. M. (1987) AIDS patent dispute settled. *Science* **236**, 17.
25. Ezzell, C. (1988) Genentech patent. *Nature* **335**, 105.
26. Ezzell, C. (1988) Genentech gets patent protection for tissue plasminogen activator. *Nature* **333**, 790.
27. Swinbanks, D. (1988) Problems over TPA patent for Genentech in Japan. *Nature* **333**, 587.
28. Swinbanks, D. (1994) Single amino-acid makes a big difference in patent court. *Nature* **372**, 123.
29. Johnston, K. (1987) TPA patent battle continues in court. *Nature* **327**, 546.
30. Gershon, D. (1990) Genentech wins round two. *Nature* **344**, 692.
31. Ezzell, C. (1987) Judge confirms injunction in sandwich assay patent suit. *Nature* **326**, 532.
32. Greene, H. E., Jr. and Duft, B. J. (1990) Disputes over monoclonal antibodies. *Nature* **347**, 117,118.
33. *Hybritech, Inc. v. Monoclonal Antibodies, Inc.*, 802 F.2d 1367 (Fed.Cir. 1986)
34. US Patent No. 4,873,191. Genetic transformation of zygotes.
35. McGourty, C. (1989) Microinjection patent granted. *Nature* **341**, 681.
36. Anonymous (1989) DNX gains rights to fundamental patent for DNA microinjection. *Biotechnology Newswatch* **9**, 1.
37. Egrie, J. (1990) The cloning and production of recombinant human erythropoietin. *Pharmacotherapy* **10**, 3S–8S.
38. Gershon, D. (1990) Amgen plays for time. *Nature* **344**, 800.
39. Gershon, D. (1990) EPO licensing talks break down. *Nature* **343**, 500.
40. *Amgen, Inc. v. Chugai Pharmaceutical Co. Ltd.*, 13 U.S.P.Q.2d 1737 (D.Mass. 1990).
41. *Amgen, Inc. v. Chugai Pharmaceutical Co. Ltd.*, 927 F.2d 1200 (Fed.Cir. 1991).
42. US Patent No. 4,703,008. DNA sequences encoding erythropoietin.
43. US Patent No. 4,677,195. Homogeneous erythropoietin.
44. Gershon, D. (1990) Market machinations. *Nature* **344**, 800.
45. Rotman, D. (1991) Xoma wins patent battle. *Chemical Week*, Nov. 6, p. 9.
46. Shnabel, J. (1992) The magic bullet that burst the bubble; monoclonal antibodies against Gram-negative sepsis. *New Scientist* **135**, 31–35.
47. Barnum, A. (1992) Xoma, Centocor settle biotech patent battle. *San Francisco Chronicle*, July 30, p. E1.
48. Anonymous (1991) Centocor infringes Xoma sepsis patent. *Biotech. Patent News* **5**, 1–2.
49. Stone, R. (1994) Search for sepsis drugs goes on despite failures. *Science* **264**, 365–367.

50. Anderson, C. (1993) Court favors drug "concept" over proof. *Science* **261**, 545.
51. Kolata, G. (1987) Imminent marketing of AZT raises problems; toxicity. *Science* **235**, 1462,1463.
52. Palca, J. (1991) Who found AZT works for AIDS? Patent dispute between the National Institutes of Health and Burroughs Wellcome. *Science* **251**, 1554.
53. Palca, J. (1991) Monopoly patents on AZT challenged. *Science* **252**, 1369.
54. Greenhouse, L. (1996) Justices reject challenge of patent for AIDS drug. *The New York Times*, Jan. 17, p. A14.
55. Ackiron, E. (1991) Patents for critical pharmaceuticals; the AZT case. *Am. J. Law Med.* **17**, 145–155.
56. Barinaga, M. (1991) Biotech nightmare: does Cetus own PCR? *Science* **251**, 739,740.
57. Barinaga, M. (1991) And the winner: Cetus does own PCR. *Science* **251**, 1174.
58. Schaefer, E. (1991) Cetus retains PCR patents. *Nature* **350**, 6.
59. *E.I. Du Pont de Nemours & Co. v. Cetus Corp.*, 19 U.S.P.Q.2d 1174 (N.D.Cal. 1990).
60. Dickman, S. (1989) Oncomouse seeks European protection. *Nature* **340**, 85.
61. Dickman, S. (1990) Mouse patent a step closer. *Nature* **347**, 606.
62. Dickson, D. (1989) No patent for Harvard's mouse? *Science* **243**, 1003.
63. Abbott, A. (1993) Protestors target European animal patents. *Nature* **361**, 103.
64. Seide, R. K. and Giaccio, A. (1995) Patenting animals. *Chem. Industry* **16**, 656–658.
65. Editorial (1992) Gene patents. *Nature* **359**, 348.
66. Anderson, C. (1992) NIH cDNA patent rejected: backers want to amend law. *Nature* **359**, 263.
67. Sgaramella, V. (1993) Lawyers' delight and geneticists' nightmares: at forty, the double helix shows some wrinkles. *Gene* **135**, 299–302.
68. Zinder, N. D. (1993) Patenting cDNA 1993: efforts and happenings. *Gene* **135**, 295–298.
69. Roberts, L. (1992) Top HHS lawyer seeks to block NIH. *Science* **258**, 209–210.
70. Healy, B. (1992) Special report on gene patenting. *New Engl. J. Med.* **327**, 664–668.
71. Kiley, T. D. (1992) Patents on random complementary DNA fragments. *Science* **257**, 915–918.
72. Adler, R. G. (1992) Genome research: fulfilling the public's expectations for knowledge and commercialization. *Science* **257**, 908–914.
73. Eisenberg, R. S. (1992) Genes, patents, and product development. *Science* **257**, 903–908.
74. Looney, B. (1994) Should genes be patented? The gene patenting controversy: legal, ethical, and policy foundations of an international agreement. *Law Policy Intl. Bus.* **26**, 231–272.
75. Lech, K. F. (1993) Human genes without functions: biotechnology tests the patent utility standard. *Suffolk Univ. Law Rev.* **27**, 1631–1660.

76. Eisenberg, R. S. and Merges, R. P. (1995) Opinion letter as to the patentability of certain inventions associated with the identification of partial cDNA sequences. *AIPLA Q. J.* **23**, 1–52.

77. Riley, P. J. (1994) Patenting Dr. Venter's genetic findings: Is the National Institutes of Health creating hurdles or clearing the path for biotechnology's voyage into the twenty-first century? *J. Contemp. Health Law Policy* **10**, 309–326.

78. Aldhous, P. (1993) PCR enzyme patent challenged. *Science* **260**, 486.

79. Abbott, A. (1996) Roche faces charges over Taq patent claim. *Nature* **382**, 660.

80. Dickson, D. (1994) Promega files court challenge to Roche's Taq enzyme patent. *Nature* **372**, 714.

81. Slind-Flor, V. (1995) Chiron challenged on hepatitis-C patent. *Science* **267**, 23.

82. *Genentech, Inc. v. Chiron Corp.*, 112 F.3d 495 (Fed.Cir. 1997).

83. Anonymous (1997) Patent law. *BioPharm*, May 1997, p. 12.

84. *Novo Nordisk of North America, Inc. v. Genentech, Inc.*, 77 F.3d 1364 (Fed.Cir. 1996).

85. *Genentech, Inc. v. Novo Nordisk, A/S*, 108 F.3d 1361 (Fed.Cir. 1997).

86. Marx, J. (1996) A second breast cancer susceptibility gene found; BRCA2. *Science* **271**, 30.

87. Marshall, E. (1997) The battle of BRCA1 goes to court; BRCA2 may be next. *Science* **278**, 1874.

88. Köhler, G. and Milstein, C. (1975) Continuous cultures of fused cells secreting antibodies of predefined specificity. *Nature* **256**, 495–497.

89. Uhr, J. W. (1984) The 1984 Nobel Prize in medicine. *Science* **226**, 1025–1028.

90. Köhler, G. (1984) Derivation and diversification of monoclonal antibodies. *Scand. J. Immunol.* **37**, 117–129.

91. Cohen, S. N., Chang, A. C. Y., Boyer, H. W., and Helling, R. B. (1993) Construction of biologically functional bacterial plasmids in vitro. *Proc. Natl. Acad. Sci. USA* **70**, 3240–3244.

92. Lehrman, S. (1993) Stanford seeks life after Cohen-Boyer patent expires. *Nature* **363**, 574.

93. Anonymous (1990) Stanford updates bottom lines on Cohen-Boyer patent users. *Biotech. Newswatch* **10**, 8.

94. US Patent No. 4,571,421. Mammalian gene for microbial expression.

95. Blumenthal, D., Campbell, E. G., Anderson, M. S., Causino, N., and Louis, K. S. (1997) Withholding research results in academic life science. Evidence from a national survey of faculty. *JAMA* **277**, 1224–1228.

96. Windman, M. (1996) Commercial interests delay publication. *Nature* **379**, 574.

97. US Patent No. 4,736,866. Transgenic non-human mammals.

98. Anderson, A. (1987) Animal patent dispute out in the open at congressional hearings. *Nature* **327**, 546.

99. Booth, W. (1988) Animals of invention. *Science* **240**, 718.

100. Hooper, C. (1987) Patenting brave new animals: religion, economics, biotech meet in Capitol Hill battle. *United Press Intl. Newswire*, Aug. 15, 1987.

101. Stone, R. (1995) Religious leaders oppose patenting genes and animals. *Science* **268,** 1126.
102. Stewart, T. A., Pattengale, P. K., and Leder, P. (1984) Spontaneous mammary adenocarcinomas in transgenic mice that carry and express MTV/myc fusion genes. *Cell* **38,** 627–637.
103. Leder, A., Pattengale, P. K., Kuo, A., Stewart, T. A., and Leder, P. (1986) Consequences of widespread deregulation of the c-myc gene in transgenic mice; multiple neoplasms and normal development. *Cell* **45,** 485–495.
104. Lehrman, S. (1993) Ruling narrows US view of animal patents. *Nature* **361,** 103.
105. Bizley, R. E. (1991) Patenting animals in Europe. *Biotechnology* **9,** 619–622.
106. Editorial (1996) One way out of a patent quagmire. *Nature* **381,** 175.
107. Bunnin, B. (1985) Protecting intellectual property: copyright for journal authors and conference speakers. *Birth* **12(suppl. 3)** 29–31.
108. Liedes, J. (1997) Copyright: evolution, not revolution. *Science* **276,** 223–225.
109. Dobkin, D. S. (1979) Copyright law undergoes major face-lift. *JAMA* **241,** 1019,1020.
110. Henry, N. L. (1974) Copyright: its adequacy in technological societies. *Science* **186,** 993–1004.
111. Frisse, M. E. and Tolva, J. N. (1996) The commerce of ideas: copyright in the digital era. *Acad. Med.* **71,** 45–53.
112. Vardy, J. (1997) Copyright move on photocopies will cost banks and lawyers dear. *Financial Post,* May 20, p. 1.
113. *American Geophysical Union v. Texaco, Inc.,* 60 F.3d 913 (2d Cir. 1995).
114. National Conference of Lawyers and Scientists (1995) How does the Texaco case affect photocopying by scientists? *Science* **270,** 1450,1451.
115. Lawler, A. (1995) Texaco offers to settle copyright case. *Science* **268,** 1127.
116. Helminski, F. (1993) Use and abuse of medical service marks. *Mayo Clin. Proc.* **68,** 1212,1213.
117. *Mayo Clinic v. Mayo's Drug and Cosmetic, Inc.,* 113 N.W.2d 852 (Minn. 1962).
118. Editorial (1995) Names for hi-jacking. *Nature* **373,** 370.
119. Chesnoff, S. (1995) The use of Taxol as a trademark. *Nature* **374,** 208.
120. Khan, N.U. (1995) Taxol trademark. *Nature* **374,** 400.
121. Wani, M. C., Taylor, H. L., Wall, M. E., Coggon, P., and McPhail, A. T. (1971) Plant anti-tumor agents. VI. The isolation and structure of Taxol. A novel anti-leukemic and anti-tumor agent from Taxus brevifolia. *J. Am. Chem. Soc.* **93,** 2325–2327.
122. Nicolaou, K. C., Liu, J. J., Ueno, H., Nantermet, P. G., Guy, R. K., Claiborne, C. F., Renaud, J., Couladouros, E. A., Paulvannan, K., and Sorensen, E. J. (1994) Total synthesis of Taxol. *Nature* **367,** 630–634.
123. Jack, D. B. (1997) One hundred years of aspirin. *Lancet* **350,** 437–439.
124. *Bayer Co., Inc. v. United Drug Co.,* 272 F. 505 (S.D.N.Y. 1921).
125. Wood, A. (1997) New recognition for an old name. *Chemical Week,* Sept. 10, 1997, p. 51.

16

From Laboratory to Clinic

The Story of CAMPATH-1

Geoff Hale and Herman Waldmann

1. Introduction

In 1890 it was shown that resistance to diphtheria toxin could be transferred from one animal to another by transfer of serum *(1)*. From this discovery, passive antibody therapy was developed as an effective treatment for infectious diseases and for neutralization of toxins, and continues to be used to this day. Meanwhile, there have been continued efforts to use antibodies for cancer therapy, starting with the pioneering work of Hericourt and Richet in 1895 *(2)*, which was the forerunner of the "magic bullet" concept. However, all of the early work on tumor therapy led ultimately to disappointment *(3)*. The problems were readily acknowledged, i.e., lack of specificity and reproducibility, lack of purity, and the xenogeneic immune response. Developments over the past 20 years, as described throughout this book, have effectively overcome all of these technical problems, often in very ingenious ways. The difficulty we have now is different. There are just too many potential new antibody-based treatments for them all to be properly evaluated in the clinic. Many will still fail because of factors that are hard to predict from experiments: unexpected toxicity, biological heterogeneity of the target disease, or lack of access to the appropriate tissue.

The unfortunate reality is that clinical development of new drugs is almost entirely in the hands of the pharmaceutical industry, where many factors other than strictly scientific/clinical ones influence the decision to develop a particular product. These include the availability of patent protection, the potential size of the market, the impact of new drug regulations, and the current mood of

From: *Methods in Molecular Medicine, Vol. 40: Diagnostic and Therapeutic Antibodies*
Edited by: A. J. T. George and C. E. Urch © Humana Press Inc., Totowa, NJ

investors. Profitability is the overriding concern and is an essential ingredient of success in our society. However, we do not think it is enough for academic scientists to patent a new technology, license it on to industry, and sit back with large upfront payments. Physicians and their patients are cut out of the decision process and become essentially commodities to be bought or discarded during the clinical trials. A better way is for scientists, physicians, patients, industry, and government to work together, each recognizing the different priorities of the other, but each contributing to the decision process. Biological therapies will be costly and they do carry risks of introducing dangerous new diseases. We all have an interest in their effective application.

Here we will tell the story of CAMPATH-1, just one of many hundreds of monoclonal antibodies (mAbs) developed for therapy. It illustrates several aspects of practical development that might apply to other projects and perhaps the reader will be able to avoid the pitfalls that we encountered. CAMPATH-1 was one of the first therapeutic mAbs to be assigned for commercial development and it was licensed to one of the best equipped UK biotech companies of the time. However, were it not for the dedication of teams of clinicians worldwide, who continued to pursue independent trials with our academic group, we are convinced that it would by now have disappeared without trace.

2. A Search for Efficient Complement Activation

The original impetus for development of CAMPATH-1 came from bone marrow transplantation. Since mAb technology was invented by immunologists, it was not surprising that they looked to immunological diseases for some of the first applications. Graft-versus-host disease (GvHD) was a good target, since it was known to be caused by T cells, which inevitably contaminated donor bone marrow. If the T cells were removed before transplantation, GvHD and its potentially lethal effects could be eliminated. Monoclonal antibodies specific for T-cell antigens were discovered by several groups in the late 1970s and early 1980s. Antibodies alone are not usually toxic to cells, and they needed to be used with a second reagent to kill or separate the unwanted T cells (4,5). An obvious choice was complement, well known as the natural effector arm of humoral immunity. However, unlike polyclonal antisera, the majority of mAbs were poor at activating complement and it was particularly difficult to kill human cells with human complement. Now we know that there are several reasons: the choice of antibody isotype, the limited density of most cell-surface antigens, the propensity of some antigens to patch and cap, and the presence of cell-surface inhibitors of complement, like decay-accelerating factor and CD59. At the time, these problems were partly overcome using heterologous serum (e.g., from rabbit) as a source of the complement because the human cell-surface inhibitors failed to inactivate the heterologous complement cascade. However, this introduced an unwanted source of heterogeneity and it was difficult to procure reliable and nontoxic batches of rabbit serum. Accordingly, our group continued to search for an antibody that would activate human complement, bind to T cells, and spare stem cells. The goal was "operational" specificity, not necessarily lineage restricted; a novel concept at the time.

3. The First CD52 Antibodies

In 1979, Herman immunized a rat with human lymphocytes and carried out a fusion that was to yield an amazing diversity of antibodies. The choice of rats rather than mice for the fusion was made for a number of technical reasons (*6*), but it turned out to be truly serendipitous. Antibodies were identified by a range of assays carried out by many team members, and many of the reagents discovered have been used in basic research and human therapy. Several antibodies were found that lysed T cells with human complement. At this point Geoff joined the lab, a young protein chemist given the task of characterizing the structure of these new antigens—a task in which he was singularly unsuccessful for many years. It turned out that all of the lytic antibodies recognized the same antigen, which we now know as CD52. The majority of other antibodies from the fusion were rat IgG2a or IgG2b, but the CD52 antibodies were mostly IgM, with one IgG2c and one IgG2a (YTH34.5). There is a strong isotype bias in the rat antibody response; IgG2a and IgG2b are commonly made against surface protein antigens, IgG1 against soluble protein antigens, and IgM or IgG2c against T-cell-independent antigens (which we originally equated with carbohydrates, incorrectly in this case). Since then, other IgM and IgG2c CD52 antibodies have been obtained but the YTH34.5 clone is still unique. It later proved to be absolutely crucial for clinical success. However, one of the IgM antibodies (clone YTH66.9, CAMPATH-1M) was originally chosen because it activated complement more efficiently and gave virtually complete elimination of T cells in vitro.

At that time our lab was fortunate to have two postdocs from the leading centers of progenitor cell biology: Sue Watt from Don Metcalf's lab in Melbourne and Trang Hoang from Norman Iscove's lab in Lausanne. Using their respective culture systems, we showed that the CAMPATH-1 antigen was not expressed on bone marrow colony-forming cells (*7,8*). CAMPATH-1 antibodies crossreacted with lymphocytes from nonhuman primates and safety studies were initiated in baboons and cynomolgus monkeys (*8,9*). It was not until the first animals were injected that we realized that the antigen was also expressed on the red cells. There was hemagglutination and hematuria, but animals remained well! Further studies showed that the red-cell antigen is polymorphic, expressed in only some monkeys, whereas it is always found on lymphocytes; a fortunate situation that allowed the safety studies to proceed but is still not explained. Screening of all available human blood groups by our colleagues in the transfusion center showed that the CD52 antigen is never expressed on human red cells. At the same time David Swirsky working with Frank Hayhoe in the Hematology Department next door to us treated a patient suffering from end stage non-Hodgkin's lymphoma (9). The clinical effect was minimal, just like all the other mAbs being tested at that time. There was temporary clearance of tumor cells from blood, accompanied by consumption of complement, but 24 h after each dose the cells bounced back. Nevertheless, the treatment was well tolerated and we felt that the stage was set for the first trial in bone marrow transplantation. With high hopes, we submitted our first paper describing this new specificity and its potential clinical application (7). We were greatly disappointed when it was comprehensively rejected, first by the *Journal of Experimental Medicine* and then by *Blood*. It was only by a personal plea from Don Metcalf that the editors of *Blood* were persuaded to change their minds.

4. No Patent, but BTG Acquires the Rights

Our work had been funded by the UK Medical Research Council (MRC). In those days, universities had no organization for commercial exploitation of inventions, but the MRC had a commitment to pass any discoveries by their employees to the National Research and Development Council (NRDC)—a government organization devoted to technical transfer. NRDC is famous for its decision when offered the pioneering discovery of Köhler and Milstein: "It is certainly difficult for us to identify any immediate practical applications which could be pursued as a commercial venture." This probably did more than anything else to facilitate the widespread use of mAbs, but no doubt the MRC regrets the untold millions of lost royalties! Although we were not bound by the rules for MRC employees, we felt that it was right to offer CAMPATH-1 to NRDC (now renamed "British Technology Group", BTG) before the work was published. In a recapitulation of the earlier decision, BTG decided that there was no need to patent the CAMPATH-1 specificity or its proposed application. However, they did acquire all of the rights to the CAMPATH-1 cell lines. We were naive about legal agreements and did not appreciate the gulf between "assignment" and "licence." We simply imagined that a government organization set up to exploit British discoveries was the obvious way forward. There was no alternative. Fortunately we did obtain a clause allowing us to continue our own academic and clinical research with the cell lines that now belonged to BTG.

5. Bone Marrow Transplants

The first bone marrow transplant using CAMPATH-1M for T-cell depletion was carried out in 1982 at the Hammersmith hospital by Jill Hows and Ted Gordon-Smith. The outcome was a disaster from the point of view of our research plans, but the antibody treatment probably saved the life of the patient! The patient suffered from severe aplastic anemia—failure of the bone marrow, which could only be cured by a bone marrow transplant. This patient had no suitable HLA-matched sibling donor, so it was decided to try a transplant from an unrelated donor. Such transplants were very experimental at the time and it was realized that there would be a high risk of GvHD. Initial optimism on seeing the first signs of marrow recovery turned to a disappointment mixed with relief when it was found that the blood cells were solely of recipient type. Remarkably, the patient's own bone marrow had started to work again and the patient remains alive and well to this present day. Although the preclinical work had convinced us that stem cells should be spared, it was hard to explain the outcome, and the physicians, not unreasonably, called a halt to the clinical program. Now we realize that T-cell depletion increases the risk of graft rejection, which was already high in an unrelated transplant for a multiply-transfused patient suffering from anemia.

A chance meeting between Steve Cobbold and Shimon Slavin from the Hadassah hospital in Jerusalem, with some vital encouragement from Cesar Milstein, led to the next step. Shimon had been conducting experimental and clinical marrow transplantation for some years and realized that T-cell depletion was the most promising method to prevent GvHD, which was still the major clinical problem. He took the chance to evaluate CAMPATH-1M in a small series of patients transplanted from HLA-matched siblings. Although they all had poor prognosis leukemia, at least the risks of immunological complications were not so extreme. The successful results of this pilot study, published in the *Lancet* in 1984 *(10)*, were soon emulated by several other transplant groups in Europe, including teams in Ulm, Germany *(11)* and again at the Hammersmith hospital in London *(12)*. This led to the formation of the CAMPATH users group, a convivial and informal association of transplant centers worldwide, which was the prototype for many other clinical collaborations over the following 15 years.

CAMPATH-1M was remarkably effective at preventing GvHD, reducing the incidence from about 40 to 10% or less, but a new problem was seen—graft rejection—that now affected 15–20% of the patients and led to a number of fatalities *(13)*. This urgently needed to be tackled if there was to be any further progress. Since 1979, in parallel with the studies on antibodies against human cells, Steve Cobbold had been working to develop analogous antimouse antibodies to study transplantation in the laboratory. He found that certain rat mAbs, notably of the IgG2b isotype, could deplete mouse T cells very effectively *(14)*. There was no homolog of CAMPATH-1 but rat IgG2b anti-Thy-1 or anti-CD4 plus anti-CD8 could prevent GvHD, and with the same outcome as in humans—i.e., graft rejection. Reasoning that graft rejection was caused by residual host T cells that had been spared by the standard conditioning regimen, Steve pretreated the recipients with the same cocktail of depleting antibodies. This time the mice survived with full engraftment and no GvHD *(15)*. Obviously, we wanted an antibody that could produce a similar depletion in vivo in humans. The likely mechanism for cell depletion was antibody-dependent cell-mediated cytotoxicity (ADCC), mediated by antibody binding to Fc receptors on natural killer (NK) cells or macrophages. By screening a large panel of rat mAbs we found that the only isotype that gave effective ADCC with human cells was rat IgG2b *(16)*, but we had no CD52 antibodies of this isotype. However, it was known that hybrid myeloma cells could occasionally switch isotypes in vitro, in a parody of the normal physiological progress of class-switching. At the time Marianne Bruggeman had joined our lab and was starting to map the rat immunoglobulin gene locus *(17)*. She showed that the IgG2b constant region was downstream of IgG2a, so there was a chance that we could select a suitable mutant of YTH34.5. Rat hybrid myelomas are more stable than mouse and after screening about 20 million clones, Geoff found 34 that had switched to IgG2b *(18)*. Many of them showed a strong tendency to switch back again, but ultimately a stable clone was isolated. This was the antibody we named CAMPATH-1G.

6. Breakthrough in the Treatment of Leukemia

A clinical opportunity to test the new antibody was soon presented. A patient suffering from chronic lymphocytic leukemia (CLL) in prolymphocytic transformation had rapidly progressive disease that had responded only partially to chemotherapy *(19)*. His tumor cells were sensitive to CAMPATH-1G in vitro and so Martin Dyer and Frank Hayhoe decided to proceed with therapy. The initial results were beyond our most optimistic expectations. Two days of treatment with CAMPATH-1M gave only a very transient response, as before, but CAMPATH-1G immediately started to clear tumor cells. After 10 d of treatment, the blood and bone marrow were completely cleared and by normal criteria the patient was in complete remission. Many sincere prayers had been offered for this man and it did cross our minds that divine intervention might have overruled our efforts! Sadly, this was not to be the case; just a few days later, signs of florid central nervous system (CNS) disease became evident, and large numbers of tumor cells were discovered in the cerebrospinal fluid.

We knew that the antibody was unlikely to cross the blood–brain barrier, and so in a last effort, CAMPATH-1G was infused directly into the cerebrospinal fluid. This was well tolerated, but unfortunately had no impact on the tumor cells; the next day there were just as many and they were all uniformly coated with antibody. The patient did not respond to other therapies and died of progressive disease a few weeks later. Despite the tragic outcome, this single clinical experiment was very informative, showing the vital role of effector cells (absent from the CNS) and gave us hope that other patients could be successfully treated. It was a crucial turning point in the development of CAMPATH-1.

The second patient was another uniquely informative case (19). This patient was suffering from CLL and in 1985 had been treated with both YTH34.5 (the original IgG2a) and CAMPATH-1M. Both had only a very transient effect, just like other patients who had been treated with the IgM antibody alone. For 2 yr her disease had been held in check by chemotherapy, but now it had transformed and started to rapidly progress. The effects of CAMPATH-1G were again dramatic, resulting in a clearance of the majority of tumor cells from blood, but only a modest reduction of tumor infiltration in the bone marrow (from 97 to 87%). After a few weeks, tumor cells started to reappear in the blood, albeit at a much lower level than before. The patient had made an immune response against the rat mAb, which neutralized the CAMPATH-1G and limited its effectiveness. We knew that a more nearly human antibody was needed and by good fortune the technology to achieve this was being developed by Michael Neuberger and Greg Winter just across the road in the MRC Laboratory of Molecular Biology (20,21).

7. CAMPATH Licensed to Wellcome

But first, we should tell some of the other developments that had been occurring. BTG (London, UK) had been set up with the aim of enabling UK companies to exploit inventions from British academia. They started negotiations with Celltech (now Lonza, Slough, UK) in 1983 and continued for two years without reaching agreement. Then in 1985 CAMPATH-1M was licensed to Wellcome Biotech (Beckenham, UK), a small subsidiary of the giant Wellcome Foundation. We were pleased because Wellcome had an important reputation in production of biologicals, being the first company to establish a process using a continuously cultured mammalian cell line (production of α-interferon). Clinical trial material was produced and used in a small number of bone marrow transplants, but the outcome was never evaluated. CAMPATH-1G had much more promise for widespread applications: treatment of leukemia and lymphoma, as an immunosuppressive agent for organ transplantation (22) and perhaps autoimmune disease. Because the original YTH34.5 clone now belonged to BTG, we were obliged to hand over CAMPATH-1G as well, and this in turn was licensed to Wellcome Biotech. For the second time they started the process of preparing material for clinical trials.

8. The First Humanized Antibody

In 1986, Greg Winter and his team published the first humanized antibody created by genetically grafting the CDR regions from a mouse antibody (21). The antibody was directed against a chemical hapten, just a model with no therapeutic application, and in fact only the heavy chain was humanized. The obvious next step was to humanize a therapeutic antibody, and it seemed that CAMPATH-1G was an ideal choice. Lutz Riechmann, a molecular biologist in Greg Winter's lab, and Mike Clark, a postdoc who had joined our lab, worked together to engineer a whole set of chimeric and humanized antibodies (23). At the time we did not know how efficient would be the association of CDR-grafted variable regions. Also, we could not be sure which human isotype would have the best effector functions, although model studies by Marianne Bruggeman, Mike Clark, and Carol Bindon were showing IgG1 and IgG3 to be good candidates (24). Therefore, the project proceeded in painstaking steps, each intermediate construct being expressed and tested for activity. Ultimately a whole panel of chimeric and humanized antibodies were created of different IgG subclasses, which allowed Mike to confirm that IgG1 is the most potent for both activation of complement and ADCC. Subsequently many more variants have been created, including different IgG allotypes, null allotypes, domain shuffled, point mutants, and so forth, and they have allowed an ever more detailed dissection of the interaction of human IgG with physiological effector mechanisms. These rules have guided the design of all subsequent therapeutic antibodies.

Our team was hugely excited by these results and we felt this was a watershed in the development of the long-awaited "magic bullet." BTG did not agree. They were concerned that CAMPATH-1H might compromise the investment already made in CAMPATH-1G and expressed their disapproval of the collaboration with Winter's group in no uncertain terms! The only thing to do was to hand over CAMPATH-1H to them, especially since this seemed to offer the best route to commercial development via a simple extension of the existing licence to Wellcome Biotech. We had developed good relationships with the Wellcome Biotech team and felt confident that the senior management had a big commitment to the project. The company abandoned work on CAMPATH-1G and started in earnest to develop CAMPATH-1H, which they expected could reach a much wider market and perhaps break through the "billion dollar threshold" that big pharma are seeking for. Over the next seven years, Wellcome were to devote maybe £50 M to the development of CAMPATH-1H.

9. Remarkable Clinical Responses

The first patient to be treated with CAMPATH-1H was a woman suffering from non-Hodgkin's lymphoma in leukemic phase *(25)*. She had a very high white cell count, bone marrow completely packed with tumor cells, and gross splenomegaly. Six months previously, she had been treated with CAMPATH-1G, which gave a partial response but had been discontinued because of an allergic type of reaction. Only a small amount of CAMPATH-1H was available and it was administed in small doses (1–20 mg) over a period of 30 d (total 120 mg). Even to an untrained observer the response seems quite remarkable (**Fig. 1**). The spleen size was reduced from 4.5 to 0.6 kg. Tumor cells could no longer be found in the blood or bone marrow and they began to be replaced by normal blood elements. Analysis of DNA from a bone marrow aspirate before treatment showed just two restriction fragments corresponding to biallelic Ig rearrangement in the tumor clone. No germ-line fragments were visible at all. In marked contrast, a sample taken 28 d after the beginning of treatment showed only germ line genes and no sign of the Ig gene from the tumor (**Fig. 2**). This technique was sensitive to about 1 in 400 tumor cells. An even more encouraging observation was that a sample taken 11 wk after the beginning of antibody treatment still showed none of the tumor-specific fragments, but now there was a spread of new fragments, as would be expected for oligoclonal expansion of normal B cells. However, the patient still had a reservoir of tumor cells in the spleen and relapse was evident in the blood and bone marrow 3 mo after the beginning of treatment. She received a second course of treatment with CAMPATH-1H with similar response and then the spleen was surgically removed (which would have been impossible originally because of its large size). Histological examination of the spleen showed very many macrophages that appeared to have ingested tumor cells; presumably opsonized by the mAb. Fifteen months later the patient relapsed again and died shortly after. This patient had been unusual in that she had no bulky lymph nodes detectable by computed tomography (CT) scanning. Previous trials with CAMPATH-1G in 18 patients with a variety of lymphoid malignancies had shown that tumor cells could generally be cleared from blood, and frequently from bone marrow and spleen, but lymph nodes and extranodal masses were very rarely affected. We were therefore very interested to know whether the humanized antibody would be any better. The second patient to be treated with CAMPATH-1H was Ken Sander, a retired professor of electrical engineering. He had been newly diagnosed with stage IVA grade 1 non-Hodgkin's lymphoma, again with a high white cell count. Enlarged lymph nodes were visible by CT scan. Treatment with CAMPATH-1H induced a complete remission by clinical criteria, including regression of the lymph nodes. However, Bence-Jones protein

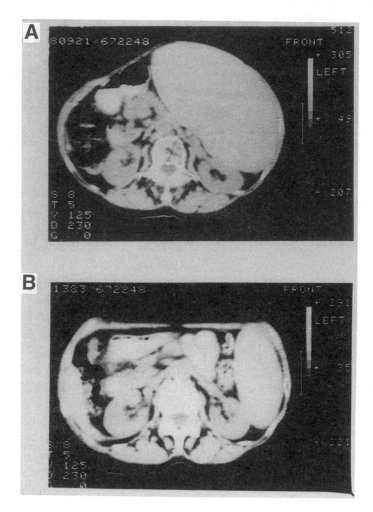

Fig. 1. Treatment of non-Hodgkin's lymphoma with CAMPATH-1H. CT scans showing the extent of splenomegaly before (**A**) and after (**B**) treatment (reproduced with permission from **ref. 25**).

(indicative of residual disease) was detectable within a few months and so he continued to be treated with conventional chemotherapy. During the coming years, Prof. Sander and his family engaged in many fund-raising activities to help our research—their commitment motivated us enormously.

10. New Center for Antibody Manufacture

The original rat mAbs had been prepared from ascitic fluid, crudely fractionated with ammonium sulfate. Quality control consisted of little more than

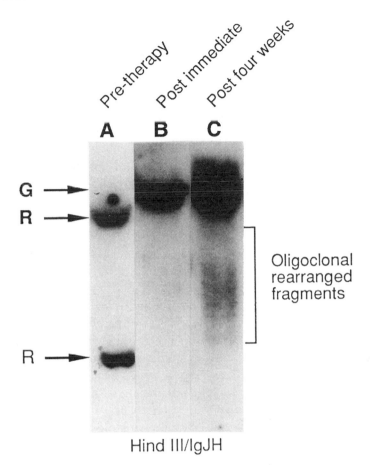

Fig. 2. Clearance of tumor cells demonstrated by Southern blotting to detect residual clonal lymphocytes following treatment with CAMPATH-1H. DNA was extracted from bone marrow mononuclear cells, digested with restriction endonuclease *Hind*III, and probed with an immunoglobulin J_H DNA probe. Lane A (before antibody therapy) shows biallelic IgJ_H rearrangement (R) with no detectable germline band (G). Lane B (directly after antibody therapy) shows germline fragment only. Lane C (4 wk later) shows oligoclonal rearranged fragments, interpreted as representing re-emergence of normal B cell progenitors. The tumour clone is still not visible (reproduced with permission from ref. 57.

measurement of binding activity and checks to ensure sterility and absence of pyrogens. In 1987 we had obtained a hollow-fiber cell-culture device (Acusyst-Jr) and started to produce CAMPATH-1G in the laboratory. This was the only way to produce CAMPATH-1H if we wanted to exclude contamination with rat proteins. There were other good reasons to avoid in vivo production—an immune response might be made against the engineered cell line with its human genes, there were concerns about the unnecessary use of animals, and the need to maintain a colony free of potential pathogens would become very onerous. However, it was becoming obvious that in an ordinary research lab we could not carry out the large amount of cell culture, processing, and quality control to make products for clinical trials. Quite aside from the scale and costs, the potential for cross-contamination was too great. Commercial production was not yet underway and there was a growing demand from our clinical colleagues to expand the scope of their trials. All of the production work was being done by one postdoctoral scientist, Jenny Phillips. In 1990, we set up a new group, the Therapeutic Antibody Centre (TAC), devoted entirely to antibody production for clinical research. We did not intend to engage in routine production or definitive clinical trials, which are more properly the role of pharmaceutical industry, but we wanted to liberate clinical research from the bottleneck of pilot scale production. Initially the TAC was based in the Blood Transfusion Centre at Cambridge, as a forerunner of what we believed to be a new and vital role for the Transfusion Service in the development of biological therapies (26). From the beginning the TAC had an emphasis on quality and with the appointment of Patrick Harrison as QA Manager we strove to meet the emerging European Community (EC) guidelines for control of manufacture of biological products. The TAC was funded by a special grant from the MRC together with a contribution from Wellcome Biotech in recognition of the growing collaboration between the commercial team and our research group. However, on the opening day of the new TAC we were told that Wellcome Biotech was to be wound up and reabsorbed into the parent company. We knew that they had suffered during a bruising patent battle with Genentech about tissue-plasminogen activator, and we were sad to hear this news, which meant that several of the senior management would shortly be moving elsewhere. Although CAMPATH-1H continued to be developed, and we enjoyed a productive relationship with many of the Wellcome scientists, the ultimate decisions were removed to a level beyond our access, and clinical trial protocols were developed with a focus on large markets, starting with non-Hodgkin's lymphoma and subsequently rheumatoid arthritis. It was unfortunate that these turned out to be two of the less favorable indications.

11. Treatment of Autoimmune Diseases

A couple of months after the TAC was opened, Martin Lockwood approached us about Nicola Cole, a young woman who was suffering from the effects of a very severe autoimmune disease, an unusual type of vasculitis characterized by T-cell infiltration of the blood vessels (27). Although Martin has

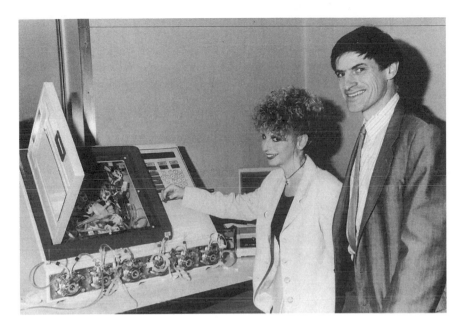

Fig. 3. Nicola Cole and Geoff Hale at the opening of the Therapeutic Antibody Centre, Oxford, December 1995.

great experience with this disease and had tried various standard and experimental therapies, there seemed to be nothing that would work. To our delight, a short course of treatment with CAMPATH-1H had a swift effect and soon it was possible to withdraw the palliative intravenous morphine. After a little while she was able to return to normal activities for the first time in several years. Over the course of the next 4 yr, she required further treatment with CAMPATH-1H on seven occasions. Each time the treatment resulted in a disease remission, but after three courses an anti-idiotype response was detected against the humanized antibody. Further courses were successfully given after temporarily removing the anti-id antibody by plasmapheresis, but eventually the titer became too high for this to be practicable. She was one of only a very few patients who have ever produced a strong antiglobulin response to CAMPATH-1H, but her antiserum has been of great value to us in defining the antigenic epitopes and guiding new developments designed to overcome this side effect. We learned a great deal from this single case, not least about the remarkable endurance and determination of patients who volunteer for clinical trials and put up with many interventions and investigations to provide data that will help others. It was a great pleasure for us when in 1995 Nicola came to open our new Therapeutic Antibody Centre in Oxford (**Fig. 3**).

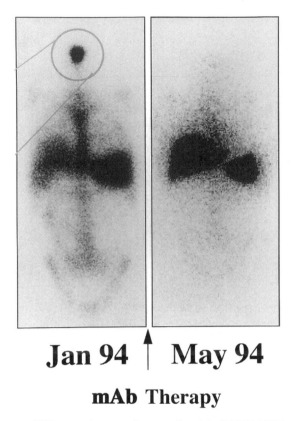

Jan 94 ↑ May 94

mAb Therapy

Fig. 4. Treatment of Wegener's granulomatosis with CAMPATH-1H. This patient suffered from severe erosion of sinus passages resulting from leukocyte infiltration, as shown by the whole body scanning after injection of ^{111}In-labeled leukocytes (area circled). Antibody treatment depleted the T cells that were driving the inflammatory process, and this resulted in a normal leukocyte scan and disease stabilization for at least 12 mo (reproduced with permission from **ref. 58**).

Since that first case, Martin Lockwood went on to treat more than 70 other patients, not only with the rare T-cell forms of vasculitis, but also including more classical cases (e.g., Wegener's granulomatosis) where autoantibodies are present *(28)*. Remissions were induced in virtually all patients, lasting from 2 mo to more than 2 yr, allowing a substantial reduction in the normal steroid therapy with obvious clinical benefits (**Fig. 4**). As a general rule, patients who relapsed have been successfully retreated and there have been few other examples of a significant antiglobulin response.

Other autoimmune diseases were potential candidates for lymphocyte depletion therapy and in 1991 John Isaacs, a clinical research fellow in our group, started a collaboration with Brian Hazleman to treat patients with rheumatoid arthritis *(29)*. Severe disease carries a substantial morbidity and mortality in addition to the pain and progressive disablement, so many investigators believe that radical treatment is justifiable if it could offer a long-term benefit. The initial clinical responses to CAMPATH-1H were quite impressive and because of the obvious large market for a new treatment, Wellcome soon started a full-scale program of clinical trials in Europe and the United States. However, the benefit proved to be relatively short-lived (about 3 mo) because a new and unpredicted problem emerged. Lymphocyte depletion by CAMPATH-1H was very profound and a single dose as low as 1 mg could reduce the blood lymphocyte count substantially. A typical course of treatment was 10 mg daily for 10 d and after this the T-cell count remained near zero for several weeks. B cells and NK cells returned to normal levels by 8 wk and CD8$^+$ T cells followed more slowly. However, CD4$^+$ T cells remained low, typically at about 200/µL (about 20–40% of normal) *(29,30)*. There have been few studies on the functional significance of these low numbers, but it was reported that proliferative capacity to mitogens in vitro was reduced *(30)* and the T-cell receptor repertoire might be diminished *(31)*. Nevertheless, immunity seems to be quite different from HIV-infected patients with similar low CD4$^+$ numbers since there have been no cases of severe opportunistic infections or malignancies during the long-term follow up (apart from 4/172 in the first 6 mo, when T cells were most profoundly suppressed). These results were being documented by Wellcome in 1994 at about the same time as data was arriving from the trials in lymphoid malignancies. The majority of patients had been treated for advanced non-Hodgkin's lymphoma, mostly with bulky lymph nodes and resistance to multiple chemotherapy. As in our previous trials using CAMPATH-1G, the responses in lymph nodes were minimal. However, some small trials were done in CLL, where the responses were more promising, and a particular subgroup of patients with T-cell proplymphocytic leukemia (T-PLL) showed remarkable responses *(32)*. T-PLL is a rare but very aggressive disease that responds very poorly to chemotherapy and has a poor prognosis. At present, it is an unexplained paradox that this disease is so uniquely responsive to CAMPATH-1H.

12. Wellcome Abandons CAMPATH but Clinicians Continue the Work

In 1994 Wellcome reviewed their clinical data and decided that, notwithstanding the good results in leukemia, there was likely to be insufficient commercial benefit for them to continue development of CAMPATH-1H. Of course, this news was very disappointing to us, especially because the TAC was receiving requests every week from physicians around the world to supply CAMPATH-1 for transplant patients and patients with a range of severe autoimmune diseases. Large trials in bone marrow transplantation were showing significant benefits (33–35) and there were case reports of good results in treatment of cornea graft rejection (36), uveitis (37), scleroderma (38), and autoimmune cytopenias (39,40). We were becoming very concerned how to support all these groups who clearly believed that CAMPATH-1 would help their patients.

One particularly interesting study was done by Alastair Compston's group at the Department of Neurology in Cambridge. In 1991 a middle-aged accountant with multiple sclerosis (MS) had insisted that something should be tried to arrest her progressive decline in mobility. By the time she received CAMPATH-1H, she was in a wheelchair. A few months later she went skiing! MS is a notoriously unpredictable disease and the placebo effect in clinical trials is considerable, so her improvement was only judged real when a series of gadolinium-enhancing magnetic resonance imaging (MRI) scans showed that inflammation was significantly diminished. Her disease remained controlled for 2 yr, providing sufficient encouragement to recruit a further six patients to a pilot study (41). New lesions were again reduced and no serious adverse effects were seen, so a larger cohort was recruited. By 1998, 29 such patients had been treated with CAMPATH-1H and monitored for 18 mo. The single treatment suppressed new MRI lesion formation by up to 90% compared to pretreatment. Patients did not experience any attacks that might indicate new cerebral inflammation. More disappointing, though informative, is that about half of the patients have progressed. That is, the disability from preexisiting lesions has steadily gotten worse. It is concluded that the mechanism underlying this deterioration is noninflammatory, possibly axonal degeneration following loss of the protective myelin sheath.

When this work started it was controversial whether MS was an autoimmune disease, but there was clearly significant immunopathology involving breakdown of the blood–brain barrier and lymphocyte infiltration. Whether antibody could reach these cells and change the course of the disease was unknown. Because of the great difficulty of measuring clinical effects, it was important to have a more objective disease marker. All of the patients had several MRI scans before treatment to establish the active and progressive nature of the lesions, followed by a series of scans afterward. Again we should remark on the important contribution of these volunteers; although MRI scanning is noninvasive, it requires complete immobility in the claustrophobic core of the scanner for 20 min and is not a procedure anyone would enjoy. Many of them had to travel long distances for these scans on a regular basis.

13. Unexpected Side Effects

Besides the reduction in new lesions detected by MRI, there were some completely unexpected results. We already knew that the first dose of CAMPATH-

1H treatment was usually accompanied by a flu-like syndrome of fever, rigors, nausea, and sometimes vomiting or marked hypotension. This is almost certainly caused by a rapid release of cytokines, including TNFα, IFNγ, and IL10, which has been well described for other anti-T-cell antibodies like OKT3 *(42)*. It can be ameliorated by prior treatment with a pulse of corticosteroids. The reaction is self-limiting and is greatly diminished on the second and subsequent doses of antibody. The MS patients suffered the same syndrome, but it was accompanied by a dramatic, though fortunately short-lived, recapitulation or exacerbation of previous neurological symptoms *(43)*. At the same time, there was physiological evidence that nerve conduction had been blocked. Pretreatment with steroids blocked both the "first-dose" syndrome and the neurologic effects. This suggested that one or more of the cytokines might have an impact on the previously damaged neurons and opened up new avenues for research into the pathology of MS.

The second unexpected complication was longer term. As in other patients, CAMPATH-1H induced a long-lasting decrease in blood CD4$^+$ T cell numbers. Between about 6 and 24 mo posttherapy about 30% of the patients developed antithyroid antibodies and hyperthyroidism (Graves' disease) *(44)*. There was no precedent for this in other patients who received CAMPATH-1H. Fortunately, the clinical symptoms have been responsive to standard therapy. One hypothesis is that the antibody treatment may have brought about a shift in immune regulation, e.g., from Th1 to Th2 type of response.

These clinical trials have helped to illuminate the underlying mechanisms of MS *(45)*. There seems to be a real possibility of arresting the inflammatory process. This gives an opportunity to test new therapies directed at remyelination *(46)*. If this should involve tissue grafting, as is currently being considered, the immunosuppressive effect of CAMPATH-1H should still be helpful.

14. Surprising Structure of the CD52 Antigen

In parallel with the clinical research on CAMPATH-1 antibodies we spent many years working on the structure and possible function of the antigen. We wanted to know why it was such a good target for cell lysis, so that similar therapeutic antibodies could be obtained against other cell types. The CAMPATH-1 antigen was very abundant, but antibodies against other highly expressed cell-surface antigens, like CD45, were by no means as lytic, particularly with human complement *(47)*. Conventional immunoprecipitation experiments with ^{125}I or [^{35}S]Met-labeled protein were unsuccessful. However, we gave samples of antibody to several other scientists and it was a chance observation by Chris Barker that identified antigenic activity in chloroform/methanol extracts. This allowed antigen to be extracted and identified as a ladder of

20–25-kDa bands by sodium dodecyl sulfate (SDS) gel electrophoresis and Western blotting *(48)*. In 1987, Meng-Qi Xia joined our laboratory as a research student. She purified the antigen by affinity chromatography and gel electrophoresis and obtained 11 residues of N-terminal sequence. This was very short, but despite repeated efforts we could go no further. We had hoped to identify a peptide that would allow synthesis of an oligonucleotide probe for DNA cloning, but the sequences predicted were too short and redundant. A new postdoc in our lab, Masahide Tone, suggested that the redundant oligo might be used as a polymerase chain reaction (PCR) primer along with a general poly-A primer to amplify the cDNA. Geoff was skeptical, but the experiment worked. We could hardly believe the DNA sequence, but it was confirmed by conventional cDNA cloning *(49)*. The surprising result was that the CAMPATH-1 antigen is a glycoprotein with only 12 amino acids. The C-terminal residue (Ser) was predicted to be attached to a glycosylphosphatidylinositol (GPI) anchor; that would account for why it was not detected by protein sequencing. We then had the good fortune to collaborate with Mike Ferguson, the doyen of GPI-anchorology, and in his laboratory the whole structure of the anchor as well as the single complex N-linked oligosaccharide were determined *(50,51)*.

As part of the preclinical testing of CAMPATH-1H, Wellcome had commissioned a study by Anthony Warford and Ian Lauder to determine its tissue crossreactivity. They saw intense staining of mature sperm and specific epithelial cells in the male reproductive tract, as well as the expected reaction with lymphocytes and macrophages throughout the body *(52)*. It turned out that the CD52 antigen is produced by cells in the epididymis and seminal vesicle, from where it is shed into the seminal fluid and acquired by sperm. The same result had been independently discovered by Christianne Kirchhoff, a reproductive biologist in Hamburg *(53)*. It is likely that the same antigen may have been examined by several teams who are looking for candidates for an intravaginal contraceptive *(54)*. We are often asked what the function of the CD52 antigen is. Its remarkable tissue distribution seems to be widely conserved. For some time we were spurred on by many discoveries of receptor-ligand pairs to look for a binding function. The best suggestion to date is from Neil Barclay, that considering its high abundance, extreme negative charge, and cell distribution, the role of CD52 may be antiadhesion, i.e., to keep the cells apart until the right time (since it is the unique role of sperm and lymphocytes to be able to migrate freely until they reach their target). As yet there are no data to support this proposition.

15. A New Start

Following Wellcome's decision to abandon CAMPATH-1H, BTG approached a range of other companies to reach a new licence agreement, but without finding any interest. In the meantime, our group was in the process of moving to Oxford, where we hoped to set up a new TAC. Its principal aim would still be to provide new biologicals for clinical research, but now we were faced with the prospect of indefinitely being the only source of CAMPATH-1 antibodies, which was clearly beyond our resources or mandate. Wellcome (soon to be bought by Glaxo) was not longer able to support our work and so we urgently needed other industrial sponsorship. A link was made with LeukoSite Inc, a small new US biotech company founded in 1993 by Tim Springer, who had worked with Herman at Cesar Milstein's laboratory in the late 1970s. Tim had pioneered the discovery of leukocyte adhesion molecules, including CD18, and this was the focus for the new company. Their chief executive, Chris Mirabelli, took a bold risk when he committed a substantial proportion of the new company's start-up capital toward the construction and running of a new center for an academic group on the other side of the Atlantic. As our hope was fading that BTG would find a new licensee, LeukoSite became persuaded that CAMPATH-1H was a genuine opportunity, even though its first application (in CLL), might be outside their original remit. There followed a long period of negotiation with BTG and Wellcome and a licence was finally agreed in April 1997. Thus began the next chapter in the story of CAMPATH-1.

16. Reflections and Lessons Learned

Our experience has been a mixture of elation, despair and simple routine. We realized that it is never a simple process to develop a new pharmaceutical; many rounds of development and refinement may be needed to overcome each hurdle. This process was only made possible by a close relationship between the research group and the clinical teams. The ability of doctors in the United Kingdom to treat individual patients as they believe best and to conduct clinical trials under the DDX system (whereby they are exempt from the more onerous regulatory requirements) has been of inestimable value. Few, if any, of the clinical developments described here could have been initiated by a pharmaceutical company. However, if we were not to abuse this system, it was important to have a production facility operating to the principles of Good Manufacturing Practice and following the relevant guidelines.

At the end of the day we know that only the pharmaceutical industry has the resources and expertise to bring a product to market. We need to work closely with them to transfer the technology and know-how in an effective way and to ensure that a fair (not extravagant) reward flows back to the academic institution when a potential product is marketed. In our experience it has been very much easier to interact with small biotech companies where the ethos is more akin to our academic culture and the management is closer to our level. To us, the big pharma like

Glaxo/Wellcome seems daunting and impersonal; our main point of contact is with lawyers who appear obsessed with details we find trivial. We still do not know whether CAMPATH-1H will prove to be as widely useful for human therapy as we hope. We do know that it has been hugely enjoyable to be part of its development, sharing with literally thousands of scientists, physicians, nurses, and patients world-wide. Along the way we have discovered many new aspects of therapeutic immu-nology relevant to other projects. We are just starting work in the lab on the next generation of CAMPATH-1 antibodies *(55)* and the physicians are continuing to find new applications *(56)*.

Acknowledgments

We estimate that more than 2000 scientists, physicians, nurses, and lawyers have been involved in the characterization and development of CAMPATH-1 antibodies, and any success we have obtained is the result of their cumulative collaborative efforts, as well as the incalculable contribution of over 3000 patients who have volunteered for clinical trials. However, we are solely responsible for the opinions expressed in this chapter. Over the last 20 years we have received financial support from the UK Medical Research Council, the Kay Kendall Leukaemia Fund, the Wellcome Foundation Ltd, LeukoSite Inc., and several other charitable and industrial sources. G. H. is currently funded by the EP Abrahams' Trust.

References

1. von Behring, E. and Kitasato, S. (1890) Dtsch. Med. Wochenshe. **16,** 1113–1114.
2. Hericourt, J. and Richet, C. (1895) "Physologie Pathologique"—de la serotherapie dans la traitement du cancer. *Comptes Rendus Hebd. Seanc. Acad. Sci.* **121,** 567.
3. Currie, G. A. (1972) Eighty years of immunotherapy: a review of immunological methods used for the treatment of human cancer. *Br. J. Cancer* **26,** 141–153.
4. Prentice, H. G., Blacklock, H. A., Janossy, G., Bradstock, K. F., Skeggs, D., Goldstein, G., and Hoffbrand, A. V. (1982) Use of anti-T cell monoclonal anti-body OKT3 to prevent acute graft versus host disease in allogeneic bone marrow transplantation for acute leukemia. *Lancet* **1,** 700–703.
5. Filipovitch, A. H., Vallera, D. A., Youle, R. J., Haake, R., Blazar, B. R., Arthur, D., Neville, Ramsay, N. K., McGlave, P., and Kersey, J. H. (1987) Graft-versus-host disease prevention in allogeneic bone marrow transplantation from histo-compatible siblings. A pilot study using immunotoxins for T cell depletion of donor bone marrow. *Transplantation* **44,** 62–69.
6. Clark, M., Cobbold, S., Hale, G., and Waldmann, H. (1983) Advantages of rat monoclonal antibodies. *Immunol. Today* **4,** 100–101.
7. Hale, G., Bright, S., Chumbley, G., Hoang, T., Metcalf, D., Munro, A. J., and Wald-mann, H. (1983) Removal of T cells from bone marrow for transplantation: a mono-clonal antilymphocyte antibody that fixes human complement. *Blood* **62,** 873–882.

8. Hale, G., Hoang, T., Prospero, T., Watt, S. M., and Waldmann, H. (1983) Removal of T cells from bone marrow for transplantation: comparison of rat monoclonal anti-lymphocyte antibodies of different isotypes. *Mol. Biol. Med.* **1,** 305–319.

9. Hale, G., Swirsky, D. M., Hayhoe, F. G. J., and Waldmann, H. (1983) Effects of monoclonal anti-lymphocyte antibodies in vivo in monkeys and humans. *Mol. Biol. Med.* **1,** 321–334.

10. Waldmann, H., Or, R., Hale, G., Weiss, L., Cividalli, G., Samuel, S., Manor, D., Brautbar, C., Polliack, A., Rachmilewitz, E. A., and Slavin, S. (1984) Elimination of graft versus host disease by in vitro depletion of alloreactive lymphocytes using a monoclonal rat anti-human lymphocyte antibody (CAMPATH-1). *Lancet* **2,** 483–486.

11. Heit, W., Bunjes, D., Weisneth, M., Schmeiser, T., Arnold, R., Hale, G., Waldmann, H., and Heimpel, H. (1986) Ex vivo T-cell depletion with the monoclonal antibody Campath-1 plus human complement effectively prevents acute GvHD in allogeneic bone marrow transplantation. *Br. J. Haematol.* **64,** 479–486.

12. Goldman, J. M., Apperley, J. F., Jones, L., Marcus, R., Goolden, A. W. G., Batchelor, R., Hale, G., Waldmann, H., Reid, C. D., Hows, J., Gordon-Smith, E., Catovsky, D., and Galton, D. A. G. (1986) Bone marrow transplantation for patients with chronic myeloid leukemia. *New Engl. J. Med.* **314,** 202–207.

13. Hale, G., Cobbold, S., and Waldmann, H. (1988) T cell depletion with CAMPATH-1 in allogeneic bone marrow transplantation. *Transplantation* **45,** 753–759.

14. Cobbold, S. P., Thierfelder, S., and Waldmann, H. (1983) Immunosuppression with monoclonal antibodies: a model to determine the rules for effective serotherapy. *Mol. Biol. Med.* **1,** 285–304.

15. Cobbold, S. P., Martin, G., and Waldmann, H. (1986) Monoclonal antibodies for the prevention of graft-versus-host disease and marrow graft rejection: the depletion of T-cell subsets in vitro and in vivo. *Transplantation* **42,** 239–247.

16. Hale, G., Clark, M., and Waldmann, H. (1985) Therapeutic potential of rat monoclonal antibodies: isotype specificity of antibody-dependant cell-mediated cytotoxicity with human lymphocytes. *J. Immunol.* **134,** 3056–3061.

17. Bruggemann, M., Free, J., Diamond, A., Howard, J., Cobbold, S. P., and Waldmann, H. (1986) Immunoglobulin heavy chain locus of the rat: striking homology to mouse antibody genes. *Proc. Natl. Acad. Sci. USA* **83,** 6075–6079.

18. Hale, G., Cobbold, S. P., Waldmann, H., Easter, G., Matejtschuk, P., and Coombs, R. R. A. (1987) Isolation of low-frequency class-switch variants from rat hybrid myelomas. *J. Immunol Methods* **103,** 59–67.

19. Dyer, M. J. S., Hale, G., Hayhoe, F. G. J., and Waldmann, H. (1989) Effects of CAMPATH-1 antibodies in vivo in patients with lymphoid malignancies: influence of antibody isotype. *Blood* **73,** 1431–1439.

20. Neuberger, M. S., Williams, G. T., Mitchell, E. B., Jouhal, S. S., Flanagan, J. G., and Rabbitts, T. N. (1985) A hapten specific chimaeric IgE antibody with human physiological effector function. *Nature* **314,** 268–270.

21. Jones, P. T., Dear, P. H., Foote, J., Neuberger, M. S., and Winter, G. (1986) Replacing the complementarity-determining regions in a human antibody with those from a mouse. *Nature* **321,** 522–525.
22. Friend, P. J., Waldmann, H., Hale, G., Cobbold, S., Rebello, P., Thiru, S., Jamieson, N. V., Johnston, P. S., and Calne, R. Y. (1991) Reversal of allograft rejection using the monoclonal antibody CAMPATH-1G. *Transplant. Proc.* **23,** 1390–1392.
23. Riechmann, L., Clark, M., Waldmann, H., and Winter, G. (1988) Reshaping human antibodies for therapy. *Nature* **332,** 323–327.
24. Bruggemann, M., Williams, G. T., Bindon, C. I., Clark, M. R., Walker, M. R., Jefferies, R., Waldmann, H., and Neuberger, M. S. (1987) Comparison of the effector functions of human immunoglobulins using a matched set of chimeric antibodies. *J. Exp. Med.* **166,** 1351–1361.
25. Hale, G., Dyer, M. J. S., Clark, M. R., Phillips, J. M., Marcus, R., Riechmann, L., Winter, G., and Waldmann, H. (1988) Remission induction in non-Hodgkin lymphoma with reshaped human monoclonal antibody CAMPATH-1H. *Lancet* **2,** 1394–1399.
26. Hale, G. (1993) Small scale production of novel therapeutic products: a new challenge for the transfusion service? (editorial) *Transfus. Med.* **3,** 1–5.
27. Lockwood, C. M., Thiru, S., Isaacs, J. D., Hale, G., and Waldmann, H. (1993) Humanised monoclonal antibody treatment for intractable systemic vasculitis. *Lancet* **341,** 1620–1622.
28. Lockwood, C. M., Thiru, S., Stewart, S., Hale, G., Isaacs, J. D., Wraight, P., Elliott, J., and Waldmann, H. (1996) Treatment of refractory Wegener's granulomatosis with humanised monoclonal antibodies. *Q. J. Med.* **89,** 903–912.
29. Isaacs, J. D., Watts, R. A., Hazleman, B. L., Hale, G., Keogan, M. T., Cobbold, S. P., and Waldmann, H. (1992) Humanised monclonal antibody therapy for rheumatoid arthritis. *Lancet* **340,** 748–752.
30. Brett, S., Baxter, G., Cooper, H., Johnston, J. M., Tite, J., and Rapson, N. (1996) Repopulation of blood lymphocyte sub-populations in rheumatoid arthritis patients treated with the depleting humanized monoclonal antibody, CAMPATH-1H. *Immunology* **88,** 13–19.
31. Jendro, M. C., Ganten, T., Matteson, E. L., Weyand, C. M., and Goronzy, J. J. (1995) Emergence of oligoclonal T cell populations following therapeutic T cell depletion in rheuamtoid arthritis. *Arthritis Rheum.* **38,** 1242–1251.
32. Pawson, R., Dyer, M. J. S., Barge, R., Matutes, E., Thornton, P. D., Emmett, E., Kluin-Nelemans, J. C., Fibbe, W. E., Willemze, R., and Catovsky, D. (1997) Treatment of T-cell prolymphocytic leukaemia with human CD52 antibody. *J. Clin. Oncol.* **15,** 2667–2672.
33. Jacobs, P. Wood, L., Fullard, L., Waldmann, H., and Hale, G. (1993) T-cell depletion by exposure to CAMPATH-1G in vitro prevents graft-versus-host disease. *Bone Marrow Transplant.* **13,** 763–769.
34. Hale, G. and Waldmann, H. for CAMPATH users (1994) Control of graft-versus-host disease and graft rejection by T cell depletion of donor and recipient with

CAMPATH-1 antibodies. Results of matched sibling transplants for malignant diseases. *Bone Marrow Transplant.* **13,** 597–611.

35. Hale, G. and Waldmann, H. for CAMPATH users (1994) CAMPATH-1 monoclonal antibodies in bone marrow transplantation. *Hematotherapy* **3,** 15–31.

36. Newman, D. K., Isaacs, J. D., Watson, P. G., Meyer, P. A., Hale, G., and Waldmann, H. (1995) Prevention of immune-mediated corneal graft destruction with the anti-lymphocyte monoclonal antibody, CAMPATH-1H. *Eye* **9,** 564–569.

37. Isaacs, J. D., Dick, A. D., Haynes, R., Watson, P., Forrester, J. V., Myer, P., Hale, G., and Waldmann, H. (1996) Monoclonal antibody therapy of chronic intraocular inflammation using CAMPATH-1H. *Br. J. Ophthalmol.* **79,** 1054,1055.

38. Isaacs, J. D., Hazleman, B. L., Chakravarty, K., Grant, J. W., Hale, G., and Waldmann, H. (1996) Monoclonal antibody therapy of diffuse cutaneous scleroderma with CAMPATH-1H. *J. Rheumatol.* **23,** 1103–1106.

39. Lim, S. H., Hale, G., Marcus, R. E., Waldmann, H., and Baglin, T. P. (1993) CAMPATH-1 MoAb in the treatment of refractory autoimmune thrombocytopenic purpura *Br. J. Haematol.* **84,** 542–544.

40. Killick, S. B., Marsh, J. C. W., Hale, G., Waldmann, H., Kelly, S. J., and Gordon-Smith, E. C. (1997) Sustained remission of severe resistant auto-immune neutropenia with Campath-1H. *Br. J. Haematol.* **97,** 306–308.

41. Moreau, T., Thorpe, J., Miller, D., Moseley, I., Hale, G., Waldmann, H., Clayton, D., Wing, M., Scolding, N., and Compston, A. (1994) Preliminary evidence from magnetic resonance imaging for reduction in disease activity after lymphocyte depletion in multiple sclerosis. *Lancet* **344,** 298–301.

42. Chatenoud, L., Ferran, C., Legendre, C., Thouard, I., Merite, S., Reuter, A., Gevaert, Y., Kreis, H., Franchimont, P., and Bach, J.-F. (1990) In vivo cell activation following OKT3 adminstration. Systematic cytokine release and modulation by corticosteroids. *Transplantation* **49,** 697–702.

43. Moreau, T., Coles, A., Wing, M. G., Isaacs, J., Hale, G., Waldmann, H., and Compston, A. (1996) Transient increase in symptoms associated with cytokine release in patients with multiple sclerosis *Brain* **119,** 225–237.

44. Coles, A. J., Wing, M. G., Smith, S. I., Corradu, F., Greer, S., Taylor, C. J., Weetman, A. P., Hale, G., Chatterjee, V. K., Waldmann, H., and Compston, A. (1998) Pulsed monoclonal antibody treatment and autoimmune thyroid disease in multiple sclerosis. *Lancet* **354,** 1691–1696.

45. Coles, A. J., Molyneux, P., Wing, M. G., Paolillo, A., Davie, C. M., Hale, G., Miller, D., Waldmann, H., and Compston, A. (1998) Monoclonal antibody treatment exposes three mechanisms underlying the clinical course of multiple sclerosis. *Ann. Neurol.* **46,** 296–304

46. Compston, A. (1994) Future prospects for the management of multiple sclerosis. *Ann Neurol.* **36,** S146–S150.

47. Bindon, C. I., Hale, G., and Waldmann, H. (1988) Importance of antigen specificity for complement mediated lysis by monoclonal antibodies. *Eur. J. Immunol.* **18,** 1507–1514.

48. Hale, G., Xia, M.-Q., Tighe, H. P., Dyer, M. J. S., and Waldmann, H. (1990) The CAMPATH-1 antigen (CDw52). *Tissue Antigens* **35,** 118–127.
49. Xia, M.-Q., Tone, M., Packman, L., Hale, G., and Waldmann, H. (1991) Characterization of the CAMPATH-1 antigen: biochemical analysis and cDNA cloning reveal an unusually small peptide backbone. *Eur. J. Immunol.* **21,** 1677–1684.
50. Xia, M.-Q., Hale, G., Lifely, M. R., Ferguson, M. J., Campbell, D., Packman, L., and Waldmann, H. (1993) Structure of the CAMPATH-1 antigen, a GPI-anchored glycoprotein which is an exceptionally good target for complement lysis. *Biochem. J.* **293,** 633–640.
51. Treumann, A., Lifely, R., Schneider, P., and Ferguson, M. A. J. (1995) Primary structure of CD52. *J. Biol. Chem.* **270,** 6088–6099.
52. Hale, G., Rye, P. D., Warford, A., Lauder, I., and Brito-Babapulle, A. (1993) The GPI-anchored lymphocyte antigen CDw52 is associated with the epididymal maturation of human spermatozoa. *J. Reprod. Immunol.* **23,** 189–205.
53. Kirchhoff, C., Krull, N., Pera, I., and Ivell, R. (1992) A major mRNA of the human epididymal principal cells, HE5, encodes the leucocyte differentiation CDw52 antigen peptide backbone. *Mol. Repr. Dev.* **34,** 11–15.
54. Diekman, A. B., Westbrook-Case, A., Naaby-Hansen, S., Klotz, K. L., Flickinger, C. J., and Herr, J. C. (1997) Biochemical characterization of sperm agglutination antigen-1, a human sperm surface antigen implicated in gamete interactions. *Biol. Reprod.* **57,** 1136–1145.
55. Gilliland, L. K., Walsh, L. A., Frewin, M. R., Wise, M., Tone, M., Hale, G., Kioussis, D., and Waldmann, H. (1998) Elimination of the immunogenicity of therapeutic antibodies. *J. Immunol.* **162,** 3663–3671.
56. Calne, R., Moffatt, S. D., Friend, P. J., Jamieson, N. V., Bradley, J. A., Hale, G., Firth, J., Bradley, J., Smith, K. G., and Waldmann, H. (1999) CAMPATH-1H allows low-dose cyclosporin monotherapy in 31 cadaveric renal allograft recipients. *Transplantation* **68,** 1613–1616.
57. Dyer, M. J. S., Hale, G., Marcus, R., and Waldmann, H. (1990) Remission induction in patients with lymphoid malignancies using unconjugated CAMPATH-1 monoclonal antibodies. *Leukemia Lymphoma* **2,** 179–193.
58. Reuter, H., Wraight, E. P., Qasim, F. J., and Lockwood, C. M. (1995) Management of vasculitis: the contribution of scintigraphic imaging to the evaluation of disease activity and classification. *Q. J. Med.* **88,** 509–516.

IV

PRODUCTION AND PURIFICATION

17

Production of Monoclonal Antibodies

Jóna Freysdóttir

1. Introduction

The discovery of monoclonal antibodies (mAbs) produced by "hybridoma technology" by George Köhler and Cesar Milstein in 1975 has had a great impact both on basic biological research and on clinical medicine. However, this impact was not immediately recognized. It took around 10 years to appreciate the importance of using these mAbs in various fields of science other than immunology, such as cell biology, biochemistry, microbiology, virology, parasitology, physiology, genetics, and molecular biology; and also in areas of clinical medicine, such as pathology, hematology, oncology, and infectious disease. The contribution of mAbs to science and clinical medicine was recognized in 1984 by the award of the Nobel Prize for Medicine to Köhler and Milstein.

The hybridoma technology was based on two facts: the antibody producing lymphocytes from immunized animals have a very short life when cultured under in vitro conditions; and the individual myeloma cell lines can be grown permanently in culture, but the antibody they produce does not express a predefined specificity. When both types of cells are fused, hybrids can be derived that will retain the two essential properties; namely, the production of an antibody with a predefined specificity and continuous growth. In order to obtain hybridoma cells that have the ability to produce immunoglobulins and survive in culture, spleen cells from an immunized host (e.g., a mouse) can be fused with myeloma cells. Among the spleen cells are the antibody-producing B lymphoblasts, which will provide the hybridoma cells with the ability to produce immunoglobulins. The fusion partner is a myeloma cell line (from the same species) that will provide the hybridoma cells with immortality. The myeloma

From: *Methods in Molecular Medicine, Vol. 40: Diagnostic and Therapeutic Antibodies*
Edited by: A. J. T. George and C. E. Urch © Humana Press Inc., Totowa, NJ

cells have a mutation in the gene encoding hypoxanthine-guanine phosphoribosyl transferase (HPRT), an enzyme of the salvage pathway of purine nucleotide biosynthesis. By using a fusogen (e.g., polyethylene glycol, PEG) the plasma membranes of adjacent myeloma and/or antibody-secreting cells are fused together, forming a single cell with two or more nuclei. During subsequent mitosis the individual chromosomes are segregated into the daughter cells. The hybridoma cells are cultured in medium containing hypoxanthine, aminopterin, and thymidine (HAT). Aminopterin blocks the main pathways of DNA and RNA synthesis. A salvage pathway can, however, be used; a pathway that depends on the presence of hypoxanthine and thymidine for the RNA and DNA pathways, respectively. Since the myeloma cells have a defect in the HPRT enzyme, which is required for the salvage pathway, these cells cannot grow in HAT-containing medium, so all unfused myeloma cells will hence die. Even though B cells are able to use the salvage pathway they do not survive for long in culture. Therefore, the only proliferating cells will be the hybridoma cells. These cells can then be cloned to produce single-cell clones that can generate antibodies directed against very well-defined antigenic determinants (**Fig. 1**).

The way the immunogen is prepared, the type of immunization procedure selected, and the choice of animal to be immunized will all depend on the purpose of the antibody production. Monoclonal antibodies can either be generated against a known antigen whose structure and function are to be investigated further, or against yet undiscovered novel molecules.

Before the fusion it is very important to have a screening method available, the choice of which will depend on the potential use of the mAbs. Several screening systems can be used, such as immunostaining of tissue sections/cytospins, Western blotting, flow cytometry, and enzyme-linked immunosorbent assay (ELISA). These will be described in Chapters 30 and 32–34. The main objective of this chapter is to summarize the steps necessary to generate a novel mAb and to serve as a practical manual that contains several troubleshooting notes that may be helpful to the nonspecialist.

2. Materials

2.1. Immunization

1. The immunogen (*see* **Subheading 3.1.**).
2. The adjuvant (*see* **Subheading 3.1.**).
3. Two glass syringes with a special connector.
4. 25-gage needle.
5. The animal to be immunized.

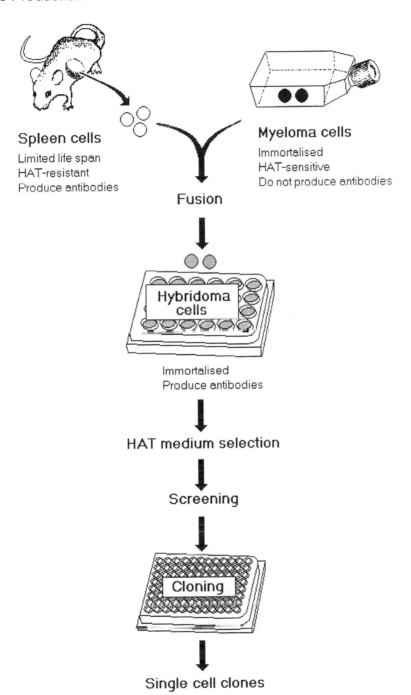

Fig. 1. Schematic representation of the steps involved in hybridoma technology.

2.2. Testing Efficiency of Immunization

1. The immunized animal.
2. Scalpel blade.
3. 0.5-mL Eppendorf tube.
4. Centrifuge.
5. Screening protocol (*see* **Note 1**).

2.3. Culturing Myeloma Cells

1. Myeloma cells from the same species as the immunized animal.
2. 10% fetal calf serum (FCS) medium: RPMI medium, sodium bicarbonate buffered, containing 10% FCS.
3. 175 cm² flasks.

2.4. Fusion

1. Immunized animal.
2. Myeloma cells (approx 1/10 spleen cells).
3. 50% polyethylene glycol (PEG) in RPMI medium (1 g PEG 1500 autoclaved, 1 mL serum-free medium added while PEG is molten). This is now commercially available.
4. Serum-free medium: RPMI medium, buffered with HEPES.
5. 15% FCS medium: RPMI medium, buffered with sodium bicarbonate, containing 15% FCS.
6. HAT medium: RPMI medium, sodium bicarbonate buffered, containing 10% FCS and 1X HAT.
7. Petri dish.
8. Tissue-culture plates (e.g., 24-well plates).
9. Syringe plunger (2 mL).
10. Nylon membrane sieve (0.7 µm).
11. Improved Neubauer counting chamber.
12. 1% acetic acid in phosphate-buffered saline (PBS).
13. 0.2% trypan blue in PBS.
14. Dissection instruments, such as forceps and scissors.
15. A beaker with water.
16. A timer.
17. 70% ethanol.

2.5. Preparation of Macrophages

1. Nonimmunized animal of the same strain as that for macrophage preparation.
2. Dissection instruments, such as forceps and scissors.
3. A 5 mL syringe containing RPMI medium (cold).
4. 21- and 25-gage needles.
5. 70% ethanol.

2.6. Cloning

1. HAT medium: RPMI medium, sodium bicarbonate buffered, containing 10% FCS and 1X HAT.
2. HT medium: RPMI medium, sodium bicarbonate buffered, containing 10% FCS and 1X HT.
3. 10% FCS medium: RPMI medium, sodium bicarbonate buffered, containing 10% FCS.
4. Tissue-culture plates (96-well plates).
5. Nonimmunized animal for macrophage preparation.
6. Dissection instruments, such as forceps and scissors.
7. 70% ethanol.
8. Two 5-mL syringes.
9. 21- and 25-gage needles.
10. Improved Neubauer counting chamber.
11. 0.2% Trypan blue in PBS.

2.7. Freezing Down Cells

1. Freezing medium: 90% FCS and 10% dimethylsulfoxide (DMSO).
2. Improved Neubauer counting chamber.
3. 0.2% Trypan blue in PBS.
4. Cryotubes.
5. Ice.
6. Freezing machine or a bubble plastic sheet, cottonwool padded box, and −70°C freezer.
7. Liquid nitrogen storage.

3. Methods

3.1. Immunization

The immunogen can be whole cells or solutions of crude tissue extracts, purified proteins, or peptides. The immunogen is not always available in a pure form, and purification (if possible) can be both expensive and time-consuming. Therefore, whole cells, crude tissue extracts, or protein mixtures are often used. This puts a great demand on a good screening method to be available that can distinguish the specific antibody required. Small proteins or peptides are often too small to provide an immune response and have to be linked to larger carrier proteins, such as bovine serum albumin and keyhole limpet hemocyanin.

For most proteins, a dose of 1–50 µg/injection is sufficient. If whole cells are used, 2×10^6 to 7×10^7 cells/injection are usually used. If these cells are tumorigenic they have to be irradiated. To increase the likelihood of successful immunization and fusion, more than one animal should be included in the immunization protocol.

For most immunogens, addition of adjuvants is used, providing an enhanced immunological response to the immunogen by delaying the clearance of the immunogen and hence prolonging the immune response. The most commonly used adjuvant is Freund's adjuvant, which consists of oil and emulsifying agent (incomplete) or oil, emulsifying agent, and killed mycobacteria (complete). Other adjuvants are available, such as aluminum hydroxide, used to produce IgE antibodies. Strict regulations govern the use of adjuvants in the United Kingdom and update advice should always be obtained from the Home Office in the United Kingdom or appropriate regulatory authorities in other countries prior to use.

There are several routes of immunizations; intravenous, intraperitoneal, intramuscular, intradermal, and subcutaneous. Whole cells used as the immunogen are usually injected intraperitoneally, whereas soluble immunogens, mixed with Freund's adjuvants to form an emulsion, can be injected via all the above routes except for intravenously. The last immunization for soluble immunogens is usually intravenous, ensuring formation of B lymphoblasts in the spleen.

The timing of immunization depends on the antibody class expected. For IgM antibodies one immunization is enough. If IgG antibodies are wanted several boosts have to be given with at least 3 wk interval to allow class switching and affinity maturation to occur. The first immunization is usually performed in the presence of complete adjuvant, whereas incomplete adjuvant is used in subsequent immunizations. The final injection is performed intravenously (if possible) 3–4 d before immunization, without any adjuvant.

When antibodies against human molecules are to be produced mice are the most common host, whereas if the antibodies will be directed against a mouse molecule the host is most commonly a rat. BALB/c mice and Lou rats are inbred strains commonly used for antibody production. Using F1 hybrids (of BALB/c or Lou origin) will increase the number of major histocompatibility complex (MHC) molecules involved in the immune response and hence may increase the chance of obtaining antibodies against different epitopes. Myeloma cell lines of both BALB/c and Lou origin are available. It is important to select lines that no longer produce functional immunoglobulins. Among such lines are NSO/1 and Sp2/0-Ag14 for mouse and YB2/0 and IR983F for rat.

3.1.1. Preparation of the Immunogen

1. Put 1 vol of immunogen (5–250 µg for 5 mice or rats) into one of the glass syringes.
2. Into the other glass syringe put 1 vol of Freund's adjuvant; complete if this is the first immunization, otherwise incomplete.
3. Link the two glass syringes with the special connector.
4. Push the immunogen solution into the Freund's adjuvant and then push the mixture between the two syringes until a white emulsion has been produced.

5. With a 25 gage needle, inject one-fifth of the emulsion into appropriate site of each of the five host animals.

3.1.2. The Immunization Protocol

1. Immunize each animal with the immunogen (whole cells intraperitoneally or immunogen mixed with complete Freund's adjuvant intraperitoneally, intramuscularly, intradermally, or subcutaneously).
2. Leave the animals for at least 3 wk.
3. If IgG antibodies are required, repeat the immunization at least two more times, replacing complete Freund's adjuvant with incomplete Freund's adjuvant.
4. Test the efficiency of the immunization (*see* **Subheading 3.1.3.**).
5. Four days before the fusion, boost one of the animals with the immunogen without the use of any adjuvants.

3.1.3. Testing the Efficiency of the Immunization

1. Warm the animals for few minutes under a heat lamp.
2. Snip off the end of the tail with a scalpel blade.
3. Massage the tail and collect few drops of blood into a test tube, e.g., a 0.5 mL Eppendorf tube.
4. Let the blood clot at room temperature for 1 h.
5. Spin in a microfuge for 10 min.
6. Collect the sera.
7. Test the sera with the screening protocol that has been set up for screening the antibodies (*see* **Note 1**).
8. Choose one of the animals for the fusion.

3.2. Fusion

When a successfully immunized animal and a screening protocol are ready the fusion can be performed.

3.2.1. Preparation of the Spleen Cells

1. Place the 50% PEG, the beaker with water, and all the media in a 37°C incubator to heat.
2. Sacrifice the immunized animal by cervical dislocation or in a CO_2 chamber.
3. Place it on the right side and soak the skin with 70% ethanol.
4. Using a pair of fine forceps and scissors, cut a snip of the skin just under the rib cage and tear the skin open. Cut the peritoneum open, just over the spleen, and carefully remove the spleen and place it in a Petri dish containing serum-free medium. Remove all excess fat and fibrous tissue.
5. Place a nylon sieve on a 50-mL tube. Transfer the spleen into the sieve and add some serum-free medium. With the plunger of a 2 mL-syringe, press the spleen through the sieve, rinsing every now and then with serum-free medium.
6. Let the solution stand for several minutes to allow bits to settle. Transfer the solution to a 50 mL tube and fill with serum-free medium.

7. Spin for 10 min at 250g at room temperature. Discard the supernatant and resuspend the cells in 10 mL serum-free medium.
8. Repeat **steps 6** and **7**.
9. Count the cells. Prepare the Neubauer counting chamber by applying a coverslip tightly over the chamber. Take 50 µL of cell suspension and mix it with 450 µL 1% acetic acid in PBS and 500 µL 0.2% trypan blue in PBS. Pipet some of the suspension into the space between the counting chamber and coverslip. The counting chamber is divided into 9 large squares, each having the volume of 0.1 µL. The corner squares are subdivided into 16 squares each. Choose one of the corners and count all live cells (i.e., exclude blue cells, which are dead) in the 16 small squares. This gives you a number (N cells/0.1 µL) that you multiply by 10^4 (converts 0.1 µL into mL), the dilution factor (20, i.e., 50 µL into 1000 µL), and the total volume (10 mL). This gives you the total number of splenocytes (X_s).

3.2.2. Preparation of the Myeloma Cells

1. Obtain the myeloma cells required for the fusion (most likely from liquid nitrogen).
2. Culture the cells in 10% FCS medium for at least a week before the fusion.
3. The day before the fusion the myeloma cells have to be divided into fresh medium so they will be in an exponential growth phase at the time of fusion. If you plate the cells at 5×10^5 cell/µL in 50 mL medium in a 175 cm^2 flask, one flask is enough.
4. On the day of fusion, harvest the myeloma cells into a 50 mL tube. Fill with serum-free medium.
5. Centrifuge at 250g for 10 min. Discard supernatant and resuspend the cells in 50 mL serum-free medium.
6. Repeat **step 5**.
7. Count the cells. Take 50 µL of the cell suspension and mix with 50 µL 0.2% Trypan blue. Count in a Neubauer counting chamber as described in **Subheading 3.2.1.** This time you multiply your number (N) with 10^4 and 2 (the dilution factor). This gives you the number of myeloma cells per milliliter (X_m). Calculate how many milliliters (V) of myeloma cell suspension you need to obtain 1/10 the number you have of spleen cells (X_s, *see* **Subheading 3.2.1.**) using this formula; $V = X_s/10 \times 1/X_m$.

3.2.3. The Fusion

1. Transfer the calculated volume of myeloma cells into the tube with the spleen cells. Spin for 10 min at 250g. Discard the supernatant. Gently resuspend the cell pellet. The cells are now ready for fusion.
2. Put the tube into a beaker with water at 37°C.
3. Add 1 mL warm PEG slowly to the cells over a period of 1 min, stirring the mixture continuously with the pipet tip. The PEG is toxic for the cells so they should not be in the concentrated PEG for more than 2 min. Immediately after the

PEG, add 1 mL warm serum-free medium over a period of another minute. Then add 4 mL of serum-free medium over 3–4 min, this time without stirring, letting the medium run slowly down the side of the tube.
4. Add carefully a further 20 mL serum-free medium and then 20 mL 15% FCS medium. Invert the tube once and leave at 37°C for 1–2 h to allow the cell membranes to stabilize.
5. Meanwhile, prepare macrophages.

3.2.4. Preparation of Macrophages

You will need 0.5 mL macrophage suspension/50 mL hybridoma cell suspension (*see* **Subheading 3.2.5.**).

1. Sacrifice an animal of the same species as the immunized animal.
2. Soak it thoroughly in 70% ethanol.
3. With sterile scissors, cut the skin open over the abdomen without tearing the peritoneum.
4. Inject carefully the 5 mL cold RPMI medium into the peritoneal cavity, using the 25 gage needle. Take care not to pierce any of the internal organs.
5. Massage the abdomen lightly.
6. With a 21 gage needle collect as much of the medium as possible into the 5-mL syringe.

3.2.5. Culturing the Hybridoma Cells

1. When the hybridoma cells have been at 37°C for 1–2 h centrifuge them at 250g for 10 min. Discard the supernatant and resuspend the cells in HAT medium at a concentration of 1–2.5×10^5 cells/mL. (Use the myeloma cell count because that is your limiting factor). Add 0.5 mL macrophage suspension into each 50 mL of hybridoma cell suspension.
2. Plate the cells out on either 96-well plates (200 µL/well) or 24-well plates (2 mL/well) (*see* **Note 2.**)
3. Incubate the plates in a humidified incubator at 37°C with 5% CO_2.
4. After 1 wk, remove 1 mL or 100 µL of medium from each well of the 24-well plates or the 96-well plates, respectively. Replace the old medium with the same amount of fresh HAT medium.
5. After a further week, repeat the procedure in **step 4**, except this time replace the old medium with fresh HT medium.
6. After yet another week, repeat the procedure in **step 4**, except this time the old medium is replaced with fresh 10% FCS medium, without any HAT or HT.
7. From now on the hybridoma cells can be cultured in 10% FCS medium because all other cells (unfused spleen cells or myeloma cells) will have died.
8. There is always a possibility that there are many unfused B cells in the wells. Therefore, you may choose to change the medium more frequently (*see* **Note 3**).

3.3. Screening and Cloning

After 1 wk you can start looking for the presence of hybridoma cells. These cells look like a bunch of grapes. Each grape-like cluster of cells represents cells growing from one hybridoma cell. Mark each well with a clone in it and when there are approx 50 cells present (you need quite a large clone to produce enough antibody to be detected in your screening), you can start collecting supernatant for screening. The different methods for screening will be described in Chapters 30 and 32–34.

You may see more than one cell cluster in some of the wells, indicating that you have more than one hybridoma clone growing in the well. Some hybridoma cells are not producing antibodies, and these may outnumber the hybridoma cells that are producing antibodies. Hence, it is very important to screen the wells regularly. When a well with hybridoma cells secreting the appropriate antibody has been detected it is important to immediately clone the cells from that well.

Cloning by limiting dilution is one way of cloning the cells and can be performed by either using set concentration (first 6 cells/well, followed by two times 0.3 cells/well) or by using titration, where you start with 10 cells/well and then titrate the cells out across the microtiterplate so that in the last column you have <1 cell/well. After the titration cloning you may want to repeat the cloning using set concentration cloning at 0.3 cells/well to ensure your hybridoma cells are a single clone. Another quick way of cloning is to take a fixed volume of cells, do several 1/3 dilutions, and plate each dilution onto a 96-well plate. To be sure your hybridoma cell is from a single clone, you need to inspect the plates every day to make sure that only one clone is growing in each well. You may also want to repeat the cloning.

3.3.1. Set Concentration Cloning

The choice of medium depends on the time since fusion was performed (*see* **Subheading 3.2.5.**).

1. Harvest all the cells in the well.
2. Count the cells and adjust them to 30 cells/mL for 6 cells/well, or to 1.5 cells/mL for 0.3 cells/well. This has to be done in steps (serial dilution). You will need 20 mL medium for each plate; hence, you will need 600 cells for 6 cells/well or 30 cells for 0.3 cells/well. It is not possible to use all the cells from the well for cloning. The remaining cells should be frozen as a back-up (*see* **Subheading 3.3.3.**).
3. Prepare macrophages as described in **Subheading 3.2.4.** You will need 0.2 mL/ plate, i.e., per 20 mL.
4. Add 200 µL of the cell suspension into each well on a 96-well plate. The number of plates depends on the screening method you are using (*see* **Note 2**).

5. When the clones of cells can be seen and the medium has turned quite yellow it is time to screen the supernatants. If you were using 6 cells/well you will have to repeat the cloning twice, using 0.3 cells/well. Remember to freeze the cells at each cloning stage (*see* **Subheading 3.3.3.**).
6. When you have ensured you have fully cloned the hybridoma cells you can transfer them to 24-well plates for freezing and growing them for bulk antibody production.

3.3.2. Titration Cloning

The choice of medium depends on the time since fusion was performed (*see* **Subheading 3.2.5.**).

1. Harvest all the cells in the well.
2. Count the cells and adjust them to 160 cells/mL. You can make 10 mL medium for each plate; hence you will need 1600 cells. It is not possible to use all the cells from the well for cloning. The remaining cells should be frozen as a back-up (*see* **Subheading 3.3.3.**).
3. Prepare macrophages as described in **Subheading 3.2.4.** You will need 0.2 mL/ plate; hence add 0.2 mL into 10 mL medium.
4. Add 100 μL medium into each well except in columns 1 and 2. You are going to do each dilution in two columns. The number of plates depends on the screening method you are using (*see* **Note 2**).
5. Add 200 μL of the cell suspension into columns 1 and 2.
6. Titrate the cells across the plate by transferring 100 μL from the wells in column 1 into wells in column 3, mixing, and then transferring 100 μL from wells in column 3 into wells in column 5, and so forth. Discard the last 100 μL from wells in column 11. Repeat this titration for column 2.
7. Add 100 μL macrophage suspension into each well.
8. When the clones of cells can be seen and the medium has turned quite yellow it is time to screen the supernatants. It is important to repeat the cloning at least twice by set concentration using 0.3 cells/well. Remember to freeze the cells at each cloning stage (*see* **Subheading 3.3.3.**).
9. When you have ensured you have fully cloned the hybridoma cells you can transfer them to 24-well plates for freezing and growing them for bulk antibody production.

3.3.3. Fixed Volume Cloning

This is a quick way of cloning and does not require counting the cells.

1. Transfer 100 μL of cell suspension from a well on a 96- or a 24-well plate into 2 mL of medium (dilution 1). The remaining cells should be frozen as a back-up (*see* **Subheading 3.3.3.**).
2. From dilution 1 make threefold dilutions four times by transferring 1 mL dilution 1 into 2 mL medium (dilution 2), mixing, and then transferring 1 mL of that dilu-

tion into 2 mL medium (dilution 3), and so on. Throw away 1 mL from the last dilution (dilution 5).

3. Prepare macrophages as described in **Subheading 3.2.4.** You will need 0.4 mL/ dilution.
4. Add 18.6 mL medium and 0.4 mL macrophage suspension into each dilution.
5. Plate the cells from each dilution onto a 96-well plate, 200 µL/well.
6. Analyze plate 5 for the presence of clones and when the medium has turned quite yellow it is time to screen the supernatants. If you are unsuccessful with plate 5 (no clones present or no positive clones) then screen plate 4. Plates 1 and 2 do usually have more than one clone/well and can be used as a back-up.
7. When you have ensured you have fully cloned the hybridoma cells you can transfer them to 24-well plates for freezing and growing them for bulk antibody production.

3.3.4. Freezing the Hybridoma Cells

At each cloning stage, it is very important to freeze some hybridoma cells as a back-up. Also, when a positive clone has been obtained, freezing cells is very important. Sometimes hybridoma cells stop producing antibodies, and then it is important to be able to go back to cells that were frozen soon after the cloning.

1. Transfer the cells into a 24-well plate. These cells can be expanded to obtain substantial number of cells.
2. Harvest the cells, count them, and centrifuge at 250g for 5 min.
3. Discard the supernatant and resuspend the cells in freezing medium so the concentration becomes $0.5–5.0 \times 10^6$ cells/mL.
4. Transfer 1 mL aliquots into cryotubes and place the tubes on ice.
5. If you do not have a freezing machine, keep the cells on ice for 2 h. Then wrap them in a bubble plastic sheet (acting as an insulator) and place them in cottonwool padded box. Store the box in a –70°C freezer overnight and then transfer the tubes into liquid nitrogen. If you have a freezing machine, the cells can be frozen immediately and then later transferred into liquid nitrogen.

4. Notes

1. Before the fusion it is very important to have a screening method available. Several screening systems can be used, such as immunostaining of tissue sections/ cytospins, Western blotting, flow cytometry, and ELISA. These will be described in Chapters 30 and 32–34. The choice of screening method depends on the intended use the mAbs.
2. Some screening methods, such as immunohistochemistry, can be very time-consuming. Therefore, it is important to minimize the number of wells you have to screen and plate the fused cells into 24-well plates, not 96-well plates. On the other hand, if a quick screening method, such as ELISA, is being used, plating

out in 96-well plates is reasonable. The same principle applies for cloning. If you are using a time-consuming screening method, take care not to use too many plates per cloning.

3. Unfused B cells can produce antibodies and secrete them into the supernatant. This can give rise to a false-positive results during your screening. To avoid that problem you can change medium after half a week (HAT medium), a week (HT medium), and a week and a half (HT medium). This will dilute any antibodies produced by B cells.

Further Reading

Goding, J. W., ed. (1996) *Monoclonal Antibodies: Principles and Practice: Production and Application of Monoclonal Antibodies in Cell Biology, Biochemistry and Immunology*, 3rd ed., Academic, New York.

Ritter, M. A. and Ladyman, H. M., eds. (1995) *Monoclonal Antibodies: Production, Engineering, and Clinical Application*, Cambridge University Press, Cambridge, UK.

Springer, T. A., ed. (1985) *Hybridoma Technology in the Biosciences and Medicine*, Plenum, New York.

McMichael, A. J. and Fabre, J. W., ed. (1982) *Monoclonal Antibodies in Clinical Medicine*, Academic, New York.

Köhler, G. and Milstein, C. (1975) Continuous cultures of fused cells secreting antibody of predefined specificity. *Nature* **256,** 495–497.

18

Purification of Monoclonal Antibodies Using Protein A/G

Bridget Heelan

1. Introduction

A major breakthrough in immunology came with the discovery that large amounts of relatively pure monoclonal antibodies (mAbs) could be prepared from the fusion of B cells (secreting the relevant mAb) with a nonsecreting myeloma cell line *(1)*. Since then mAbs have become a central tool for researchers, enabling them to investigate previously unknown molecules. More recently mAbs have also gained an important role in medicine, e.g., in helping to prevent allograft rejection and in the treatment of digoxin poisoning.

Simple methods are available that enable us to purify large amounts (tens of milligrams) of mAbs from tissue culture supernatant in vitro, and in this chapter I will focus on the purification of mAbs using either protein A or protein G coupled to sepharose beads.

Protein A and protein G are both bacterial antibody-binding proteins found in *Staphylococci* and *Streptococci*, respectively. Although these two proteins lack sequence or structural similarity, both bind to nonidentical though overlapping areas in the heavy-chain constant domains of the Fc region of immunoglobulins (Igs) *(2)*. Binding to this region of Igs prevents FcR and C1q binding by the Ig. These molecules inhibit the effector function of Ig molecules in vivo, thereby enabling the infecting organisms to evade the host's immune response.

Although both protein A and protein G bind to most mammalian Ig Fc regions, they differ in their affinities for different Ig isotypes *(3,4)*. Thus, the choice of which one to use will depend on the isotype of the mAb to be purified. However, since both these proteins when bound to sepharose beads can

From: *Methods in Molecular Medicine, Vol. 40: Diagnostic and Therapeutic Antibodies*
Edited by: A. J. T. George and C. E. Urch © Humana Press Inc., Totowa, NJ

be used interchangeably in the techniques I describe below, I will concentrate on protein G throughout this chapter. The principle of mAb purification using protein G bound to Sepharose beads is very simple. The secreted mAb in the tissue culture supernatant is bound by protein G, which in turn is attached to solid-phase Sepharose beads (**Fig. 1**). After incubation the beads with attached protein G, the mAbs are washed and then finally eluted, thereby leaving the Sepharose-bound protein G available for further use. The mAb is then quantified, suspended at the desired concentration and its purity is checked with one of a large number of techniques, such as sodium dodecyl sulfate-polyacrylamide gel electrophoresis (SDS-PAGE), high performance liquid chromatography (HPLC), or immunoassay.

2. Materials
2.1. Tissue Culture, Growth of Hybridoma Cell Lines, and Preparation of Supernatant

1. An mAb-secreting hybridoma cell line.
2. Tissue culture medium (RPMI).
3. Additives for RPMI: L-glutamine (final concentration of 2 mM), 2-mercaptoethanol (2-ME) (final concentration of $2 \times 10^{-5} M$), penicillin, streptomycin, and kanamycin (at final concentrations of 75 U/mL, 45 mg/mL and 90 mg/mL, respectively).
4. Fetal calf serum (FCS).
5. Dimethlysulfoxide (DMSO).
6. Tissue culture flasks.
7. Freezing vials (1.5 mL).
8. Equipment: water bath, tissue culture incubator (humidified at 37°C with 5% CO_2), –80°C freezer, liquid nitrogen and container (not absolutely necessary), phase contrast microscope, and tissue culture hood.

2.2. Purification of mAb from Tissue Culture Supernatant

1. Protein G (or protein A)-coupled sepharose beads.
2. 0.1 M glycine, pH 2.7.
3. 20% ethanol (filtered through a 0.22-μm filter).
4. 1 M Tris-HCl, pH 8.0.
5. Sodium azide.
6. Phosphate buffer: 20 mM sodium phosphate, pH 7.0.
7. Bottle-top sterile filters (0.22 μm).
8. 100- or 200-mL columns with fiber glass filters at the end.
9. Quills and plastic tubing and syringes.
10. Dialysis tubing.
11. Concentrators.
12. Equipment: spectrophotometer (280 nm), quartz cuvets, and centrifuge.

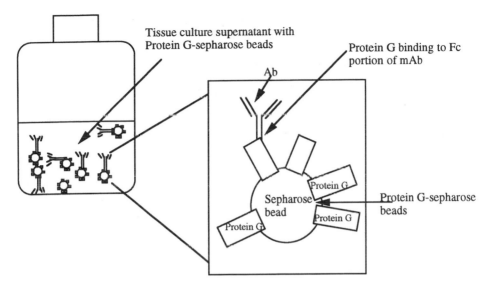

Fig. 1. Principle of antibody purification using protein G Sepharose beads.

3. Methods

3.1. Preparation of Tissue Culture Medium

1. Set a water bath to 56°C.
2. Heat the FCS to 56°C for 30 min. (This inactivates complement, an observation made when complement was originally discovered *(5)*, thus avoiding the risk of toxic effects mediated by bovine complement.)
3. Add the heat-inactivated FCS to a final concentration of 10% to the RPMI (It may be possible to use concentrations of FCS as low as 2–5% for some hybridomas.)
4. Add L-glutamine and 2-ME at final concentrations of 2 mM and 5 × 10^{-5} M, respectively. Both these additives degrade at 4°C. Because of this it is always best to use freshly made medium. (L-glutamine, a necessary though labile amino acid, degrades slowly to ammonia, which itself can inhibit cell growth *[6]*. It is not clear how 2-ME acts to enhance cell growth in vitro, but it is known to improve growth in a variety of cell types, such as murine blastocysts *[7]* and T lymphocytes *[8]*)
5. If required, add penicillin, streptomycin, and kanamycin (at final concentrations of 75 U/mL, 45 µg/mL, and 90 µg/mL, respectively). Although the use of antibiotics in tissue culture is common practice, cells tend to fare better without them. When dealing with cells, such as a mAb-secreting hybridoma (for which there should be numerous frozen vials available as backups), it is worth growing them without antibiotics, because the yield of mAb can be higher.

6. If the complete medium is not used immediately, it can be stored at 4°C for a short period of time (but preferably for <2 wk).

3.2. Growth of the mAb-Secreting Hybridoma

1. Prewarm the complete medium to room temperature.
2. Remove the frozen cells from liquid nitrogen.
3. Thaw the hybridoma cells rapidly by placing the vial in a 37°C water bath or by simply clasping the vial in the hand.
4. When the contents become liquid, use a syringe and quill to transfer them gently into a 50 mL plastic tube.
5. Slowly, drop by drop, add 5 mL of complete medium with constant swirling of the contents over a 5 min period. (This prevents rapid shifts in tonicity, which are toxic to the cells.)
6. Add another 5 mL over 2 min.
7. Spin the cells at 1200*g* for 5 min.
8. Decant the supernatant by inverting the tube (the cell pellet remains at the bottom).
9. Resuspended the cell pellet in the remaining volume (approx 100 µL) by tapping the tube vigorously.
10. Add 10 mL of complete medium to the cells and repeat **steps 7–9**. (This ensures that all the DMSO is washed out.)
11. Resuspend the cells at 5×10^5/mL in a 10 mL tissue culture flask.
12. Place the flask in the incubator with the lid slightly loose (this ensures aeration with 5% CO_2). The lid can be tightened fully 4–6 h later.
13. Monitor the growth of the cells daily and as the cell numbers increase split the cells into larger flasks with larger volumes of medium (*see* **steps 7–9**).
14. Allow the cells in one small flask to grow to confluence. When 70–80% of the cells are dead, harvest the supernatant. After spinning the cells (*see* **steps 7–9**), decant the supernatant into a second 50 mL tube and filter it (0.22 µm filter). This supernatant should have 2–15 µg of mAb/mL.

    At this point it is important to ensure that antibody is being secreted into the supernatant before expanding the hybridoma into large numbers of flasks. There are numerous ways of testing it, largely dependent on availability. Ideally, both the specificity and concentration of the antibody should be tested each time a new vial of frozen cells is thawed. Vials can be mislabeled, cells can be in poor condition when frozen, and freezers also break down—all good reasons for being meticulous at this point. Moreover, it is important to freeze some of the cells at this stage for future use (*see* **Subheading 3.4.**).
15. Because most of the mAb secretion is toward the end of the lifespan of the hybridoma cells, it is best to wait until ~ 80% of the cells have died (*9*). The 20% viability time point works well for most cell lines, but it is worth testing the cell lines you decide to use to see if it is possible to improve on the mAb yield. At this point, the cells should be spun down at 1200*g* × 5 min, the cells discarded, and the supernatant collected. The supernatant is then filtered (0.22 µm) and ready

for use. If desired, 0.02% sodium azide may be added to the filtered supernatant. This helps to prevent bacterial contamination. However, caution must be used when handling solutions containing azide because it is toxic.

3.3. Preparation of Tissue Culture Medium Free of Bovine Immunoglobulin

The importance of growing mAb-secreting hybridomas in tissue culture medium that is free from bovine Igs is that protein G binds to Igs from a variety of mammals, including that present in FCS. Therefore, the final purified antibody preparation will contain both the mAb of interest and bovine IgG. For most purposes this will not matter, but there are instances in which a very highly purified mAb is required.

There are two ways to avoid this problem. Both approaches ensure that the final purified Ig contains only the mAb required. The first approach is to use serum-free medium, which contains the necessary factors for cell growth but contains no FCS (and therefore no bovine Igs). The second approach, using protein G Sepharose beads, involves removing bovine Ig from the FCS prior to adding it to the tissue culture medium *(10)*.

3.4. Freezing Hybridoma Cell Lines

1. Make up fresh freezing mix (50% FCS, 35% complete tissue culture medium, and 15% DMSO).
2. Take a tissue culture flask in which the cell viability is more than 90%.
3. Transfer the contents to a 50-mL tube and spin the cells as in **Subheading 3.2., steps 7–9**.
4. When the cells have been resuspended in the residual volume of medium at the bottom of the tube add the freezing mix (1 mL to approx 5×10^6 cells).
5. Gently transfer this into a prelabeled freezing vial.
6. Place the vial into a box containing cotton wool and then place it immediately into the −80°C freezer. The cotton wool ensures a slow rate of cooling for the cells (approx 1°C/min).
7. After a minimum of 4 h at −80°C, the vial can then be transferred into liquid nitrogen for long-term storage. It is worth noting that cells will remain viable at −80°C for approx 6 mo, though they are stable for much longer (many years) in liquid nitrogen.

3.5. Purification of mAb from Tissue Culture Supernatant

1. Filter all solutions (PBS; supernatant; 20% ethanol; 0.1 *M* glycine) through 0.22 µm bottle-top filters.
2. Prenumber 20 × 1 mL tubes (1–20) and put 100 µL of 1 *M* Tris-HCl (pH 8.0) in each of them.
3. Take protein G Sepharose beads (in PBS) and pour them into a column with a fiber glass filter at the bottom, followed by 50 mL of prefiltered PBS. The quan-

tity of beads used depends on the antibody concentration in and volume of the supernatant to be purified. (The binding capacity of 1 mg of protein G is 6–7 mg rodent IgG. If one assumes that the average hybridoma secretes 5–15 µg/mL, then 2 L would contain 10–30 mg IgG. In this example 7 mg/protein G bound to Sepharose beads would be the correct amount to use.) Do not allow the beads to dry at any point in the procedure.

4. Ensure that no beads are stuck to the edges of the column and that they have all settled to the bottom. If necessary, wash the edges of the column with more PBS.

5. Run the supernatant through the column at a rate of 0.5 mL/min. This will give the mAb time to bind to the protein G. The supernatant should be collected and stored after running it through the column because there may be some mAb left. It is always worth checking this for any remaining mAb.

6. When all the supernatant has run through, wash the column by running 4×20 mL PBS. This ensures that all nonspecifically bound proteins (e.g., albumin) are washed through.

7. Elute the bound mAb by running 4×5 mL aliquots of 0.1 M glycine (pH 2.7) and collecting the eluant (1 mL fractions) into the prenumbered tubes containing Tris-HCl buffer.

8. Quantitate the amount of antibody in each fraction by spectrophotometry (using as a blank 1 mL of glycine in a separate tube with Tris-HCl buffer).

9. Wash the column with 3×20 mL PBS and store it at 4°C in PBS, 0.02% azide in PBS, or 20% ethanol.

10. Coalesce all the fractions that contain antibody and dialyse overnight against PBS at 4°C.

11. Using any concentrator device, suspend the mAb at the desired concentration and assess the purity. This can be done in a variety of ways, but one of the fastest is by HPLC. If this is not possible, another reliable technique involves labeling the antibody with a radioactive isotope, such as ^{125}I. After labeling, the antibody can then be run on an SDS gel. The gel should be dried and autoradiography performed. Although these approaches provide information about the purity of the mAb, what is most important is the immunoreactivity of the mAb. Radioimmunoassay, ELISA immunohistology, or flow cytometry analysis are techniques commonly used to assess immunoreactivity.

3.6. Purification of mAb from Large Volumes of Tissue Culture Supernatant

When very large volumes of tissue culture supernatant (e.g. 3–4 L) are being purified, running such volumes even through a large column is a lengthy process. A slight modification, which although faster does not compromise on mAb binding by protein G, is described below and shown in **Fig. 2**.

1. Add 7–8 mg protein G Sepharose beads (prewashed with PBS) to 3 L prefiltered supernatant in a large flask filled to capacity.

2. Incubate at room temperature for 2–4 h with gentle mixing.

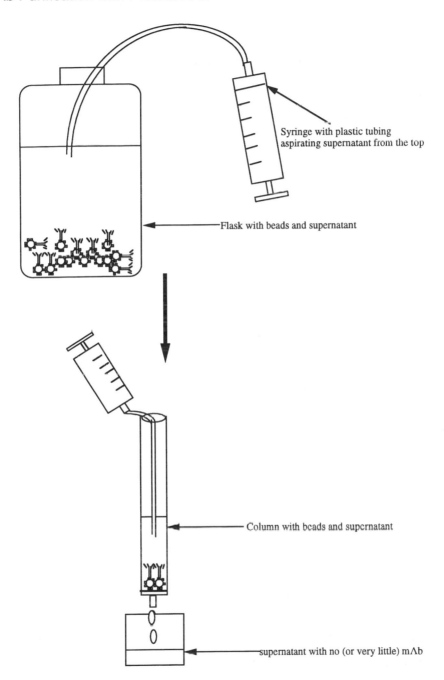

Fig. 2. Quick method for mMAb purification using protein G-coupled Sepharose beads.

3. Leave the mixture undisturbed for 1–2 h to allow the beads to settle to the bottom of the flask.

4. Using a 60 mL syringe with attached plastic tubing aspirate the supernatant from the top of the flask without disturbing the sediment and run it through a 200-mL column (with a glass fiber filter at the bottom). Because this part of the supernatant should be relatively free from Sepharose beads, it will run through the column very quickly. However, by running it through the column no Sepharose beads will be lost.

5. Continue aspirating from the top until all the supernatant has been run through the column. Toward the end of the aspiration, the supernatant at the bottom of the flask will have a high concentration of Sepharose beads and therefore the rate of flow through the column will slow down.

6. Wash the flask with 3 × 50 mL PBS to ensure that no beads are lost. Then follow **Subheading 3.5., steps 6–11**.

References

1. Köhler, G. and Milstein, C. (1975) Continuous cultures of fused cells secreting antibody of predefined specificity. *Nature* **256,** 495–497.

2. Kato, K., Lian, L., Barsukov, I., Derrick, J., Kim, H., Tanaka, R., Yoshino, A., Shiraishi, M., Shimada, I., Arata, Y., et al. (1995) Model for the complex between protein G and an antibody Fc fragment in solution. *Structure* **3,** 79–85.

3. Jones, R., Rademacher, T., and Williams, P. (1996) Bias in murine IgG isotype immobilisation. Implications for IgG glycoform analysis ELISA procedures. *J. Immunol. Methods* **197,** 109–120.

4. Guss, B., Eliasson, M., Olsson, A., Uhlen, M., Frej, A.-K., Jornvall, H., Flock, J.-I., and Lindberg, M. (1986). Structure of the IgG-binding regions of Streptococcal Protein G. *EMBO J.* **5,** 1567–1575.

5. Bordet, J. (1898) Sur l'agglutination et la dissolution des globules rouges par le serum d'animaux injectes dee sang definrine. *Annales de l'Institute Pasteur* **12,** 688–695.

6. Butler, M. and Christie, A. (1994) Adaptation of mammalian cells to non-ammoniagenic media. *Cytotechnology* **15,** 87–94.

7. Spindle, A. (1980) An improved culture medium for mouse blastocysts. *In Vitro* **16,** 669–74.

8. Flad, H., Ulmer, A., Claesson, M., and Opitz, H. (1979) Role of serum factors and adherent cells in cloning of human T lymphocytes in agar culture. *Acta Haematol.* **62,** 326–330.

9. Ker-hwa, O. and Patterson, P. (1997) A more efficient and economical approach for monoclonal antibody production (letter). *J. Immunol. Methods* **209,** 105–108.

10. Darby, C., Hamano, K., and Wood, K. (1993) Purification of monoclonal antibodies from tissue culture medium depleted of IgG. *J. Immunol. Methods* **159 (1–2),** 125–129.

19

Preparation of Monoclonal Antibodies Using Ion Exchange Chromatography

Maureen Power

1. Introduction

One of the most successful methods for the preparation of pure monoclonal antibodies (mAbs) is ion exchange chromatography. It is not dependent on the reaction of immunoglobulins with immobilized ligands, as is the case of adsorption chromatography, which uses either protein A or G, but on the charge of the biomolecules. Some immunoglobulins bind only weakly or not at all to protein A or G, and for these molecules ion exchange is the method of choice. Additional advantages of ion exchange are its high resolving power, high capacity (capable of large scale purification), and the relative ease with which it can be controlled.

The principle of ion exchange chromatography is dependent on the adsorption of charged molecules to an immobilized ion exchange group that possesses the opposite charge. As the electrostatic interaction is reversible; this allows the mAb to be readily eluted from the exchanger, in most cases by increasing the salt concentration.

The procedure can be simplified into the following stages.

1. Preparation of the starting material (ascitic fluid or culture supernatant) so that it can be applied to the column for purification.
2. Applying the material to the column under conditions in which the molecule of interest binds to the ion exchanger. An alternative approach is the reverse of this, in which the molecule of interest passes through the exchanger, whereas the contaminants are bound. The first method allows a greater degree of fractionation, together with some concentration of the substance of interest. The second approach is, however, simpler and will be used in the example given in this chapter.
3. Collection of the purified material from the ion exchanger.

From: *Methods in Molecular Medicine, Vol. 40: Diagnostic and Therapeutic Antibodies*
Edited by: A. J. T. George and C. E. Urch © Humana Press Inc., Totowa, NJ

2. Materials

2.1. Reagents

1. Ion exchange resin, Whatman DEAE 52 (Whatman International, Maidstone, UK).
2. TE8 (2 M stock pH 8.0) 2 M Tris-HCl, 100 mM ethylenediamine tetra-acetic acid (EDTA). Prepare 0.2 M TE8 and 50 mM TE8 from 2 M stock.
3. Saturated ammonium sulfate made up in 0.2 M TE8.
4. Sodium chloride for step gradient (if needed).

2.2. Equipment

1. Glass chromatographic columns of approx 3 cm diameter by approx 25 cm length. Homemade type or Pharmacia K (Pharmacia, Uppsala, Sweden) series approx 2.5 cm wide and 30–60 cm in length with one flow adaptor. Jacketed columns are not needed because runs are at room temperature.
2. UV monitor, chart recorder, and fraction collector.
3. Stirred concentration cell or disposable single-use concentrators. Either method uses 10 kDa molecular weight cutoff.
4. Electrophoresis system.
5. Centrifuge (bench type nonrefrigerated).
6. Coarse membrane filters.
7. Laboratory stirrer.
8. Sintered funnel and Buchner flask.
9. Vacuum pump.
10. pH meter.
11. Conductivity meter (not always essential).

3. Methods

The protocol describes the procedure to prepare a typical mAb from culture supernatant.

3.1. Collection and Concentration of Culture Supernatant

1. If starting with culture supernatant, material grown from several flasks can be harvested over a period of time and pooled.
2. The material is passed through a coarse membrane filter to remove any debris that may still remain (*see* **Note 1**).
3. Concentrate this material using a stirred concentration cell or disposable concentrator to a smaller volume (e.g., 2–3 L of material down to 100–200 mL). To avoid loss of product always overconcentrate and wash residue from the device with a small volume of buffer.

3.2. Precipitation of the Immunoglobulin

The procedure is carried out at room temperature to ensure maximum recovery of the mAb.

1. Slowly add an equal volume of saturated ammonium sulfate to the stirred antibody solution (*see* **Note 2**).
2. Leave stirring for a further 15 min.
3. Recover the precipitated fraction by centrifugation (approx 1700*g* for 25 min).
4. Suspend pellet in 0.2 *M* TE8 and reprecipitate it using the same protocol as above (**steps 1–3**).
5. Suspend the final pellets in 50 m*M* TE8 in as small a volume as possible and extensively dialyse against this buffer at 4°C.

3.3. Preparation of Exchanger

Whatman DEAE 52 comes already preswollen and only needs to be transferred to the running buffer 50 m*M* TE8.

1. Attach a scintered funnel to a Buchner flask connected to a vacuum pump.
2. Add exchanger to the scintered funnel.
3. Wash with 10 L 50 m*M* TE8.
4. Check that the pH and ionic strength of the buffer coming through the exchanger are the same as that being added. If so, the exchanger is ready for use. If not, add more 50 m*M* TE8 (*see* **Note 3**).

3.4. Packing the Column

1. Estimate the volume of exchanger that will be needed (*see* **Note 4** for guidelines).
2. Add this volume of DEAE in 50 m*M* TE8 to the chromatographic column.
3. Attach a container containing 1 L of 50 m*M* TE8 to the column, and raise it about 20 cm above the top of the column. This will provide enough "head of pressure" to allow the column to be packed. The exact manner in which you connect the column to the buffer will depend on the nature of your apparatus; please refer to appropriate instruction manuals.
4. Adjust the height of the buffer container so that an adequate flow rate is achieved (typically 10 mL/min, though the flow rate is not critical for DEAE columns).

3.5. Purification of IgG

1. Add the sample onto the column. The way in which you can do this will depend on the setup of your apparatus.
2. Pass 50 m*M* TE8 through the column.
3. Using a 200 mL column the majority of antibodies will elute quite early, after 150–250 mL (**Fig. 1**).
4. However, occasionally an immunoglobulin will bind under these conditions and it is necessary to use a step salt gradient for its elution.
5. Change the buffer to 0.025 *M* sodium chloride/50 m*M* TE8. In most cases this will cause the antibody to elute (*see* **Fig. 2**). If the antibody still fails to elute then further increase in the sodium chloride concentration. A suggested progression would be 0.025 *M*, 0.05 *M*, 0.1 *M*, 0.2 *M* NaCl.

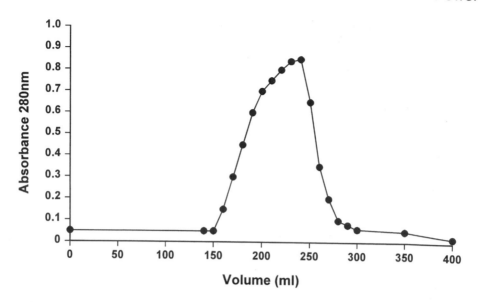

Fig. 1. Simple purification of a mAb by ion exchange. The sample containing the antibody is added at 0 mL. The column is then washed with 50 m*M* TE8 and the absorbance at 280 nm monitored (to detect protein). The volume of buffer passed through the column is shown on the *x* axis. The antibody is seen eluting after about 150 mL of buffer has passed through the column.

3.6. Testing of Eluted mAb

Fractions are taken from the above column run and assessed by electrophoresis for purity of the mAb recovered. This can be compared with the original concentrated starting material, which should show a distinct monoclonal band of immunoglobulin.

Only those fractions demonstrating a single band with a mobility the same as the original starting material should be taken and pooled. Any material that shows impurities can be rerun using a freshly equilibrated column (*see* **Notes 5** and **6**).

4. Notes

1. All normal debris can be removed by adequate centrifugation. However, when ascites is used as the starting material this is often contaminated with pristane, which can only be removed by filtration through a coarse membrane.
2. Saturated ammonium sulfate solution is made from 770 g salt/1 L 0.2 *M* TE8. The upper layers of this stored solution are often not fully saturated if the storage bottle has been standing for any length of time. It is therefore best to shake the solution vigorously and then filter to ensure a fully saturated solution is used.

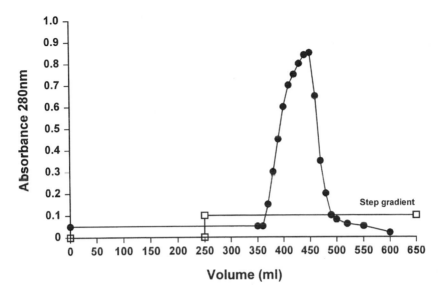

Fig. 2. Use of a step gradient to elute antibody. The setup is similar to **Fig. 1**. However, in this case the antibody did not elute in 50 m*M* TE8. The buffer was changed after 250 mL to 0.025 m*M* NaCl in 50 m*M* TE8. This causes the antibody to be eluted, as seen with the peak between 350 and 500 mL.

3. The use of a conductivity meter can be avoided by passing a large (>10 L) volume of 50 m*M* TE8 buffer through the exchanger.
4. A suitable size column for 2–3 L supernatant containing approx 10 μg/mL antibody would be 200 mL Whatman DEAE 52.
5. Impure fractions can also indicate a failure (at some point) to equilibrate fully in appropriate buffer, typically insufficient dialysis of the precipitated fraction or insufficient equilibration of the exchanger. These runs should be pooled, concentrated, and redialysed and applied to a new fully equilibrated column of exchanger.
6. Exchange can be used many times and can be cleaned by addition of 0.5 *M* NaOH for 30 min only, followed by extensive washing with distilled water until pH is neutral. Storage can be in concentrated Tris buffer at 4°C.

20

Quality Control of Raw Materials

Patrick Harrison and Geoff Hale

1. Introduction

High-quality starting materials are a prerequisite for any scientific method to be reliable and reproducible, but for the production of monoclonal antibodies (mAbs) for human diagnostics or therapy, and for successful preclinical studies, this is of paramount importance. Standard laboratory chemicals are normally perfectly satisfactory and it should not be necessary for a research laboratory to invest substantial effort in setting up in-house testing procedures. Nevertheless, according to current good manufacturing practice, all raw materials that come into contact with medicinal products need to be controlled and tested for purity and identity. In producing antibodies for clinical trials we find that the best way to do this is to specify pharmacopoeia-grade chemicals whenever possible (these are labeled BP, USP, or EuPh and many are available from Merck, Lutterworth, UK) and to require the supplier to send a certificate of analysis with all raw materials. Any supplier who cannot provide a certificate should be avoided. When goods are delivered, check the labels for conformity with the certificate to check that the tests listed were those actually carried out on the product. Few research laboratories are equipped to carry out formal chemical tests for identity, so we suggest that you critically test the functionality of the final reagent. For example, prepare buffers by mixing calculated weights of components (rather than pH adjustment), then measure the final pH and conductivity to check that they conform to your specification.

The more difficult reagents to control are those that are most important for cell culture, namely water, culture medium, and serum (here we will use "serum" to include serum replacements of whatever sort). The purpose of this chapter is to describe some simple and practical methods for ensuring that these ingredients are suitable for production of clinical trial material. They must meet

From: *Methods in Molecular Medicine, Vol. 40: Diagnostic and Therapeutic Antibodies*
Edited by: A. J. T. George and C. E. Urch © Humana Press Inc., Totowa, NJ

two main requirements: promote reliable cell growth and antibody production, and avoid introducing undesirable contaminants, particularly endotoxins, microbes, or viruses. Many tests can be carried out using standard commercial kits, or contracted to a suitable testing laboratory. However, we have found that a simple quantitative cell growth test is an invaluable functional assay for complete medium (*see* **Note 1**). The principle of this assay is to set up a series of cell cultures in both the test and control media, with different numbers of input cells ranging from about 5×10^5/mL down to about 4×10^3/mL. The cells used should be representative of the final antibody-producing cell line(s). After a suitable period of growth (e.g., 3–7 d), the number of viable cells in each culture is measured by a standard method, conversion of MTT dye [(4,5-dimethylthiozol-2-yl)-2,5 diphenyl tetrazolium bromide] (*see* **Note 2**) *(1,2)*. MTT is converted to an insoluble, blue/brown product by the activity of mitochondrial dehydrogenases present in living cells. The color change can be measured spectrophotometrically, allowing a sensitive comparison of growth-supporting activity of the test and control media.

2. Materials
2.1. Water

In the past there has been a lot of superstition about water for tissue culture. In our experience any of the standard laboratory methods of making purified water are suitable, i.e., distillation or reversed osmosis plus ion exchange (RO/DI). The most important parameter that needs control is the level of bacterial endotoxin. Traditionally in the pharmaceutical industry, water is purified by distillation and stored at 80°C to prevent microbial growth. This is very expensive and most laboratories would use RO/DI systems with storage at ambient temperature. We recommend that the system include continuous recirculation through the storage tank via a disinfection system, which is normally a tube containing a high-intensity UV lamp flanked by 0.2 μm filters. It is also possible to install an endotoxin-removing ultrafilter at the point of use, but this is not essential if the water is kept free from bacteria. In use, it is important to sanitize the system on a regular basis (especially RO membranes), and to dump the contents of the tank if the water is not used regularly. We strongly recommend routine monitoring and recording of the water quality (e.g., weekly); this should include measurement of resistivity, bioburden, and endotoxin. Suggested specifications are: resistivity never <1 MΩ/cm, on average >5 MΩ/cm; bioburden never >100 organisms/mL, on average <10 organisms/mL; endotoxin never >10 EU/mL, on average <1 EU/mL.

2.2. Culture Medium

A crucial decision is whether to purchase ready-made liquid media or powder. Powder is more stable and more economical because it can be purchased in large batches. Besides the advantage of bulk purchase, there is much less batch testing. However, liquid media are less trouble because you do not need to control your own water supply, nor allow for in-house work mixing, filtering, and batch testing. The cost of liquid media in the 20–1000 L scale is now becoming very competitive.

In either case, the well-known suppliers pay a lot of attention to the quality of their products. Nevertheless, it is worth checking the formulation very carefully. The availability of some ingredients (e.g., amino acids) changes from time to time and so the supplier may change e.g., from a hydrated to anhydrous salt, or from a hydrochloride to a free base. Even if the appropriate change in formula weight is made, there might be subtle differences in solubility that affect the performance of the media. We recommend that the exact bill of ingredients be examined carefully and that no changes be allowed to the formula without prior approval. This is particularly important for custom formulations. At a sufficient scale, a custom formulation is no more costly than a standard one, and it may be cheaper. For example, media for use in a controlled pH fermentor does not require HEPES buffer, which is one of the most costly and least pure ingredients of standard formulations. Other useful changes can be made that save the need to add supplements (e.g., amino acids, selective drugs) or reduce possible downstream problems. Many investigators like to eliminate phenol red (pH indicator) from large scale media formulations because it can bind to proteins and might copurify with antibodies. We prefer to keep it in any situation in which the cultures can still be observed visually; the check on pH is a useful monitor of cell viability or possible microbial contamination.

2.3. Serum

Probably the single most important factor about serum is the country of origin. This is not because of major biological differences in cattle from different countries, but because of political and regulatory issues that will affect the ultimate use of the products you make. The most topical problem is BSE. There is little, if any, evidence that this can be transmitted by serum, let alone fetal serum, but since there is no in vitro test for the causative agent, the only way to minimize risk is to use serum from animals in a country where BSE has not been reported. New Zealand is the origin preferred by regulatory authorities. However, there is a considerable import/export market in both live cattle and fetal serum, and it is not always easy to trace the ultimate origin of any batch. It is said that more "New Zealand" serum is sold than actually produced in that country. We are very dependent on the suppliers and we recommend that you establish good relationships with a reputable supplier who can provide comprehensive documentation. Avoid "bargain discounts" if you plan to export your antibodies or use them in clinical trials.

The US Department of Agriculture is very concerned about importation of any products that might carry diseases like foot and mouth virus. They require a permit for all biological materials, like mAbs, which will usually specify that all serum used in production (at any time), must have originated in the United States (some other countries are acceptable if specifically nominated). This regulation is strictly enforced. Other countries have different concerns, e.g., the United Kingdom has strict rules to ensure that the maternal history of any fetal serum is thoroughly documented in order to prevent the reintroduction of BSE.

More likely and more troublesome contaminants of serum are bovine diarrhea virus and mycoplasma. Both of these should be tested for by the supplier (Microbiological Associates, Stirling, UK) and the test results included on the certificate of analysis. Since one devastating experience with mycoplasma contamination that was not detected in culture tests, we like to confirm that serum is free from mycoplasma by independent tests, including DNA hybridization. We have found the Gen-Probe Mycoplasma T.C. rapid detection system to be effective and easy to use (Gen-Probe Inc, San Diego, CA); alternatively independent companies can carry out these tests (e.g., Microbiological Associates; Q-One, Glasgow, UK).

The following are our minimal recommendations for serum specifications:

Hemoglobin: <0.2 mg/mL (20 mg/dL)
Bovine IgG: <0.25 mg/mL (lower is better)
Endotoxin: <5 EU/mL
Bacteria and fungi: negative
Mycoplasma: negative
Bovine adventitious agents: negative (bovine diarrhea virus, bovine
    rhinotracheitis and parainfluenza 3)
Growth promoting activity: At least 80% compared with a standard batch

Even if all the checks done by the supplier are satisfactory, it is still important for you to test that the serum batch is suitable for your cell line(s). That is the purpose of the assay described below. All reputable suppliers will send small samples for testing on approval and reserve the main batch. The number of samples and reserves is not as great as it used to be, but on the other hand, batches seem to be more reproducible. We recommend that you reserve the largest batch you can afford to cover foreseeable use in order to ensure long-term reproducibility and minimize the need for further testing.

Suppliers will carry out further processing on serum, e.g., dialysis, heat inactivation, gamma irradiation. Any of these might be useful, but it may be necessary to commit funds to a batch before it is processed. You would need to check growth promoting activity after the treatment, so it is advisable to carry out the preliminary tests yourself on a suitably treated aliquot.

Similar considerations may apply to many types of serum-free media and serum replacements, since some of these may ultimately have been derived from bovine or other animal products. In our experience, suppliers may be reluctant to disclose the ingredients and sources. They should be able to certify that certain sources are not used, but it is best to enter a suitable confidentiality agreement and obtain all the information if you want to use this type of material for clinical trial production.

2.4. Reagents for Culture Assay

1. Test cell line: Use the final production cell line or one that represents it. In a group working with numerous production lines, we normally use one NS0 (mouse myeloma), one Y3 (rat myeloma), and one CHO (hamster fibroblast) cell line. Prepare working cell banks specifically for these tests so that identical cell samples can be used each time. Handle mammalian cell lines in accordance with your local safety requirements.
2. Test and control culture media and sera. Store frozen aliquots of suitable reference samples of media and sera for the controls.
3. MTT (e.g., Sigma M-5655)—This chemical may cause inheritable genetic damage. Wear protective clothing, including gloves and a dust mask, when handling. Prepare a stock solution at 2 mg/mL in PBS, sterile filter, and store frozen in 3 mL aliquots.
4. Acid propanol: Mix 0.8 mL of 5 M HCl with 100 mL propan-2-ol.
5. Microtiter plate reader with 570 nm filter (we use a multiscan Plus Mark II).
6. Standard tissue culture equipment and supplies, including safety cabinet, CO_2 incubator, sterile pipets, and multichannel pipeters, tubes, and flat-bottomed sterile 96-well microtiter plates (e.g., Falcon 3072).

3. Methods

1. Use sterile materials and aseptic culture technique throughout.
2. Ensure that you have suitable viable cultures of the test cells in exponential growth.
3. Take 20 mL samples of test and control complete media. Prepare an assay plan. You can test three samples on each 96-well microtiter plate (*see* **Note 3**).
4. Pour a few milliliters of the first medium into a trough. Add 100 μL to columns 2–4 of a microtiter plate. Take a fresh trough and tips, and transfer 100 μL of the second sample to columns 6–8. Likewise add the third sample to columns 10–12.
5. Calculate the number of cells required (6×10^5 cells/test, 3 tests/plate) and harvest a suitable quantity. Check their viability, which should be at least 70% (*see* **Note 4**).
6. Label a set of 15 mL tubes, according to the test/control samples, and add suspension containing 6×10^5 viable cells to each tube. Pellet the cells by centrifugation. Remove the supernatant and resuspend each cell pellet in 1.2 mL of its appropriate medium sample.

7. Add 125 µL of the first cell suspension to column 1. Make fivefold serial dilutions by transferring 25 µL to column 2, mix and transfer 25 µL to column 3, mix and transfer 25 µL to column 4, mix and discard 25 µL. Repeat the procedure for each subsequent sample (**Note 5**).

8. Incubate the samples at 37°C in a suitable CO_2 humid incubator for 3 d (**Notes 6–9**).

9. Thaw sufficient MTT solution (3 mL/plate). Add 25 µL to rows A–F on each plate. Return the plates to the incubator for 3 h. Keep the remaining MTT solution away from bright daylight.

10. Add 100 µL acid propanol to all wells. Then add 25 µL MTT to rows G and H (**Note 10**).

11. Thoroughly mix the contents of each well to resuspend the colored product.

12. Measure the absorbance of each well at 570 nm.

13. Calculate the mean of wells A–F in each column and subtract the mean of wells G and H. Calculate the standard deviation of wells A–F. Compare the test and control samples of media at each cell dilution. The mean of the test results should lie within 2 SD of the control result (**Note 11**).

4. Notes

1. The important features of this test are that it is quantitative and it tests the media at different cell densities. Cells are often more fastidious at low density, whereas lack of a common ingredient (like glutamine) may only be evident at high density.

2. This protocol illustrates one implementation as used in our laboratory. No doubt numerous modifications could be made according to the local requirements, especially in the plate layout and the cell dilutions. Other methods (e.g., radioisotope incorporation) might be used to measure cell viability, but we found MTT to be convenient.

3. For testing new batches of serum, it is a good idea to prepare a number of different dilutions spanning the desired range. This assay is a good way to optimize serum concentration.

4. Though we normally use a growing culture of test cells, it may also be possible to use cells directly after thawing if the viability is adequate. This would save time and trouble if an adequate cell bank is prepared.

5. Multichannel pipeters are very useful for all repetitive additions and for mixing the final precipitate.

6. The CO_2 level in the incubator needs to be adjusted to suit the media. If media with different buffering properties are tested (e.g., ± HEPES), it may be necessary to first add some buffer to all of them. In any event, proper pH control is important as in all cell culture.

7. Wells with high input cell density may overgrow and die by 3 d and show little color change with MTT. This is normal and a useful indication of media quality as long as adequate growth is measured at lower cell densities.

8. The assay can be extended for up to 7 d if the division rate of your test cell line is low and there is little color change at low cell input density.

9. Check for the presence of any microbial contamination and discard results from any contaminated wells.

10. The reason for including the wells G and H where no growth with MTT is allowed is to control for differences in color between media samples. Any background reading in these wells can be subtracted from the corresponding test wells.

11. We have used this assay over the past 7 yr to test more than 500 batches of media and serum. It is useful to determine the shelf life of liquid media in the laboratory, especially since it is inconvenient to store large volumes (thousands of liters) in the cold. For example, we found that standard IMDM (containing glutamine) still gives results within 80% of control with Y3 and CHO cells after 3 mo storage at 20°C.

References

1. Mosmann, T. (1983) Rapid colorimetric assay for cellular growth and survival: application to proliferation and cytotoxicity assays. *J. Immunol. Methods* **65,** 55–63.

2. Denizot, F. and Lang, R. (1986) Rapid colorimetric assay for cell growth and survival. Modifications to the tetrazolium dye procedure giving improved sensitivity and reliability. *J. Immunol. Methods* **89,** 271–277.

21

Cell Banks and Stability of Antibody Production

Pru Bird and Geoff Hale

1. Introduction

The original and fundamental appeal of monoclonal antibodies (mAbs), compared with polyclonal antisera, is the possibility for indefinite production of the same product. However, even well-established cell lines have limited stability in long-term culture and it is necessary to establish a control system to ensure continuity of product supply. This is normally done by a seed lot system. A pool of cells derived from a single clone is frozen in a number of vials (say 100) to create a master cell bank (MCB). This MCB is carefully stored in liquid nitrogen. As required, individual vials are thawed and expanded to provide working cell banks, which might also consist of about 100 vials. Thus up to 10,000 production runs can be initiated before the original cell stock is exhausted. Obviously the number of vials in a bank can be adjusted to meet individual requirements. Working cell banks may not be necessary for experimental or preclinical projects, but you should at all costs avoid depletion of a clinically important master cell bank.

There are extensive guidelines for the testing of master and working cell banks that will be used for production of therapeutic products (e.g., *1,2*) and it is not our purpose to reiterate them here. Those tests are designed primarily to check the identity of the cell line and to characterize any microbial or viral contaminants. They must be carried out by expert virologists and are usually contracted to suitable commercial organizations. Because the testing process is costly and time consuming, it is important to establish cell banks as early as possible in a new project. However, for the same reasons, it is equally important to choose the optimal cell line, which is both a high producer and is clonally stable.

From: *Methods in Molecular Medicine, Vol. 40: Diagnostic and Therapeutic Antibodies*
Edited by: A. J. T. George and C. E. Urch © Humana Press Inc., Totowa, NJ

It is a *sine qua non* that cell lines must be truly clonal before making a master cell bank. When receiving a hybridoma or transfectant from another laboratory, the wise production laboratory will first check its mycoplasma status and then reclone it. Many mouse and hetero- hybridomas are notoriously unstable regarding antibody production, and we have found the same to be true of transfectants, particularly several made using the glutamine synthetase (GS) expression system *(3,4)*. It is laborious and time-consuming to check and compare the stability of different clones or transfectants; the normal procedure being to carry out analytical cloning after an appropriate period of continuous culture. Many subclones have to be assessed for antibody secretion to obtain an accurate measure of the heterogeneity of the cell line. Here we describe a simpler procedure whereby the cytoplasmic immunoglobulin within the antibody-producing cells is measured by flow cytometry *(5)*. The concentration of cytoplasmic Ig correlates well with the capacity to secrete Ig, and provides a useful quantitative marker for the distribution of cells in a sample (*see* **Note 1**).

2. Materials

1. Rigid round-bottom microtiter plates (e.g., Falcon 3910) or sample tubes suitable for the flow cytometer (*see* **Note 2**).
2. Wash buffer: Phosphate-buffered saline (PBS) containing 0.5% bovine serum albumin (BSA, e.g., Sigma [St. Louis, MO] A-9647) and 0.1% sodium azide. Store at 4°C for up to 1 mo.
3. Permeabilizing buffer: PBS containing 0.5% BSA, 0.1% sodium azide, and 0.5% saponin (Sigma S-2149). Saponin is an irritant; wear gloves and a mask when weighing out the powder. Store at 4°C for up to 1 mo.
4. Detection reagent, as appropriate for the target antigen, e.g.:
   Polyclonal FITC-conjugated goat antimouse IgG (Fc specific) (Sigma F-0257).
   Polyclonal FITC-conjugated goat antirat IgG (Fc specific) (Sigma F-6258).
   Polyclonal FITC-conjugated goat antihuman IgG (Fc specific) (Sigma F-9512).
5. 2% formaldehyde: Add 1 mL formalin (37% formaldehyde, e.g., Sigma F-1268) to 17.5 mL PBS. Formaldehyde is toxic; handle with care.
6. Standard laboratory equipment, including a centrifuge equipped with microtiter plate carriers.
7. Negative and positive cell controls of the same cell type as the test samples.
8. Test samples, typically $0.2–2 \times 10^6$ viable cells (*see* **Note 3**).
9. Reference beads for flow cytometer (e.g., Quantum fluorescence kit, Sigma cat. no. QMF-2) (*see* **Note 4**).

3. Methods

1. Transfer samples containing a minimum of 2×10^5 cells into the microtiter wells according to a predetermined plan. It is best to place the negative control cells first, followed by the positive control and then the test samples. Test all samples in duplicate.

2. Centrifuge the microtiter plates (200*g* for 2 min) to pellet the cells, and remove the supernatant.
3. Add 100 µL 2% formaldehyde to each well and incubate at room temperature for 15 min to fix the cells.
4. Pellet the cells again, resuspend in 200 µL wash buffer, pellet, and resuspend in 100 µL wash buffer.
5. Add 100 µL permeabilizing buffer to each well, pellet, and discard the supernatant.
6. Resuspend the cells in 50 µL permeabilizing buffer and incubate at room temperature for 30 min to make the pores in the cell membrane.
7. Dilute the FITC-conjugated antibody to the optimal dilution in permeabilizing buffer (*see* **Note 5**).
8. Pellet the cells, discard the supernatant, and resuspend in 50 µL of the diluted FITC-conjugate. Incubate at room temperature for 30 min.
9. Add 150 µL permeabilizing buffer and pellet the cells. Discard the supernatant and resuspend in 200 µL wash buffer to close off the pores. Pellet the cells and resuspend in 100 µL wash buffer.
10. Analyze the samples by flow cytometry (*see* **Note 6**). Generally there will be two populations in the forward vs 90° scatter cytogram. Cells that were viable at the time of fixing will have higher forward scatter and should comprise the majority population. Set a gate to include these cells and exclude the others. Record the fluorescence distribution of the gated population. Compare test and control samples (compare **Fig. 1**) (*see* **Notes 8** and **9**).

4. Notes

1. Cytoplasmic Ig is measured in the assay because it is present at high concentrations in both hybridomas and immunoglobulin transfectants. Surface Ig is rarely expressed at a useful level.
2. This procedure is described at microtiter scale because we normally run the samples on a Becton Dickinson FACSscan (Becton Dickinson, San Jose, CA) equipped with a FACSmate microtiter plate sampler. It can equally well be carried out in tubes, and the volumes can be adjusted *pro rata*. Centrifugation times should be increased if necessary to ensure that the cells are pelleted at each step. If you use the microtiter method, take great care to avoid any splashing or spillover of cells from one well to another.
3. For consistent results the cell samples should all be taken from cultures in exponential growth with at least 80% viability. Samples of low viability (e.g., end of production from a fermentor run) should first be depleted of dead cells by centrifugation over a density gradient medium, such as Histopaque (e.g., Sigma H-8889).
4. It highly recommended to include a standard calibration sample with each flow cytometry run. Standard fluorescent beads can be used and/or fixed control cells can be stored for up to 4 wk in washing buffer at 4°C.
5. The optimal dilution of fluorescent detection reagent should ideally be established by experiment; the manufacturer's recommendation is generally a good

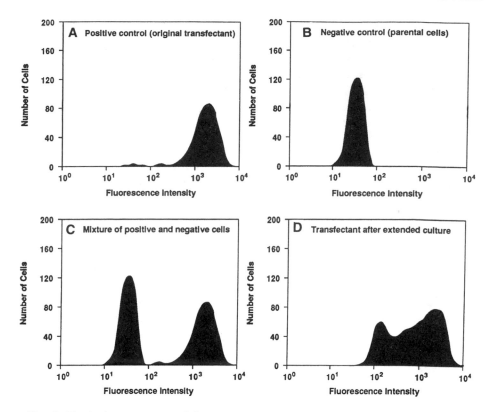

Fig. 1. Typical appearance of fluorescence histograms. (**A**) Positive control, stable transfectant cells, or cells at early passage. (**B**) Negative control, e.g., parental cell line, not transfected with Ig genes. (**C**) Positive and negative cells mixed before staining, showing no equilibration of stain. (**D**) Typical appearance of unstable cell line several months after cloning.

guide. To standardize a series of experiments over time, we suggest that you use a single batch of diluted conjugate stored frozen in small aliquots, each sufficient for one experiment. The specificity of the conjugate must obviously be chosen to suit the cell line. We recommend using goat polyclonal reagents since they should give minimal binding to Fc receptors and should be relatively unaffected by fixation of the antigen. However, other reagents may be equally suitable.

6. Stained cells can be stored at 4°C for up to 2 mo, but they should first be fixed once more with formaldehyde as in **Subheading 3., steps 3** and **4** to stabilize the antibody-Ig complex.

7. To check that there is no redistribution of stain within the cell population, you can mix positive and negative control cells either before or after staining. In both cases the fluorescence histogram should show the two clearly resolved populations (**Fig. 1C**).

8. Various patterns of low or nonproducers have been seen after extended culture of transfectants. Sometimes a discreet population of low-Ig cells appears and increases with time. In other cell lines, there is a gradual broadening of the fluorescence distribution and a downward shift in the mean fluorescence. We take either of these to indicate instability of antibody production; this has been confirmed by measurement of secreted antibody and by analytical cloning. The method can detect the early appearance of 10% low or nonproducers. Higher sensitivity may be possible with careful attention to standardization and controls.

9. Appearance of variants in a cell population is a stochastic event. The apparent stability may vary considerably in small-volume cultures. We recommend that the total cell number in test cultures never fall below 10^5 and that replicate cultures be maintained and tested.

References

1. Committee for Proprietary Medicinal Products: Ad hoc working party on Biotechnology/Pharmacy (1998) Guidelines on the production and quality control of medicinal products derived by recombinant DNA technology. *Trends Biotechnol.* **6,** G1–G4.

2. Committee for Proprietary Medicinal Products: Ad hoc working party on Biotechnology/Pharmacy (1998) Guidelines on the production and quality control of monoclonal antibodies of murine origin intended for use in man. *Trends Biotechnol.* **6,** G5–G8.

3. Bebbington, C. R., Renner, G., Thomson, S., King, D., Abrams, D., and Yarranton, G. T. (1992) High-level expression of a recombinant antibody from myeloma cells using a glutamine synthetase gene as an amplifiable selectable marker. *Bio/Technology* **10,** 169–175.

4. Bird, P., Bolam, E., Castell, L., Obeid, O., Darton, N., and Hale, G. (1998) Glutamine synthetase transfected cells may avoid selection by releasing glutamine. New developments and new applications in animal cell technology (Merten, O.-W., Perrin, P., and Griffiths, B., eds.) *15th Meeting of the European Society for Animal Cell Technology 1997*, Kluwer, Dordrecht, The Netherlands, pp. 43–49.

5. Assenmacher, M., Schmitz, J., and Radbruch, A. (1994) Flow cytometric determination of cytokines in activated murine T helper lymphocytes: expression of interleukin-10 in interferon-γ and in interleukin-4 expressing cells. *Eur. J. Immunol.* **24,** 1091–1101.

22

Measurement of Endotoxin

Jenny Phillips, Patrick Harrison, and Geoff Hale

1. Introduction

Bacterial endotoxin is probably the most common significant contaminant that might be found in antibody preparations. It is found ubiquitously in normal environments but its pyrogenic effects in vivo can be lethal. It is absolutely vital to control the level of endotoxin in therapeutic products, but its significance for experimental work must not be underestimated since it can have numerous confounding effects both in vivo and in vitro. Methods for removing endotoxin from products have been described (1–4), but in our experience, it is much better to avoid it from the beginning by scrupulous control of raw materials and use of good aseptic technique. To grow, bacteria need water; therefore, the most likely sources of endotoxin are water and any process equipment that has been wet. Water must be obtained from a controlled source that is low in endotoxin. If you do not have a suitable dedicated water purification system, then it is best to purchase purified water. Water for irrigation (from a pharmaceutical supplier) is possibly the most economic. Equipment in contact with cells or products should preferably be sterile disposable plastic. Standard tissue culture ware is usually very reliable. Plastic bags for media and process intermediates are now widely available in all sizes (e.g., Stedim, Aubagne, France) and should be used in preference to glass bottles. Silicone tubing (food or medical grade) is suitable for all fluid transfers and should not be reused. If reusable equipment is essential, it can be soaked in 0.5 M NaOH and/or baked in an oven at high temperature (steam sterilization is not sufficient) (1).

Whatever precautions are taken to reduce the risk of endotoxin contamination, it is important to carry out routine assays to check that they are effective. For small and inexpensive antibody batches destined for experimental use, it

From: Methods in Molecular Medicine, Vol. 40: Diagnostic and Therapeutic Antibodies
Edited by: A. J. T. George and C. E. Urch © Humana Press Inc., Totowa, NJ

may be sufficient only to test the final batch. For larger batches and therapeutic materials, it is much wiser to test all the process intermediates (media, buffers, and so forth) before they are actually used. This will reduce the risk of final failure of a batch.

In the past, endotoxins were measured by injecting the test substance into rabbits and measuring the temperature rise. This is costly and an unnecessary use of animals. Now there are commercial test kits based on the clotting reaction induced in horseshoe crabs (animals are still used, but from a lower order!) *(5)*. The test has been refined with an artificial chromogenic substrate, so that the results can be read in a spectrophotometer, which is technically very much more reliable than visual examination of a clot (Bio-Whittaker Inc, Walkersville, MD). At least two versions of the chromogenic test are available, an endpoint method and a kinetic method. The kinetic method is more sophisticated and suitable for precise determinations but it requires a more costly spectrophotometer that is not available in most labs. A simple modification of the endpoint method is described here. It is a scaled-down version of a standard kit. Some sensitivity is lost, but the method is still suitable for routine measurements of process intermediates and samples for experimental use. Scaling down the method enables many more samples to be tested for the same cost, which will provide an overall improvement in quality control.

2. Materials

1. LAL test kit, QCL-1000 (Bio-Whittaker cat. no. 50-647U). The kit contains:
   a. Complete instructions (*see* **Note 1**).
   b. Sterile pyrogen-free water.
   c. *Escherichia coli* endotoxin-positive control. Reconstitute in 1 mL water with very vigorous mixing as instructed (*see* **Note 2**). Use this stock to prepare a series of standards containing 0.1–1.0 EU/mL. Endotoxin is toxic! Handle with care.
   d. Chromogenic substrate. Reconstitute in 6.5 mL water as instructed.
   e. *Limulus amoebocyte* lysate. Reconstitute immediately before use in 1.4 mL water as instructed (*see* **Note 3**).
2. 25% acetic acid. Mix 25 mL glacial acetic acid with 75 mL water.
3. Disposable 96-well flat-bottomed microtiter plates (e.g., Costar 3596 or Falcon 3072).
4. Microtiter plate reader with 405 nm filter (we use a Multiskan Plus Mark II).
5. Dry block heater with microtiter plate adaptor and lid. Check the temperature continuously with an accurate thermometer.
6. Microtiter plate shaker.
7. Standard laboratory equipment, including pipets and pipeters and a stop watch (*see* **Note 4**).

3. Methods

1. Set the dry block heater to 37 ± 1°C. Allow all reagents (except LAL) and test samples to adjust to room temperature. Draw up a plate plan as follows:

   Rows A–F: Standards, controls, and test samples.

   Row G: LAL stock for preincubation.

   Row H: Substrate stock for preincubation.

   Each assay should include a set of standards (0.1–1.0 EU/mL) and negative contol(s) (e.g., pyrogen-free water) as well as test samples. Culture medium, water, and physiological buffers can generally be tested undiluted. Test samples containing high levels of endotoxin must be diluted to within the working range. It is advisable to test several different dilutions of unknown but suspect samples (*see* **Note 5** and **6**).

2. Carefully dispense 10 µL of the standards, controls, and test samples into the bottom of each well according to the plate plan.

3. Calculate the total amount of substrate required (20 µL per sample) and dispense this into Row H so that it can later be quickly transferred to the sample wells with a multichannel pipettor.

4. Calculate the amount of LAL required (10 µL per sample) and dispense it into Row G in the same way.

5. Pre-equilibrate the plate in the dry block heater for 10 min.

6. From now on, timing is critical. Use a stopwatch and add reagents smoothly in the same order, so that all wells have identical reaction times. Keep the plate in the dry block heater as far as possible to maintain constant temperature (*see* **Note 7**).

7. At 0 min, add 10 µL LAL to each well. Mix thoroughly on the plate shaker for 15 s.

8. At 30 min, add 20 µL substrate to each well. Mix as before.

9. At 36 min, add 20 µL 25% acetic acid to each well. Mix as before.

10. Measure the absorbance at 405 nm in the microtiter plate spectrophotometer. Blank with water alone. A standard containing 1 EU/mL normally gives an absorbance between 0.25 and 0.35. A negative control should be <0.05. Plot a standard curve and calculate the endotoxin level in the test samples by interpolation.

4. Notes

1. This method is scaled down for economical use of reagents. It is less sensitive than the manufacturer's standard method but adequate for experimental work providing it is done carefully. The manufacturer's full-scale method should be used for any processes under regulatory control. The method instructions contain useful background and guidelines.

2. It is important to vigorously vortex the endotoxin standard samples for 15 min when preparing the stock and making dilutions. Standards can be stored at 4°C for up to 1 mo, but should be vortexed for 3 min just before use. This is because endotoxin tends to attach to the surface of containers.

3. We have found that the LAL reagent can be stored frozen in aliquots for future use, though this is not recommended by the manufacturer.
4. Take care to avoid introducing endotoxin contamination during the assay. Use the pyrogen-free water provided for dilutions, and if possible work in a laminar flow hood or clean air environment throughout. Use sterile disposable pipets and avoid repeated sampling from stock solutions.
5. Sometimes water is not a suitable diluent for test samples (e.g., IgM antibodies will precipitate). Pyrogen-free saline may be a suitable alternative.
6. Some test samples contain substances that might inhibit the reaction (high salt concentration, extreme pH, organic solvents, detergents, and so forth) or give a false positive (colored substances). Validate the assay for a new test substance by "spiking" a sample with 1.0 EU/mL of endotoxin standard and check the recovery. If there is significant inhibition, the test sample can often be diluted to a point where there is no inhibition. Of course, the assay will then be correspondingly less sensitive. Suggested starting dilutions for test substances commonly encountered are given below:

Purified antibodies	Undiluted
Culture medium	Undiluted
PBS	Undiluted
100 mM citrate, pH 3.2	1:10
Serum	Undiluted
20% ethanol	Undiluted

7. The temperature and reaction timings are critical.

References

1. Pearson, F. (1987) Pyrogens and depyrogenation: theory and practice, in *Aseptic Pharmaceutical Manufacturing Technology for the 1990s* (Olson, W. P. and Groves, M. J., eds.) Interpharm Press, Prairie View, IL, pp. 75–100.
2. Anspach, F. B. and Hilbeck, O. (1995) Removal of endotoxins by affinity sorbents. *J. Chromatogr.* **A711,** 81–92.
3. Liu, S., Tobias, R., McClure, S., Styba, G., Shi, Q., and Jackowski, G. (1997) Removal of endotoxin from recombinant protein preparations. *Clin. Biochem.* **30,** 455–463.
4. Legallais, C., Anspach, F. B., Bueno, S. M., Haupt, K., and Vijayalakshmi, M. A. (1997) Strategies for the depyrogenation of contaminated immunoglobulin G solutions by histidine-immobilized hollow fiber membrane. *J. Chromatogr. B. Biomed. Sci. Appl.* **691,** 33–41.
5. Young, N. S., Levin, J., and Prendergast, R. A. (1973) An invertebrate coagulation system activated by endotoxin: evidence for enzymatic mechanism. *J. Clin. Invest.* **51,** 1790.

23

Aseptic Vial Filling

Kuldip Bhamra, Patrick Harrison, Jenny Phillips, and Geoff Hale

1. Introduction

Ideally, injectable drugs are sterilized in their final containers by a foolproof method like autoclaving. This is not possible for biologicals like monoclonal antibodies (mAbs), so they must be manufactured aseptically, sterilized by filtration and then filled into sterile vials or ampoules. The final filling procedure is the most critical aseptic process and should be done in a very clean environment. Automatic machines are used for large production processes and eliminate the risk of contamination associated with manual processes. However, preparing material for early clinical trials can be problematic because the batch size is normally too small for a filling machine (e.g., 500–1000 vials). Normal practice is to fill this number of vials by hand, but the vials and closures have to be washed, depyrogenated (by baking in an oven), and sterilized, and the filling has to be carried out in a very strictly controlled environment, because the vials are open throughout the process and are only stoppered and sealed in a second step.

We have developed a procedure that we believe is much simpler and safer (*see* **Note 1**). Vials are purchased ready washed, sterilized, and assembled with closure and a crimp top. They are filled using a standard pharmaceutical dispensing syringe system in a Class 100 environment. There are several advantages:

1. Costs and controls associated with washing, baking, and sterilization are eliminated;
2. Vials are always sealed, so the risk of introducing contaminants is reduced;
3. The hand sealing and crimping step is eliminated (instead this has been done by machine, which is more reliable); and
4. The filled vials are pressurized so loss of seal integrity would be evident to the user.

From: *Methods in Molecular Medicine, Vol. 40: Diagnostic and Therapeutic Antibodies*
Edited by: A. J. T. George and C. E. Urch © Humana Press Inc., Totowa, NJ

There are some potential drawbacks: the closure is punctured and it is not possible to fill the vials more than about 40% because of the pressure buildup.

Over the past 7 yr we have used this method to fill 105 batches of therapeutic antibodies, a total of over 46,000 vials. Samples from every batch were tested for sterility by aerobic and anaerobic cultures by independent laboratories. Organisms were found on only one occasion, and the testing laboratory ascribed this to contamination during the test (extensive repeats tested negative). Over the same period we have also filled more than 2000 vials with nutrient broth and exposed them to a variety of storage conditions (*see* **Note 2**). None have shown any evidence of microbial growth.

2. Materials

1. Sterile transfer bags (We use 1–5 L Bio-Pharm recovery bags from Stedim (Aubagne, France). Similar bags can be obtained from other suppliers.
2. Connector for coupling bag to syringe. Prepare a short length (approx 7 cm) of new silicone tubing (e.g., Cole Parmer H-06411-03) with a capped female luer at one end and a loose cap on the other end. Steam sterilize.
3. Syringe dispensing pump (Multi-Ad fluid dispensing system, Burron Medical Inc.).
4. Repeating syringe transfer sets for Multi-Ad system (10 mL, Product code MA 1040; Burron Medical, distributed by B. Braun Medical Ltd.).
5. 18-gage disposable sterile hypodermic needles (eg. 0.8 × 40 mm) and sharps discard bin.
6. Sterile, nitrogen-filled vials (e.g., 10 mL nitrogen filled, cat. no. N46 from Amersham). Better vials can be obtained on special order to Adelphi (Tubes) Ltd. (*see* **Note 3**).
7. Aluminum or stainless-steel trays suitable for holding 50–100 vials (inventory storage racks from New Brunswick Scientific are very suitable).
8. Calibrated balance for checking the fill volume.
9. Autoclave, suitably validated to GMP standards. Autoclave packaging materials.
10. Suitable clean working environment. We work in a Class 100 laminar flow cabinet within a Class 10,000 clean room.
11. Standard clean-room supplies (clean gowns and caps, sterile masks, gloves, wipes, chlorhexidine/alcohol spray).
12. For broth fill: Nutrient broth (e.g., Tryptic Soy Broth, Difco cat. no. 0370-88).
13. Filter integrity tester. We use a Sartocheck Junior (Sartorius Ltd.) to apply a controlled and gradually increasing pressure to a membrane filter. A wet filter will not allow gas to pass because of the surface tension of liquid in the pores. At a sufficiently high pressure (the "bubble point"), liquid is blown out and gas passes through freely. This pressure is related to the size of the pore and is used as a measure of filter integrity.

3. Methods

1. Autoclave the vials to ensure the outside surfaces are sterile. Weigh a sample of vials (up to 10%) and label them with their individual weights. Pack the vials into stainless-steel racks. Pack in a suitable autoclave bag and steam sterilize at 121°C for 20 min according to your standard procedure.

2. Make all necessary preparations for work in the clean environment according to your standard procedures, including handwashing, gowning, cleaning of working environment, establishment of correct operating conditions, and documentation of procedures.

3. Carry out the final membrane filtration of product according to your standard procedure. Filter the product direct into a sterile transfer bag with a male luer lock connector. Take a sample and check that it has the correct product concentration. Carry out an integrity test on the membrane filter.

4. Connect the dispensing system as shown in **Fig. 1**. Attach the sterile silicone tubing connector (with female luer) to the spike of a 10-mL Multi-Ad fluid dispensing system. Connect the female luer to the product bag. Attach a needle to the male luer of the dispensing tubing.

5. Attach the 10 mL syringe to the two-way check valve, set for the correct delivery volume in the range 2.0–4.0 mL, lock in place with the adjusting nut, and fine tune with the screw thread.

6. Prime the syringe until the tubing is full of product.

7. Attach the primed syringe system to the holder on the face of the Multi-Ad pump. (For full details see manufacturer's instructions.)

8. Hang up the product bag and open the first bag of prepared, autoclaved vials.

9. At this stage it is an advantage to have two people working together, one filling the vials and the other weighing. Insert the needle through the septum of the first preweighed vial and operate the pump with the foot switch. When the fluid has been fully delivered, crimp the tubing near the needle, remove the needle, and insert it into a new preweighed vial.

10. Weigh the vial and calculate the amount injected (assume 1 mL = 1 g). Adjust the syringe setting if necessary and repeat until the volume injected is within 5% of the target volume. Reject any vials outside this limit and segregate them clearly from acceptable vials.

11. Dispense antibody into the vials as in **step 9**. Never touch the top of the vials. Replace the syringe needle if necessary before it becomes blunt.

12. Repeat the check weighing at regular intervals to ensure that the fill volume remains correct.

13. If necessary, wipe the tops of the vials with a sterile wipe soaked in chlorhexidine/alcohol to remove any drops of liquid.

14. Filled vials should be individually inspected by your standard procedures for integrity, fill volume, and presence of any particulate material (e.g., fragments of the closure). We recommend viewing with a lens under polarized light. Acceptable vials will then be labeled and packaged according to your standard procedure.

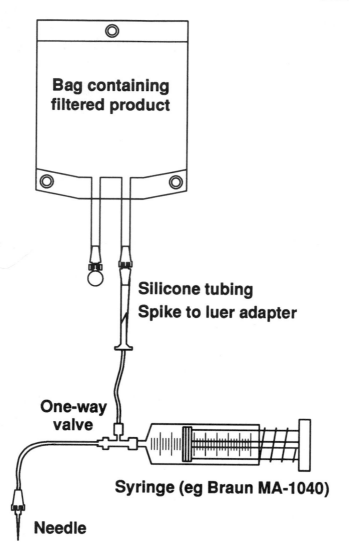

Fig. 1. Diagram of assembly for vial filling.

4. Notes

1. This is just an outline procedure to illustrate the principle of the process. If it were used as part of a regulated GMP procedure to prepare clinical trial material, it would be necessary to include local details, especially the recording of data in suitable batch record forms and the validation of critical steps. A system for approval of raw materials is an essential component of GMP and it is necessary

for users to assure themselves of the quality and suitability of the components suggested, especially the sterile vials. We recommend that you prepare a detailed user specification for your supplier and check that it is complied with.

2. The most important method of validation is to carry out the whole process using sterile nutrient broth instead of product. The filled vials are then incubated to reveal any microbial contamination. Samples would be subject to typical storage and/or transport procedures prior to incubation. We recommend that this test be repeated whenever new operators are trained and when a new lot of vials is obtained.

3. Commercial sterile vials (e.g., Amersham, Adelphi) are normally filled with Nitrogen. This may not be essential for antibody products, but there is no disadvantage, and the inert atmostphere may contribute to product stability. We have more experience with vials from Amersham, but they have given us some problems because the crimp seal is not always very tight and the closure is relatively thick and rigid, which means that there is a significant proportion of rejects caused by "coring" by the needle. It has not always been easy to obtain batch documentation from the supplier. Tests with vials from Adelphi suggest they may be suitable for this procedure. They are also significantly cheaper, but are currently only supplied by special order.

24

Measurement of Antibody Concentrations by Hemagglutination

Jenny Phillips and Geoff Hale

1. Introduction

During every stage of development and production of diagnostic or thera-peutic antibodies, it is necessary to have an assay to measure antibody concentration. Several techniques are routine in virtually all antibody laboratories. High-performance liquid chromatograpy (HPLC) using an affinity matrix (protein A or protein G) is rapid and quantitative and measures most types of antibody, though the equipment is quite costly. Enzyme-linked immunosorbent assay (ELISA) is widely used and extremely versatile. By judicious choice of anti-Ig reagents, specific for heavy chain, light chains, or particular domains, it is possible to screen for almost any desired Ig molecule or fragment. This is specially useful when analyzing a complex mixture (1). Native gel electro-phoresis is a useful technique for screening relatively concentrated samples (e.g., from fermentors) since different antibodies can be readily distinguished by their characteristic mobilities. However, none of these methods are really suited to the rapid semiquantitative testing of huge numbers of samples that is often necessary early in a project (when screening for a rare hybridoma or transfectant, or for somatic mutants) and for routine analysis of process samples during cell culture. Instead we have found that red cell agglutination as origi-nally developed by Coombs (2,3), is convenient, quick, and very cheap.

The principle is simple. An antiglobulin specific for the test Ig is coupled to red cells (see **Note 1**). The coupled cells are mixed with various dilutions of the test substance. The highest dilution that still gives agglutination indicates the concentration of Ig in the sample. This method has enabled the screening of more than 10^7 hybridoma clones to find rare class-switch variants (4) and has been regularly used in our center to monitor productivity of fermentors as well

From: *Methods in Molecular Medicine, Vol. 40: Diagnostic and Therapeutic Antibodies*
Edited by: A. J. T. George and C. E. Urch © Humana Press Inc., Totowa, NJ

as for a variety of development work. It is extremely sensitive and by suitable choice of the antiglobulin coupled to the red cells, it is possible to test for unwanted Ig contaminants (e.g., different isotypes, other monoclonals concurrently in production) that might potentially contaminate a therapeutic product *(5)*.

2. Materials

1. Fresh human red cells, group O rhesus negative, approx 10 mL. This should preferably be obtained from a blood transfusion service and be acceptable for transfusion. Nevertheless, observe due precautions in handling human blood *(see* **Note 2**).
2. 1% chromic chloride. Dissolve 1 g $CrCl_3.6H_2O$ (e.g. Sigma [St. Louis, MO] C1896) in 100 mL normal saline (NaCl, 9 g/L). Leave overnight at room temperature. The pH should be approx 3.0. Adjust to pH 5.0 with 5 M NaOH. Leave for 3 d. The pH should drift back to 3.0. Adjust to pH 5.0 again and leave for 3 d. The pH should drift back to 3.5. Store at 4°C for up to 24 mo. The pH should remain at 3.5–3.6.
3. Anti-Ig antibody for coupling *(see* **Note 1**). This should be at least 1.0 mg/mL. Use the same batch of antibody as long as possible.
4. Normal saline (NaCl, 9 g/L) and phosphate-buffered saline (PBS).
5. Alsever's solution: 114 mM glucose, 71 mM sodium chloride, 27 mM trisodium citrate, adjusted to pH 6.1 with citric acid, e.g., Gibco cat. no. 15190-044 or -051.
6. Vortex mixer, tube shaker (or rotator), microplate shaker (optional), pipettors, dialysis tubing.
7. Small test tubes for coupling reaction. Sarstedt 500, cat. no. 55.476 are recommended.
8. Test sample and standards. Depending on the sensitivity of the coupled cells, the samples will need to be diluted with PBS to give a starting concentration of typically 1 µg/mL.
9. Rigid, round-bottomed microtiter plates (e.g., Bibby Sterilin cat. no. 611U96 or Falcon 3910).

3. Methods
3.1. Preparation of Antibody-Coated Red Cells

1. Dialyse the antibody exhaustively against normal saline at 4°C. It must not contain any trace of phosphate. At least five changes over 3 d is recommended (**Note 3**).
2. Measure the protein concentration and adjust it with normal saline to the desired concentration (e.g., 1.0 mg/mL; *see* **Note 1**).
3. Prepare the red cells by washing 10 mL of blood three times with PBS in a 50 mL tube (five times when detecting human IgG; **Note 4**). Centrifuge at 1200*g* for 5 min. Aspirate the supernatant each time, along with the top layer of cells, to

obtain a well-washed, firm pellet of cells. Transfer them to a 15 mL graduated conical tube for the final wash. Note the volume of the cell pellet and resuspend in an equal amount of normal saline. The washed cells can be kept for up to 7 d at 4°C, but should be washed at least once again before use (**Note 3**).

4. Prepare fresh 0.005% chromic chloride in normal saline (e.g. 10 µL stock in 2.0 mL saline).
5. Mix 100 µL of 50% red cells with 50 µL of the antibody samples in Sarstedt 500 tubes (*see* **Note 5**).
6. Vortex the mixture and add 400 µL of 0.005% $CrCl_3$ dropwise over 30 s. Continue to vortex during the addition and for a further 30 s. Leave the tubes on a gentle shaker or rotator for a further 5 min to keep the cells in suspension.
7. Fill the tubes with PBS and wash three times with PBS by centrifugation at 800g for 5 min (five times when detecting human IgG).
8. Coupled cells may be stored for up to 1 wk in PBS at 4°C. For longer storage, resuspend the cells in sterile Alsever's solution (2.5 mL per tube). Then they may be stored for up to 4 wk at 4°C providing they are kept free from microbial contamination. Wash out the Alsever's before use and check that positive and negative controls are acceptable before using with test samples (*see* **Note 6**).

3.2. Measurement of Ig Concentration by Hemagglutination

1. Wash the coupled red cells three times with PBS and resuspend at 2% in PBS.
2. Prepare an assay plan. Include a standard of known concentration on each plate. Make suitable starting dilutions of the test samples and the standard in PBS. Aim for end points between wells 3 and 9. A typical starting concentration is 1 µg/mL.
3. Put 25 µL of PBS into all wells of the microtiter plate.
4. Add 25 µL of the diluted test or control samples to the first well in each row according to the assay plan. Make twofold serial dilutions up to column 11 using a multichannel pipettor. Leave column 12 with PBS alone as a negative control.
5. Add 25 µL of the 2% suspension of coupled red cells to each well. It is vital to avoid contamination of the suspension of red cells by the test samples; for this reason a multichannel pipettor is not recommended for dispensing the cells. Drops from a repeating dispensor or Pasteur pipet are better.
6. Tap each side of the plate hard to mix the cells thoroughly (or use a plate shaker).
7. Wait for the cells to settle. This takes about 30 min.
8. The negative control (PBS) should show a small button of cells. Positive samples will show a homogenous mat of cells. Record the endpoint for each sample. This is the last column that shows full agglutination. Estimate antibody concentrations by comparing the sample endpoints with the standard (*see* **Notes 7** and **8**).

4. Notes

1. The mechanism by which proteins couple to red cells with chromic chloride is poorly understood. This technique has acquired a certain mystique because the coupling is not always predictable. In our experience, polyclonal antisera are more reliable than monoclonal (although some monoclonals work very well).

We have the impression that crude preparations (e.g., ammonium sulfate fraction) may work better than highly purified antibodies. It is important to optimize the coupling conditions for each antiglobulin reagent. The antibody concentration should be varied (from 0.25 to 2.0 mg/mL) and the amount of chromic chloride (from 0.004 to 0.006%) to optimize the coupling reaction. Once successful conditions are found, they should be reproducible if the same stocks of reagents are used consistently.

2. The sensitivity of coupled red cells is a function of the amount of anti-Ig coupled and the intrinsic agglutinability of the cells. Cells from different species are agglutinable to different extents and their sensitivity may be altered by changing the surface charge, e.g., by treatment with chymotrypsin, which cleaves membrane glycoproteins bearing negatively charged sialic acid residues. Chymotrypsin-treated sheep cells are very sensitive and ideal for detecting very low antibody concentration (pg/mL) *(2)*. Untreated human red cells are more convenient for routine assays.

3. Many buffer salts interfere with the coupling reaction. It is essential to dialyse the anti-Ig and wash the red cells extensively with saline.

4. Special care must be taken when using human red cells for detecting human IgG (or any similar homologous system) since traces of normal IgG from the blood could cause false hemagglutination. The number of wash steps is increased to ensure all traces of plasma are removed.

5. The coupling reaction may not work well if the volumes are increased. To prepare more coupled cells it is better to repeat the reaction in multiple tubes.

6. Coupled red cells can be stabilized almost indefinitely by treatment with glutaraldehyde, with a small loss of sensitivity *(6)*. Stablized coupled red cells specific for mouse and rat immunoglobulin isotypes are marketed by Serotec Ltd. (Kidlington, UK).

7. A special stand with mirror for viewing the plates from underneath can make it easier to score the agglutination, but is not essential.

8. Do not confuse a positive but hyperagglutinated well where the red cells have collapsed into a small pellet, with a negative button. The former will appear slightly crinkly and remain as small particles on shaking; the latter will flow into a teardrop on tilting and form a homogenous suspension on shaking.

References

1. Clark, M. R. and Waldmann, H. (1987) T cell killing of target cells induced by hybrid antibodies: a comparison of two bispecific monoclonal antibodies. *J. Natl. Cancer Inst.* **79**, 1393–1401.

2. Coombs, R. R. A., Scott, M. L., and Cranage, M. P. (1987) Assays using red-cell labelled antibodies. *J. Immunol. Methods* **101**, 1–14.

3. Clark, M. R. (1986) The detection and characterization of antigen-specific monoclonal antibodies using anti-immunoglobulin isotype antibodies coupled to red blood cells. *Methods Enzymol.* **121**, 548–555.

4. Hale, G., Cobbold, S. P., Waldmann, H., Easter, G., Matejtschuk, P., and Coombs, R. R. A. (1987) Isolation of low-frequency class-switch variants from rat hybrid myelomas. *J. Immunol. Methods* **103,** 59–67.

5. Hale, G., Drumm, A., Harrison, P., and Phillips, J. (1994) Repeated cleaning of protein A affinity column with sodium hydroxide. *J. Immunol. Methods* **171,** 15–21.

6. Cranage, M. P., Gurner, B. W., and Coombs, R. R. A. (1983) Glutaraldehyde stabilisation of antibody-linked erythrocytes for use in reverse passive and related hemagglutination assays. *J. Immunol. Methods* **64,** 7–16.

V

CLINICAL APPLICATION OF ANTIBODIES

25

Enzymatic Digestion of Monoclonal Antibodies

Sarah M. Andrew

1. Introduction

Originally, digestion of antibodies by proteolytic enzymes was used to study their structure. Many diverse structures can be obtained by fragmentation of the different classes of antibody with different enzymes, or by using the same enzyme and changing the conditions (**Fig. 1**). Not all the fragments obtained have significant binding activity; for example, in several studies by this author Fv fragments obtained by digestion have been found to have lost their binding activity. Fragmentation of antibody is now usually carried out to introduce required properties (e.g., a decrease in molecular size), or to remove undesirable properties (e.g., nonspecific Fc receptor binding).

The most usual digestions carried out are:

1. Production of bivalent $F(ab')_2$ from mouse McAb IgG;
2. Production of univalent Fab from mouse McAb IgG;
3. Production of bivalent IgMs from mouse McAb IgM; and
4. Production of bivalent $F(ab')_{2\mu}$ from mouse McAb IgM.

$F(ab')_2$ and $F(ab')_{2\mu}$ are produced by digestion with pepsin and Fab is produced by digestion with papain. One useful fragmentation uses papain that has been preactivated with cysteine. This cleaves IgG_1 to produce $F(ab')_2$, IgG_{2a} IgG_{2b} to produce Fab. It is a very stable fragmentation in which the times of incubation are not at all critical. The IgG-like subunit of IgM (IgMs) is the product of a mild reduction; this is most conveniently done using cysteine, which reduces the IgM and alkylates the subunit, thus preventing reassociation.

After digestion of the antibodies it is necessary to purify the fragments for two reasons: to separate the fragment from any remaining intact antibody; and to separate the fragments of interest from other miscellaneous fragments pro-

From: *Methods in Molecular Medicine, Vol. 40: Diagnostic and Therapeutic Antibodies*
Edited by: A. J. T. George and C. E. Urch © Humana Press Inc., Totowa, NJ

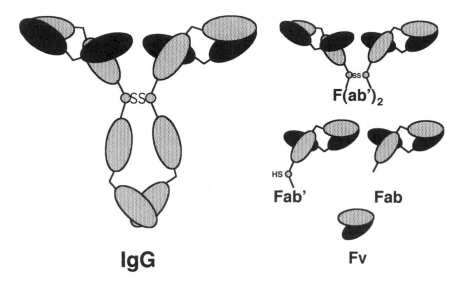

Fig. 1. Diagramatic representation of the major fragments of an IgG molecule that can be produced by enzymatic digestion, as described in the text.

duced by the process of digestion. Purification of IgG fragments by protein A affinity chromatography is possible if an intact Fc region remains after fragmentation, as it does in the case of undigested antibody and, sometimes, in digestions with pepsin. In general this method of purification is rough and ready and size exclusion chromatography is recommended as an additional step.

2. Materials

2.1. Digestion with Pepsin

1. Purified solution of mouse McAb (IgG or IgM) at a concentration of ≥1 mg/mL.
2. 0.2 *M* Sodium acetate buffer brought to pH 4.0 with glacial acetic acid.
3. 0.2 *M* Sodium acetate buffer brought to pH 4.5 with glacial acetic acid.
4. 0.1 mg/mL pepsin (Sigma [St. Louis, MO] number P6887) in acetate buffer at appropriate pH (*see* **Subheadings 3.1.** and **3.2.**).
5. 2 *M* Tris base.
6. Phosphate-buffered saline (PBS) brought to pH 8.0 using NaOH.
7. Protein A-sepharose CL-4B (Sigma number P 3391) swollen in PBS, pH 8.0, and packed into a 10 × 100 mm column, or a 1 mL HiTrap Protein A column (Sigma number 5-4838).
8. PBS.
9. A size exclusion column equivalent to 26 × 900 mm Sephacryl S-200 (Pharmacia, Uppsala, Sweden).
10. Centriprep 100 concentrator (Amicon, Beverly MA; Stonehouse, Glocestershire, UK).

2.2. Digestion with Papain

1. Purified solution of mouse IgG McAb at a concentration of ≥1 mg/mL.
2. PBS made to 0.02 *M* with respect to ethylenediaminetetra-acetic acid (EDTA) and 0.2 *M* with respect to cysteine.
3. Iodoacetamide crystals.
4. PBS brought to pH 8.0 using NaOH.
5. Protein A-sepharose CL-4B (Sigma number P 3391) swollen in PBS, pH 8.0, and packed into 10 × 100 mm column, or a 1 mL HiTrap Protein A column (Sigma number 5-4838).
6. PBS.
7. A size exclusion column equivalent to 26 × 900 mm Sephacryl S-200 (Pharmacia), optional.

2.3. Reduction and Alkylation with Cysteine

1. Purified solution of mouse IgM McAb at a concentration of ≥1 mg/mL in PBS.
2. 0.1 *M* cysteine stock solution in PBS (L-cysteine free base, Sigma number C7755)
3. Borate-buffered saline (0.015 *M* sodium borate, 0.15 *M* sodium chloride, made to pH 8.5 with sodium hydroxide).
4. A size exclusion column equivalent to 26 × 900 mm Sephacryl S-200 (Pharmacia).

3. Methods

3.1. Preparation of F(ab')₂ from IgG

The various subclasses of mouse IgG vary in their susceptibility to pepsin fragmentation. IgG_1 is quite resistant to digestion and and it is impossible to fragment IgG_{2b} to F(ab')₂ because it breaks down to Fab (*see* **Notes 1–3**). The method below is one that should work in most cases.

1. Dialyse the IgG against acetate buffer, pH 4.0, overnight at 4°C. Use any known amount of antibody between 1 and 20 mg.
2. Determine the concentration at A_{280}.
3. Add 0.1 mg/mL pepsin in acetate buffer, pH 4.0, to give an enzyme-to-antibody ratio of 1 : 20 (w : w).
4. Incubate for 6 h in a water bath at 37°C.
5. Stop the reaction by adding sufficient Tris base to bring the pH to roughly 8.0 (start by adding 50 µL Tris, mix, and test the pH with pH paper).
6. Dialyse the mixture against PBS, pH 8.0, overnight.
7. Equilibrate the protein A column with PBS, pH 8.0, and load the dialysed mixture onto it 1 mL at a time. Collect the unbound fraction that contains the F(ab')₂ fragments.
8. If further purity is desired, the mixture should be concentrated to a volume of ≤3 mL and added to a precalibrated size exclusion column (26 × 900 mm

Sephacryl S-200 or equivalent). At this stage regular PBS can be used to equilibrate the column and elute the fractions.

9. Collect 2.5-mL fractions over the molecular weight range of F(ab')$_2$ (110 kDa). The purity of the product can be assessed by sodium dodecyl sulfate-polyacrylamide gel electrophoresis (SDS-PAGE) in nonreducing conditions and in reducing conditions when a doublet at 25 kDa is seen.

3.2. Preparation of F(ab')$_{2\mu}$ from IgM

See **Note 3** for further information regarding this procedure.

1. Dialyse the IgM against acetate buffer, pH 4.5, overnight at 4°C.
2. Determine the concentration at A$_{280}$.
3. Add 0.1 mg/mL pepsin in acetate buffer, pH 4.5, to give an enzyme-to-antibody ratio of 1:20 (w:w).
4. Incubate for between 6 and 12 h in a water bath at 37°C.
5. Stop the reaction by adding sufficient Tris base to bring the pH to roughly 8.0 (start by adding 50 µL Tris, mix, and test the pH with pH paper).
6. Dialyse the mixture against PBS overnight, or concentrate and change the buffer using a Centriprep 100 concentrator.
7. Concentrate the mixture to a volume of ≤3 mL and add to a precalibrated size exclusion column (26 × 900 mm Sephacryl S-200 or equivalent). Elute fractions of between 1 and 2.5 mL. The molecular weight of F(ab')$_{2\mu}$ is 130 kDa. Assess purity on an 8% polyacrylamide gel under nonreducing conditions.

3.3. Preparation of Fab from IgG

Again, there is a variable susceptibility to the enzyme between the IgG subclasses. The method described is one that should give good results in most cases. If fragments are not obtained, variations in the concentration of enzyme or time of incubation can be tried. *See* **Notes 1, 2**, and **4** for further information.

1. Use IgG in PBS at a concentration between 1 and 5 mg/mL.
2. Dissolve sufficient papain in an equal volume of digestion buffer to the volume of antibody solution to give a papain-to-antibody ratio of 1:20 (w:w).
3. Add the two equal solutions, one containing antibody and one containing papain together; mix thoroughly but gently.
4. Incubate for 4–6 h at 37°C.
5. Stop the reaction by adding crystalline iodoacetamide to make the mixture 0.03 *M* with respect to iodoacetamide, and dissolve by mixing gently.
6. Dialyse the mixture against PBS, pH 8.0, overnight at 4°C.
7. Equilibrate the protein A column in PBS, pH 8.0, then add the dialysed mixture to it. Collect the unbound fraction. Wash the column with PBS, pH 8.0, to completely recover the Fab fragments.
8. Concentrate the Fab fragment mixture to a volume <5 mL.

9. Load the mixture containing the Fab fragments onto the size exclusion column equilibrated in PBS. Collect fractions corresponding to a molecular weight of 50 kDa.
10. Check the purity of the final product on a 10% SDS-polyacrylamide gel in nonreducing conditions.

3.4. Preparation of IgG Fragments Using Preactivated Papain

Bivalent $F(ab')_2$ fragments can be obtained from IgG_1 by this method. The protocol is also useful for producing monovalent Fab fragments from IgG_{2a} and IgG_{2b}. *See* **Note 4** for further information.

3.4.1. Preactivate the Papain

1. Make up a 2 mg/mL solution of papain in PBS with 0.05 M cysteine. Warm at 37°C for 30 min.
2. Equilibrate a PD10 column with acetate/EDTA buffer and apply the papain mixture.
3. Collect 10 × 1 mL fractions eluting with acetate/EDTA buffer. Assay the fractions at A_{280} and pool the two or three fractions containing protein.
4. Calculate the concentration of the preactivated papain using the following formula:

$$A_{280}/2.5 = \text{mg preactivated papain/mL} \tag{1}$$

3.4.2. Digest the IgG

1. Dialyse the IgG against acetate/EDTA buffer and determine the concentration after dialysis.
2. Mix the preactivated papain solution and the IgG solution in an enzyme-to-antibody ratio of 1 : 20.
3. Incubate for 6–18 h at 37°C.
4. Stop the reaction by adding crystalline iodoacetamide to a concentration of 0.03 M.
5. Dialyse the mixture against PBS, pH 8.0.
6. Purify the fragments as in **Subheading 3.3.**

3.5. Preparation of IgM Subunits from Pentameric IgM

See **Note 5** for further information regarding this method.

1. Add cysteine to IgM in PBS (up to 10 mg in 5 mL); make the solution 0.05 M with respect to cysteine.
2. Incubate the mixture for 2 h at 37°C.
3. Separate the fragments from intact antibody on a 26 × 900 mm size exclusion column or equivalent. The buffer in the column should be made 3 mM with respect to EDTA, if possible, because this prevents reassociation of the IgM fragments. Collect the fractions corresponding to a molecular weight of 180 kDa.

4. Notes

1. It is possible, but expensive, to buy kits for digestion of mouse antibody (Pierce, Warrington, UK). These kits work extremely well and can be a time-saving option. Each laboratory must consider whether the time saved in preparation is worth the extra expenditure on a kit. Fragmentation of antibodies from human and rabbit is described in **ref. 6**; generally the methods and enzymes used are similar.

2. The most common problems likely to occur when following these methods are that the antibody does not digest or that the molecule overdigests to produce small unrecognizable fragments. These can be overcome by varying the concentrations of enzyme, the times of digestion and, in the case of pepsin, the pH of the mixture *(1)*. Generally, it is unwise to embark on fragmentation of IgG if the subclass of the antibody is not known. In digestion with both pepsin and papain the susceptibility to digestion varies with subclass. The order of susceptibility has been found to be $IgG_{2b} > IgG_3 > IgG_{2a} > IgG_1$ *(2,3)*. Not all antibodies fall into this order (IgG_{2a} can be extremely sensitive to the action of papain in the presence of cysteine) and individual exceptions must be expected.

3. Digestion with pepsin has a great subclass variability. IgG_{2b} does not digest to $F(ab')_2$ fragments at all; the monovalent Fab/c (a single binding site and an intact Fc portion) is produced instead. This molecule has a very similar molecular weight to $F(ab')_2$; thus, is is easy to imagine success with the fragmentation. The reason for the problem is thought to be an asymmetric glycosylation of the heavy chains in the molecule. All IgG subclasses can be further digested by pepsin to produce monovalent Fab fragments because there is a site of secondary cleavage on the NH_2-terminal side of the disulfide bonds. Further digestion with pepsin at a pH of 3.5 can produce Fv fragments after approx 3 h of incubation. There are reports of these having activity as antigen-binding fragments *(4)*, but the personal experience of this author and colleagues suggests this is rare. It is also unfortunately true that it is difficult to produce active fragments from IgM. It has been suggested that IgM heavy chains can be truncated *(5)*, but this has not been confirmed. The method given for IgM $F(ab')_{2\mu}$ will work, but one should not be too disappointed if the affinity is low.

4. On the whole, papain fragmentations work well and the timings of the incubations are not critical. Initially, care should be taken to mix the papain as it is in suspension; it will dissolve completely at the concentration given in the method. The methods using preactivated papain work extremely well and the incubation times are not at all critical.

5. The digestion to IgMs from IgM causes dissociation of the inter subunit disulfide bonds. It is possible to reduce the intrachain disulfide bonds on further reduction. This is why cysteine is the reducing agent chosen. Reduction by dithiothreitol or mercaptoethanol can be used, but more care is required with the incubations and a separate alkylation step is required.

References

1. Andrew, S. M. and Titus, J. A. (1997) Fragmentation of immunoglobulin G, in *Current Protocols in Immunology* (Coligan, J. E., Kruisbeek, A. M., Margulies, D. H., Shevach, E. M., and Strober, W., eds.), Wiley, New York, pp. 2.8.1–2.8.10.
2. Parham, P. (1986) Preparation and purification of active fragments from mouse monoclonal antibodies, in *Handbook of Experimental Immunology, Vol. 1: Immunochemistry* (Wier, D. M., ed.), Blackwell Scientific, London, UK, pp. 14.1–14.23.
3. Parham, P. (1983) On the fragmentation of monoclonal IgG$_1$, IgG$_{2a}$ and IgG$_{2b}$ from BALB/c mice. *J. Immunol.* **131,** 2895–2902.
4. Sharon, J. and Givol, D. (1976) Preparation of the Fv fragment from the mouse myeloma XPRC-25 immunoglobulin possessing anti-dinitrophenyl activity. *Biochemistry* **15,** 1591–1598.
5. Marks, R. and Bosma, M. J. (1985) Truncated μ (μ′) chains in murine IgM: evidence that μ′ chains lack variable regions. *J. Exp. Med.* **162,** 1862–1877.
6. Stanworth, D. R. and Turner, M. W. (1986) Immunochemical analysis of human and rabbit immunoglobulins and their subunits, in *Handbook of Experimental Immunology, Vol. 1: Immunochemistry* (Wier, D. M., ed.), Blackwell Scientific, London, UK, pp. 12.1–12.45.

26

How to Make Bispecific Antibodies

Ruth R. French

1. Introduction

This protocol describes the production of bispecific $F(ab')_2$ antibody derivatives (BsAbs) by the linking of two Fab' fragments via their hinge region SH groups using the bifunctional crosslinker *o*-phenylenedimaleimide (*o*-PDM) as described by Glennie et al. *(1,2)*. The procedure is illustrated in **Fig. 1**. The first step is to obtain $F(ab')_2$ from the two parent IgG antibodies. Methods for digestion of IgG to $F(ab')_2$ are described in Chapter 25. Fab' fragments are then prepared from the two $F(ab')_2$ species by reduction with thiol, thus exposing free SH groups at the hinge region (three SH-groups for mouse IgG1 and IgG2a antibodies) (*see* **Note 1**). One of the Fab' species (Fab'-A) is selected for alkylation with *o*-PDM. Because *o*-PDM has a strong tendency to crosslink adjacent intramolecular SH-groups, two of the three hinge SH-groups will probably be linked together, leaving a single reactive maleimide group available for conjugation (**Fig. 1**; *see* **Note 2**). Excess *o*-PDM is then removed by column chromatography, and the Fab'-A(mal) is mixed with the second reduced Fab' (Fab'-B) under conditions favoring the crosslinking of the maleimide and SH groups. When equal amounts of the two parent Fab' species are used, the major product is bispecific $F(ab')_2$, resulting from the reaction of one Fab'-A(mal) with one of the SH groups at the hinge of Fab'-B. Increasing the proportion of Fab'-A(mal) in the reaction mixture results in a significant amount of $F(ab')_3$ product by the reaction of two molecules of Fab'-A(mal) with two free SH-groups at the hinge of a single Fab'-B molecule (*see* **Note 3**). The remaining free SH groups on Fab'-B are alkylated, and the $F(ab')_2$ bispecific antibody product (Fab'-A × Fab'-B) is separated by gel filtration chromatography. Each stage of the procedure is checked by HPLC.

From: *Methods in Molecular Medicine, Vol. 40: Diagnostic and Therapeutic Antibodies*
Edited by: A. J. T. George and C. E. Urch © Humana Press Inc., Totowa, NJ

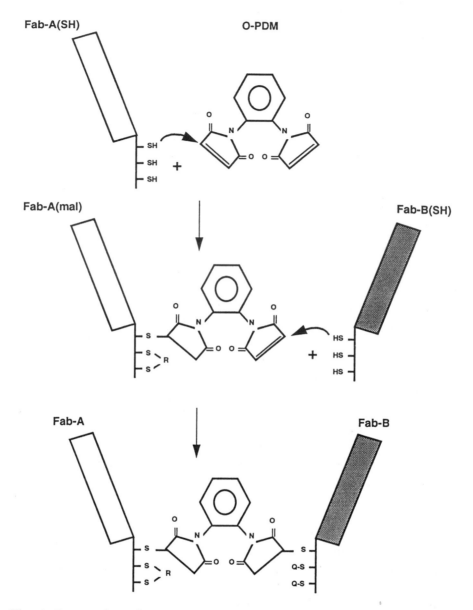

Fig. 1. Preparation of BsAb using *o*-PDM as crosslinker. The F(ab')$_2$ BsAb illustrated is produced from Fab' fragments derived from mouse IgG1 or IgG2a antibody. Two adjacent hinge SH-groups of Fab'-A are crosslinked by *o*-PDM (R, *o*-phenylenedisuccinimidyl linkage), leaving one with a free maleimide group for crosslinking with an SH-group at the hinge of Fab'-B. Unconjugated SH-groups at the Fab'-B hinge are blocked by alkylation (Q, carboxyamidomethyl). Increasing the ratio of Fab'-A(mal) to Fab'-B(SH) will favor the production of bispecific F(ab')$_3$, in which two molecules of Fab'-A(mal) are linked to one molecule of Fab'-B.

Using this method, well-defined derivatives are produced with good yield, and the products are easily isolated; starting with 10 mg each of two parent F(ab′)$_2$ species, expect to obtain 5–10 mg BsAb. The derivatives can be produced at relatively low cost, and quickly. It is possible to obtain the BsAb product from the parent IgG in five working days. The protocols can be scaled up to produce larger amounts (100–150 mg) of derivative for therapeutic applications if required. However, bear in mind that the derivatives produced by this procedure are almost always contaminated with trace amounts of parent IgG antibody or Fc fragments, which are coharvested with the parent F(ab′)$_2$ and the final product. If the presence of Fc is likely to be a problem, preparations can be tested for Fc by enzyme-linked immunosorbent assay (ELISA), and, if necessary, Fc removed by immunoaffinity chromatography *(2)*.

2. Materials

2.1. Reagents

1. 2 *M* TE8: 2 *M* Tris-HCl, pH 8.0, 100 m*M* ethylenediaminetetra-acetic acid (EDTA). Prepare 0.2 *M* TE8 from 2 *M* stock.
2. F(ab′)$_2$ reducing solution: 220 m*M* 2-ME, 1 m*M* EDTA. Make up 10 mL. Use a fume cupboard.
3. Sephadex G25 (Pharmacia, Uppsala, Sweden) and Ultragel AcA44 (Biosepra S. A., Villeneuve la Garenne, France) gel filtration media.
4. G25 column buffer (50 m*M* AE); 3.35 g sodium acetate, 526 µL glacial acetic acid, 0.186 g EDTA, made up to 1 L. Degas before use under vacuum or using nitrogen.
5. High performance liquid chromatography (HPLC) buffer (0.2 *M* phosphate, pH 7.0): Add 0.2 *M* Na$_2$HPO$_4$ to 0.2 *M* NaH$_2$PO$_4$ to obtain the required pH.
6. *o*-PDM/DMF for Fab′(SH) alkylation: 12 m*M* *o*-PDM in dimethylformamide. Make up just prior to use. Chill in a methylated spirit/ice bath. Caution: *o*-PDM is toxic and should be handled with care.
7. NTE8, 1 *M*: 1 *M* NaCl, 0.2 *M* Tris-HCl, pH 8.0, 10 m*M* EDTA.
8. Iodoacetamide: 250 m*M* in 0.2 *M* TE8 and 50 m*M* in 1 *M* NTE8.

2.2. Chromatography Equipment

1. Two chromatography columns packed with Sephadex G25 (*see* **Subheading 2.1.**) and equilibrated and run in 50 m*M* AE are required. The first (column 1) should be 1.6 cm in diameter, packed to a height of 25 cm with gel, and pumped at approx 60 mL/h. The second (column 2) should be 2.6 cm in diameter, packed to a height of 20 cm with gel, and pumped at approx 200 mL/h. The columns must be fitted with two end-flow adaptors and water jackets to allow chilling throughout the procedure. Pharmacia K Series columns are ideal.
2. Two larger columns packed with polyacrylamide agarose gel (Ultragel AcA44; *see* **Subheading 2.1.**) and run in 0.2 *M* TE8 are used for the size exclusion chro-

matography of the BsAb products. These should be 2.6 cm in diameter, and packed to a height of 80 cm with gel. The two columns should be joined in series using Teflon capillary tubing and pumped at approx 30 mL/h. Chilling is not required at this stage of the preparation, and the columns can be run at room temperature.

3. Two peristaltic pumps capable of rates between 15 and 200 mL/h for column chromatography.
4. Chiller/circulator to cool columns. A polystyrene box containing water and crushed ice and a submersible garden pond pump (rate approx 10 L/min) can be used as an alternative to a commercial chiller.
5. UV monitor, chart recorder, and fraction collector.
6. Amicon stirred concentration cell (Series 8000, 50 or 200 mL) with a 10,000 Mr cutoff filter for concentration of products.
7. HPLC system fitted with Zorbex Bio series GF250 column (Du Pont Company, Wilmington, DE) or equivalent gel-permeation column capable of fractionation up to approx 250,000 Mr.

3. Methods

3.1. Preparation of Bispecific F(ab')$_2$ Derivatives

The method described here is for the preparation of F(ab')$_2$ BsAb starting with 5–20 mg of each parent F(ab')$_2$ to obtain 1–8 mg of BsAb product.

1. Use equal amounts of F(ab')$_2$ from the two parent antibodies. The F(ab')$_2$ should be in 0.2 M TE8 at 5–12 mg/mL in a final volume of 1–3 mL. Keep a 50 µL sample of both F(ab')$_2$ preparations for HPLC analysis (*see* **Subheading 3.3.**).
2. Reduce both parent F(ab')$_2$ preparations to Fab'(SH) using 1/10 vol F(ab')$_2$ reducing solution (final concentration 20 mM 2-ME). Incubate at 30°C for 30 min and then keep on ice. Maintain the tempterature at 0–5°C for the rest of the procedure unless stated otherwise.
3. Select the species to be maleimidated [Fab'-A(SH)] (*see* **Note 3**). Remove 2-ME by passing through the smaller Sephadex G25 column (column 1). Collect the protein peak, which elutes after approx 8–10 min, in a graduated glass tube in an ice bath (*see* **Note 4**). Take a 45 µL sample from the top of the peak for HPLC analysis (*see* **Subheading 3.3.**). Keep the column running to completely elute 2-ME, which runs as a small secondary peak.
4. When the chart recorder has returned to baseline, load the second Fab'(SH) species [Fab'-B(SH)] onto the column, and separate as for Fab'-A(SH), again taking a sample for HPLC analysis (*see* **Subheading 3.3.**).
5. After the Fab'-B(SH) has been loaded onto the G25 column, the Fab'-A(SH) partner can be maleimidated. Rapidly add a 1/2 vol (normally 4–5 mL) of cold o-PDM/DMF to the Fab'-A(SH), seal the tube with Parafilm or similar, and mix by inverting two to three times (*see* **Note 5**). Stand in an ice bath for 30 min.
6. When the Fab'-B(SH) has been collected, connect the larger Sephadex G25 column (column 2) to the chart recorder. After the 30 min incubation, load the

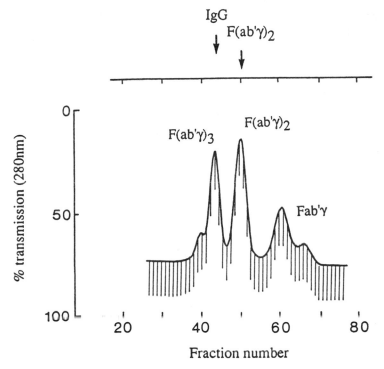

Fig. 2. Chromatography profile showing the separation of parent Fab′ and bispecific F(ab′)$_2$ and F(ab′)$_3$ products on AcA44 columns. In this case, Fab′-A(SH) and Fab′-B(mal) were mixed at a ratio of 2 : 1 to increase the formation of bispecific F(ab′)$_3$. The unreacted Fab′ fragments and the F(ab′)$_2$ and F(ab′)$_3$ products are indicated. The arrows show the points at which protein standards eluted from the same columns.

Fab′-A(SH)/*o*-PDM/DMF mixture onto this column. Collect the Fab′-A(mal) protein peak (elutes after 8–10 min) (*see* **Note 6**).

7. Pool the Fab′-A(mal) and the Fab′-B(SH). Immediately concentrate in a stirred Amicon concentration cell to around 5 mL, and then transfer to a tube for overnight incubation at 4°C (*see* **Note 7**).

8. During conjugation, in addition to the required BsAb, disulfide bonded homodimers may also form. To eliminate these, after overnight incubation add 1/10 volume 1 *M* NTE8 to the mixture to increase the pH, and then 1/10 volume F(ab′)$_2$ reducing solution to reduce the homodimer disulfide bonds. Incubate at 30°C for 30 min.

9. Alkylate to block sulphydryl groups by the addition of 1/10 vol 250 m*M* iodoacetamide in 0.2 *M* TE8 (*see* **Note 8**). Check the composition of the mixture by HPLC (*see* **Subheading 3.3.**).

10. Separate the products on two AcA44 columns run in series. Collect 10–15 min fractions. A typical elution profile is shown in **Fig. 2**.

11. Pool the fractions containing the BsAb product. To minimize contamination, only take the middle two-thirds of the peak. Concentrate and dialyze into appropriate buffer.
12. If required, check the final product by HPLC (*see* **Subheading 3.3.**).

3.2. Preparation of Bispecific F(ab′)₃ Derivatives

This is as for the preparation of bispecific F(ab′)$_2$ except that the ratio of Fab′(mal) to Fab′(SH) is increased from 1:1 to 2:1 or greater. Therefore, start with at least twice as much of the F(ab′)$_2$ which is to provide two arms of the F(ab′)$_3$ product.

3.3. HPLC Monitoring

For rapid analysis of products during the preparation, an HPLC system is used as described in **Subheading 2.2.** This will resolve IgG, F(ab′)$_2$, and Fab′ sized molecules in approx 20 min, and can be performed while the preparation is in progress. The parent F(ab′)$_2$ and the alkylated reaction mixture can be loaded directly onto the column and the eluted product monitored at 280 nm. However, we have found that F(ab′)SH rapidly reoxidizes back to F(ab′)$_2$ while on the column. This can be overcome by alkylating the free SH-groups by the addition of 5 μL 50 m*M* iodoacetamine in 1 *M* NTE8 to the 45-μL sample from the G25 column.

Fab′ will elute from the column later than F(ab′)$_2$ resulting in a shift in the position of the peak on reduction. In most cases >95% of the F(ab′)$_2$ is reduced. Following alkylation and overnight incubation, the reaction mixture typically elutes from HPLC as a triplet, containing a mixture of alkylated Fab′ and Fab′(mal), which elute in a similar postion to Fab′(SH), bispecific F(ab′)$_2$ product, which elutes similarly to the parent F(ab′)$_2$, and a smaller amount of bispecific F(ab′)$_3$, which elutes similarly to IgG.

4. Notes

1. Two SH groups may also be produced by the reduction of the heavy/light chain disulfide bond. However, under the conditions used, this bond is not fully reduced, and any SH groups that are produced are less likely to be available for conjugation (*1,2*). This procedure relies on one maleimidated hinge SH-group remaining free for conjugation after the intramolecular crosslinking of adjacent SH-groups with *o*-PDM. It follows that the Fab′ species chosen to be maleimidated must be derived from IgG with an odd number of hinge region disulfide bonds. Of the mouse IgG subclasses, IgG1 and IgG2a (three bonds), and IgG3 (one bond) qualify, whereas IgG2b (four bonds) does not. F(ab′)$_2$ derived from rabbit Ig (one bond) and rat IgG1 (three bonds) can also be employed. However, rat IgG2a and IgG2c both have two, and rat IgG2b has four and so cannot be used as the maleimidated partner.

2. If F(ab′)₃ derivatives are required, the number of SH-groups at the hinge of the unmaleimidated partner should be at least two and preferably three, because this determines the number of Fab′(mal) arms that can be conjugated.

3. We have found that a few antibodies give consistently low yields of BsAb when used as the maleimidated partner. If large quantities of a derivative are required, it is worthwhile performing small scale pilot preparations to determine which maleimidated partner gives the optimal yield.

4. It is very important to avoid contamination of the Fab′-A(SH) with 2-ME. In order to minimize the risk, stop collecting when the recorder has returned two-thirds of the way back to the baseline. In order to ensure that Fab′-B(SH) is not contaminated with 2-ME left over from the first run, make sure that it is not loaded until the chart recorder has returned to the baseline.

5. Sometimes the mixture becomes slightly cloudy.

6. To avoid contamination with *o*-PDM/DMF, which elutes as a second large peak, stop collecting when the chart recorder has returned halfway to baseline.

7. To avoid loss of product, slightly over concentrate, then wash the cell with a small volume of chilled buffer.

8. It is very important to add excess iodoacetamide at this stage; otherwise the BsAb derivative can precipitate.

References

1. Glennie, M. J., McBride, H. M., Worth, A. T., and Stevenson, G. T. (1987) Preparation and performance of bispecific F(ab′γ)₂ antibody containing thioether-linked Fab′γ fragments. *J. Immunol.* **139,** 2367–2375.

2. Glennie, M. J., Tutt, A. L., and Greenman, J. (1993) Preparation of multispecific F(ab′)₂ and F(ab′)₃ antibody derivatives, in *Tumour Immunobiology, A Practical Approach* (Gallagher, G., Rees, R. C., and Reynolds, C. W., eds.), Oxford University Press, Oxford, UK, pp. 225–244.

27

Radiolabellng of Monoclonal Antibodies

Calvin S. R. Gooden

1. Introduction

Radiolabeling of monoclonal antibodies (mAbs) is often one of the principal methods for the in vitro and in vivo assessment of these reagents, whether this is determining the affinity of a new reagent, preparing for preclinical testing, or clinically for diagnostic or therapeutic use.

The basis of a good radiolabeling technique is speed, efficiency, and robustness. Most of the methods described below have been chosen because they are the most commonly used and generally applicable. Alternative methods, possibly better suited to the chosen antibody or application, are available elsewhere; the techniques described are intended as a good starting point.

Appropriate radiation safety precautions must be taken at all times when working with radioisotopes. If you have any doubts about the safe use and disposal of radioactivity, seek advice from an appropriately qualified person. Any safety advice given in this chapter should only be used as a guide—local safety rules must be followed at all times.

2. Materials

2.1. Gel Filtration Chromatography

1. Sephadex G50.
2. 20 mL syringe.
3. Sterile surgical gauze or polypropylene.

2.2. Filter Sterilization

1. Millex GV filter (or similar) (Millipore S.A., Molshein, France).
2. Syringe (Luer-fit).
3. Needles (22 gage).
4. Sterile glass vial with rubber stopper and aluminum crimp lid.

From: *Methods in Molecular Medicine, Vol. 40: Diagnostic and Therapeutic Antibodies*
Edited by: A .l T. George and C. E, Urch © Humana Press Inc., Totowa, NJ

2.3. Concentration of Antibodies (Molecular Weight Cutoff Filters)

1. Protein concentrator units (appropriate molecular weight cutoff).

2.4. Ascending Paper Chromatography/Instant Thin-Layer Chromatography

1. 25 mL Universal bottle.
2. Whatman 3MM paper (radioiodine) or silica-impregnated strips (Gelman Sciences, Ann Arbor, MI) (^{99m}Technetium).
3. 15% Trichloroacetic acid (TCA)(radioiodine) or 0.9% saline (^{99m}Tc).

2.5. Radiolabeling with Iodine (^{125}I or ^{131}I)

1. Iodo-Gen (Pierce, Oud-Beijerland, The Netherlands).
2. Chloroform.
3. Cryovials, 1.8 mL capacity.
4. Antibody solution concentrated to ≥ 1 mg/mL (pH 7.4–8.0).
5. Phosphate-buffered saline (PBS), pH 7.4.
6. Sephadex G50 column equilibrated in PBS.
7. Radioiodine–high specific activity in 0.1 M NaOH (Amersham International, Amersham, UK).

2.6. Antibody Labeling with ^{111}Indium (^{111}In)

1. Antibody solution concentrated to ≥ 10 mg/mL.
2. 1 M NaHCO$_3$.
3. Diethylenetriaminepenta-acetic acid anhydride (DTPA) (Sigma, Poole, Dorset, UK).
4. Dimethylsulfoxide (DMSO).
5. ^{111}InCl$_3$ in 0.04 M HCl (Amersham).
6. 3.8% Sodium citrate for injection.
7. Sephadex G50 column equilibrated in PBS.
8. Sephadex G50 column equilibrated in either 0.1 M sodium citrate, pH 6.0, or 0.1 M sodium acetate, pH 6.0).

2.7. Antibody Labeling with ^{99m}Tc

1. Antibody solution concentrated to ≥ 10 mg/mL.
2. 2-Mercaptoethanol.
3. Sephadex G50 column equilibrated in PBS.
4. Methylene diphosphonate (MDP) bone-scanning kit (Amersham).
5. 0.9% Saline.
6. ^{99m}Tc pertechnetate.

2.8. Antibody Labeling with ⁹⁰Yttrium (⁹⁰Y)

1. Antibody solution concentrated to ≥80 mg/mL.
2. *p*-Isothiocyanatobenzyldiethylenetriaminepenta-acetic acid (CITC-DTPA).
3. Saturated trisodium phosphate solution.
4. Sephadex G50 column equilibrated in 0.1 M ammonium acetate, pH 5.5.
5. 1 M Sodium acetate, pH 5.5.
6. 50 mM Ethylenediaminetetra-acetic acid (EDTA) in 0.1 M sodium acetate pH 5.5.
7. Sephadex G50 column equilibrated in PBS.

3. Methods
3.1. General Methods

Throughout this chapter several techniques are quoted that are common to more than one radiolabeling process. These universal techniques are described in this section (*see* **Notes 1–3**).

3.1.1. Gel Filtration Chromatography

A 2 × 6 cm Sephadex G50 column is prepared in the barrel of a 20 mL syringe using a thin layer of surgical gauze or precut polypropylene as the frit. The Sephadex is allowed to swell overnight in the appropriate elution buffer before careful pouring the gel into the syringe barrel up to the 20 mL mark. Ensure that there are no visible air bubbles or cracks in the column matrix. The column is then thoroughly washed with elution buffer (5–10 column volumes). After all of the wash has eluted from the column, the bottom of the column is capped and the reaction mixture is carefully loaded on to the top of the column, taking care not to disturb the column resin (**Note 4**). The cap at the bottom of the column is then removed and the displaced column buffer is allowed to elute before loading and collecting 10 × 2 mL fractions. The radioactivity (or absorbance at 280 nm) in each fraction is measured, and the fractions containing purified antibody are combined (antibody-containing fractions elute first, free radiolabel/chelate elutes in the later fractions). The radiolabeling efficiency can then be determined by comparing the activity in the antibody-containing fractions with the total activity loaded onto the column and the free radioactivity peak.

3.1.2. Filter Sterilization

Sterile filtration should be done reasonably quickly, using a syringe shield to minimize any radiation doses to the operator. All radiolabeled antibody preparations to be used in preclinical and clinical studies must be filter-sterilized prior to use. It is also advisable to filter-sterilize any radiolabeled antibody that will not be used immediately after preparation.

1. Attach the filter unit to a syringe large enough to contain the volume of the radio-labeled antibody.
2. Attach a sterile needle to the filter unit and slowly draw up the radiolabeled anti-body solution through the filter into the syringe.
3. The filtered solution may now be dispensed into a sterile glass vial, stoppered, and overcrimped until required for use. The required individual dose should be dispensed from this stock.

3.1.3. Concentration of Antibodies (Molecular Weight Cutoff Filters)

The principle of this technique is centrifugation through a porous membrane. Various membranes are available, each with different molecular weight cut-offs. Careful choice of membrane will ensure that buffer passes through the membrane to the lower chamber (waste), leaving more concentrated antibody solution in the top chamber. The Centricon, Amicon system is a good example of this type of system. In all cases, the manufacturer's instructions must be followed. These systems are generally not suitable for the preparation of clini-cal grade reagents.

3.1.4. Ascending Paper Chromatography and Instant Thin-Layer Chromatography

Ascending paper chromatography and instant thin-layer chromatography (ITLC) are used to assess the radiolabeling efficiency of antibodies with radioiodines and ^{99m}Tc, respectively. In each case a tiny amount of radiola-beled antibody solution is spotted at the origin of the paper. Using the appro-priate mobile phase, radiolabeled antibody is separated from free radiolabel (radiolabeled antibody at the origin and free radiolabel at the solvent front) and the proportion of radioactivity in each portion is used to calculate the radiola-beling efficiency.

1. Cut a piece of Whattmann 3MM paper (radioiodine) or silica-impregnated strip (^{99m}Tc) measuring approx 1.5 × 9 cm.
2. Add 1.5 mL of the mobile phase (15% trichloroacetic acid for radioiodine, 0.9% NaCl for ^{99m}Tc) in the bottom of a 25-mL Universal bottle. Do not allow the liquid to moisten the sides of the bottle.
3. Place a 3-μL spot of radiolabeled antibody at the origin (about 1 cm from the bottom of the strip).
4. Immediately place the ITLC strip into the Universal, with the origin at the bot-tom in the mobile phase. Allow the ascending chromatography to run.
5. When the solvent has reached about 1 cm from the top of the strip, stop the chro-matography by removing the ITLC strip from the universal bottle.

6. Cut the ITLC strip in half (4.5-cm intervals) to give two equally sized sections and measure the radioactivity in each section.

3.2. Radiolabeling with Iodine (^{125}I or ^{131}I)

A simple and generally applicable technique for radioiodination is the Iodo-Gen™* method *(1)*. In this method, radioiodine is introduced onto tyrosine residues in the antibody molecule by an oxidation, catalyzed by 1,3,4,6-tetrachloro-3α, 6α-diphenylglyco/uril (Iodo-Gen).

Antibody and radioiodine are mixed in a tube that has previously been coated with Iodo-Gen. Labeled antibody is separated from free radiolabel by gel filtration chromatography.

1. Preparation of Iodo-Gen-coated tubes: Iodo-Gen (Pierce, UK) is dissolved in chloroform at a concentration of 2 mg/mL. Aliquots of 25 μL (50 mg) are then transferred to plastic reaction tubes. The solvent is allowed to evaporate overnight, leaving a thin coat of Iodo-Gen in the tube. These Iodo-Gen-coated tubes are then capped and can now be stored at –20°C for up to 6 mo until required for use (**Note 5**).
2. Reaction mixture: In a typical reaction 400 mg antibody (pH 7.4–8.0) is mixed with 15 MBq radioiodine in an Iodo-Gen–coated tube (**Note 6**).
3. The reaction is allowed to proceed at room temperature for approx 10 min (**Note 7**).
4. The radiolabeled protein is then purified by gel filtration chromatography (**Notes 8–11**).

3.3. Antibody Labeling with ^{111}Indium (^{111}In)

Preparation of antibodies labeled with radiometals (^{111}In, ^{99m}Tc, and ^{90}Y) in most cases requires the covalent attachment of metal-binding moiety to the antibody, which is able to bind or chelate the radiometal. In this simple method, DTPA is the chosen chelating agent *(2)*.

3.3.1. Preparation of Antibody-DTPA Conjugates

1. Concentrate antibody (if necessary) to approx 10 mg/mL.
2. Adjust the pH of the antibody to pH 8.5 using 1 *M* $NaHCO_3$ by adding 10 μL at a time and testing the resulting solution with indicator strips.
3. For the reaction, a molar ratio of 10:1 (DTPA:antibody) is required. Weigh out a *small* amount of dry DTPA anhydride (about 0.0002 g). From this calculate how much concentrated, buffered antibody would be required for the 10:1 molar ratio and add this to the dry DTPA anhydride. Incubate the reaction mixture for 1 min at room temperature.

---

*Iodo-Gen is a trademark of Pierce Chemical Co. for 1,3,4,6-tetrachloro-3α, 6α-diphenylglyco/uril.

Alternatively, the DTPA anhydride may be dissolved in dry DMSO to give a concentrated solution. This allows very low DTPA:antibody ratios to be obtained. A small sample of the reaction mixture (about 5 µL) should be retained for estimation of the number of DTPA molecules bound per antibody (**Note 12**).

4. Purify the DTPA-conjugated antibody by Sephadex G50 gel filtration using 0.1 *M* sodium citrate, pH 6.0 (0.1 *M* sodium acetate, pH 6.0) as the elution buffer.
5. Combine antibody-containing fractions (determined by absorbance at 280 nm) and filter-sterilize.
6. The antibody:DTPA conjugate should now be aliquoted and may be stored at –20°C for several months.
7. The immunoreactivity of the antibody-DTPA conjugate should be tested by enzyme-linked immunosorbent assay (ELISA)—*see* Chapters 28 and 30.

3.3.2. Estimation of the Number of DTPA Molecules Bound per Antibody Molecule

This procedure is performed using the sample of reaction mixture saved from the coupling reaction (**Subheading 3.3.1.**). This sample contains antibody-DTPA, free DTPA, and unmodified antibody. When reacted with a trace amount of ^{111}In, the isotope will distribute itself between the protein-bound DTPA and free DTPA. This calculation assumes *incorrectly* that the binding affinity of DTPA for ^{111}In is not compromised by attachment to a protein molecule; hence, only an approximate answer can be calculated. Subsequent separation of the two radiolabeled species by Sephadex G50 gel filtration gives an estimate of the percentage of loaded ^{111}In that is bound to the protein. Since the DTPA:antibody molar ratio is known, the number of DTPAs per antibody can be estimated.

3.3.3. Estimation of Available Antibody-Bound DTPA Molecules for Radiolabeling

This procedure is carried out using a vast excess of ^{111}In and a known, small amount of purified antibody-conjugate, allowing the maximum specific activity to be calculated.

1. The pH of ^{111}In in 0.04 *M* HCl is increased to pH 6.0 using 3.8% sodium citrate, pH 7.4. Antibody-DTPA conjugate (approx 100 µg) is mixed with ≥74 MBq ^{111}In citrate. The reaction is allowed to proceed for 15 min at room temperature.
2. Free radiolabel is removed by Sephadex G50 gel filtration column equilibrated in PBS.
3. Pool fractions containing radiolabeled antibody.
4. Calculate the labeling efficiency and the specific activity.

3.3.4. Antibody-Labeling Procedure

1. Thaw the frozen antibody aliquot (if necessary).
2. Adjust the pH of the isotope (^{111}InCl$_3$ in 0.04 *M* HCl) to pH 6.0 using sodium citrate. Typically 18.5–74 MBq ^{111}In is used.
3. Add the antibody-DTPA conjugate and mix.
4. Incubate for 15 min at room temperature.
5. Purify the antibody-DTPA-^{111}In from the unbound ^{111}In by gel filtration using a 20 mL Sephadex G50 column equilibrated in PBS.
6. Pool the radiolabeled protein fractions, and filter-sterilize.
7. The required doses are dispensed from this stock.

3.4. Antibody Labeling with ^{99m}Tc

In the method described, no metal chelator is used. Instead, disulfide bridges within the antibody are cleaved using 2-mercaptoethanol (2ME), and methylene diphosphonate (MDP) from a bone scanning kit is used as a transchelator to mediate ^{99m}Tc labeling of high-affinity thiol groups within the reduced antibody molecule *(3)*.

3.4.1. Reduction of Antibody with 2ME

1. Concentrate antibody (if necessary) to approx 10 mg/mL.
2. Add 2ME to the antibody solution to provide a molar ratio of 1000:1 2ME:antibody and mix well.
3. Incubate at room temperature for 30 min.
4. Purify the reduced antibody by Sephadex G50 gel filtration on a 20 mL column, using PBS as the elution buffer.
5. Combine the antibody fractions (determined by absorbance at 280 nm) and filter-sterilize.
6. Divide into 0.5 mg aliquots and freeze immediately at –20°C (**Note 13**).

3.4.2. Antibody-Labeling Procedure

1. Reconstitute Amerscan MDP with 2 mL 0.9% saline injection BP.
2. Thaw the frozen antibody aliquot.
3. Add 35 µL MDP solution to the antibody aliquot, then mix.
4. Add the required amount of ^{99m}Tc pertechnetate (approx 1000 MBq) to the antibody/MDP mixture. Mix, and then leave for 5 min at room temperature.
5. Assess the labeling efficiency by ITLC using a silica-impregnated strip and 0.9% saline as the mobile phase. (^{99m}Tc-antibody at origin; ^{99m}Tc-MDP at the solvent front.)
6. If the labeling efficiency is < 95%, the labeled antibody can be further purified by gel filtration on a Sephadex G50 column.
7. Filter-sterilize the radiolabeled antibody aliquot and dispense the required dose from this stock. The labeled antibody is stable for some hours after preparation.

3.5. Antibody Labeling with ^{90}Y

Antibodies can be radiolabeled with ^{90}Y using chelate and techniques similar to those quoted for ^{111}In *(4)*. However, the technique described below uses the chelate CITC-DTPA, which retains yttrium much more stably than DTPA *(5)* (**Note 14**).

3.5.1. Method for Coupling CITC-DTPA to Antibody

1. Concentrate the antibody to 80 mg/mL in 0.1 M phosphate buffer, pH 8.2.
2. Add CITC-DTPA to a final concentration of 2 mM at a molar ratio of ≥2 : 1 chelate to antibody.
3. Adjust to pH 9.0–9.5 using saturated trisodium phosphate.
4. React for 2 h at 37°C.
5. Purify antibody-CITC-DTPA from unreacted chelate by Sephadex G-50 gel filtration using an elution buffer of 0.1 M ammonium acetate, pH 5.5.
6. Pool and filter-sterilize antibody-containing fractions.

3.5.2. Radiolabeling of Antibody-CITC-DTPA

1. Raise the pH of the ^{90}Y to pH 5.5 by adding 1 M sodium acetate solution (pH 5.5) to a final concentration of approx 0.2 M sodium acetate.
2. Add the required amount of antibody-CITC-DTPA to the required amount of ^{90}Y acetate.
3. Incubate for 15 min at room temperature.
4. Add EDTA (from a 50 mM stock solution in 0.1 M sodium acetate, pH 5.5) to a final concentration of 5 mM EDTA.
5. Incubate for 5–10 min at room temperature.
6. Separate ^{90}Y-labeled antibody from ^{90}Y-EDTA by Sephadex G50 gel filtration eluting in PBS.
7. Pool the antibody-containing fractions and filter-sterilize. Dispense required doses from this stock.

4. Notes

4.1. General Methods

1. Only reagents of the highest quality should be used, and where possible, these should be of an appropriate pharmacopoeia (or similar) standard. Reagents that are not available to pharmacopoeia standards must be stringently tested for sterility, pyrogenicity, particulates and pH *at the very least,* prior to use.
2. All clinical preparations must be made in a clinical radiopharmacy or an environment suitable for the preparation of radiopharmaceuticals.
3. Syringes, filters, and needles comprising the Luer-lock system should be used to minimize the risk of a radioactive spillage.

4. When small amounts of antibody are radiolabeled, protein losses owing to non-specific binding of the antibody to the purification column may become significant. Preblocking the column with a 1–5% solution of albumin helps to reduce these losses (not suitable for clinical preparations).

4.2. Iodinations

5. Appropriate safety precautions must be taken when using flammable chloroform—evaporation must be conducted in an approved fume-hood.
6. Antibody concentrations of ≥1 mg/mL should be used to achieve the best labeling efficiencies.
7. Incubation times longer than those stated may lead to damage to the antibody molecules.
8. For antibodies containing tyrosine residues within or in close proximity to the antigen-binding region, immunoreactivity may be impaired when radiolabeled using this method.
9. Typically, a radiolabeling efficiency of >90% is achieved using this method. However, a more efficient method, such as the *N*-bromosuccinimide *(6)* method, may be required where, for instance, large quantities of radioactivity are being used for radioimmunotherapy. In this case, the column purification step should be avoided to reduce operator exposure.
10. The efficiency of the radiolabeling reaction can also be measured by ascending paper chromatography using 15% TCA as the mobile phase.
11. Radioiodines are very volatile and are concentrated in the thyroid if inhaled—take appropriate safety precautions and work only in an environment approved by radiation safety personnel.

4.3. ^{111}In

12. Metal-containing objects (spatulas, pipet tips), containers (glass bottles), and solutions *must* be avoided at all steps prior to addition of the ^{111}In. This entails using low-metal plastic tips and plastic containers for all buffers. Where the use of glass containers is unavoidable, the containers must be prewashed with concentrated hydrochloric acid and then thoroughly rinsed with water for injection BP.

4.4. ^{99m}Tc

13. After the reduction step, the antibody should be frozen (–20°C) as quickly as possible to avoid reoxidation of free sulfydryl groups.

4.5. ^{90}Y

14. As with radiolabeling with ^{111}In, the use of metal-containing substances and containers must be avoided until after the addition of the EDTA solution.

References

1. Fraker, P. J. and Speck, J. C., Jr. (1978) Protein and cell membrane iodinations with a sparingly soluble chloramide, 1,3,4,6-tetrachloro-3α,6α-diphenylglycoluril. *Biochem. Biophys. Res. Commun.* **80,** 849–857.
2. Hnatowich, D. J., Childs, R. L., Lanteigne, D., and Najafi, A. (1983) The preparation of DTPA-coupled antibodies radiolabeled with metallic radionuclides: an improved method. *J. Immunol. Methods* **65,** 147–157.
3. Mather, S. J. and Ellison D. (1990) Reduction-mediated technetium-99m labelling of monoclonal antibodies. *J. Nucl. Med.* **31,** 692–697.
4. Hnatowich, D. J., Snook, D., and Rowlinson, G. (1988) Preparation and use of DTPA-coupled antibodies radiolabeled with yttrium-90, in *Antibody-Mediated Delivery Systems* (Rodwell, J. D., ed.), Marcel Dekker, New York, pp. 353–363.
5. Meares, C. F., McCall, M. J., Reardan, D. T., Goodwin, D. A., Diamanti, C. I., and McTigue, M. (1984) Conjugation of antibodies with bifunctional chelating agents: isothiocyanate and bromoacetamide reagents, methods of analysis, and subsequent addition of metal ions. *Anal. Biochem.* **142,** 68–78.
6. Zorzos, J., Pozatzidou, P., Pectasides, D., Bamias, A., Sivolapenko, G., Tsalta, K., Skarlos, D. V., Koutsioumba, P., and Lincourinas, M. (1993) Biodistribution and immunolocalization of intravesically administered ^{131}I-labeled antibody in urothelial cell carcinomas, in *Monoclonal Antibodies 2* (Epenetos, A. A., ed.), Chapman and Hall, London, UK, pp. 513–517.

28

Determination of the Immunoreactivity of Radiolabeled Monoclonal Antibodies

Gail Rowlinson-Busza

1. Introduction

Radiolabeled monoclonal antibodies (mAbs) are in use for numerous immunoassays and localization studies both in vitro and in vivo. It is often important to determine to what extent the radiolabeling procedure has affected the immunoreactivity of the antibody. If, for example, the radioisotope was inserted in the antigen-binding site, this would adversely affect the ability of the antibody to bind to its antigen. It is possible that, by changing the labeling technique or the radioisotope, this loss of immunoreactivity could be minimized. For example, if the antigen-binding site contains tyrosine, then the usual oxidation methods of labeling with radioiodine (1,2) may iodinate this important tyrosine residue. Other labeling methods may be more appropriate for these antibodies. For example, Bolton-Hunter reagent (3) can be used to iodinate antibodies on a lysine residue. Most chelating agents used for radiolabeling with metals are linked to the protein via a lysine residue, so if there is lysine in the antigen-binding site of the antibody, radiometals may not be the most appropriate isotope to use. However, the antibody is likely to contain a number of tyrosine and lysine residues that can be labeled, so the reduction in immunoreactivity caused by radiolabeling may not be too great. The magnitude of the effect will depend on the particular antibody.

The immunoreactive fraction of a mAb, after radiolabeling with various isotopes, can be tested in a live cell radioimmunoassay, using the method of linear extrapolation to binding at infinite antigen excess (4). A cell line expressing the relevant antigen is necessary for the assay.

From: *Methods in Molecular Medicine, Vol. 40: Diagnostic and Therapeutic Antibodies*
Edited by: A. J. T. George and C. F. Urch © Humana Press Inc., Totowa, NJ

2. Materials

1. Tissue culture medium.
2. Antigen-positive cell line.
3. Dibutyl phthalate.
4. Dioctyl phthalate.
5. Microfuge tubes (30 × 5 mm).
6. Solid carbon dioxide.
7. Radiolabeled antibody to be tested.
8. Clippers for cutting microfuge tubes (e.g., dog's claw clippers).
9. Appropriate facilities for counting radioactivity (will depend on isotope being used).

3. Methods

A 60/40 (v:v) mixture is prepared of dibutyl phthalate and dioctyl phthalate and the relative density corrected to 1.017 g/mL by small adjustments in the ratio of the two oils, which have different relative densities (dibutyl phthalate higher and dioctyl phthalate lower than 1.017 g/mL). The relative density is determined by weighing 1 mL of the oil mixture. At the correct relative density, cells, but not supernatant, pass through the oil when centrifuged, avoiding the need for repeated washing of the cell pellet and the subsequent loss of cells *(5)*.

3.1. Immunoreactivity

Cells in the exponential phase of growth are harvested and resuspended at several (at least 6–8) different cell concentrations spanning 2 logs (e.g., 3×10^5–3×10^7 cells/mL) in the appropriate tissue culture medium but without fetal calf serum, which tends to make the cells clump together. Two-hundred microliter aliquots of each cell concentration are pipeted into eight small tubes (such as LP3 tubes), and 50 µL of either unlabeled antibody, at a concentration of 300 or 30 µg/mL, or tissue culture medium added to each in duplicate and mixed well (**Fig. 1**). The tubes are incubated at 4°C for 30 min before the addition of 50 µL radiolabeled antibody at a concentration of 0.6 µg/mL or 0.06 µg/mL. In the total incubation volume of 300 µL, the final radiolabeled antibody concentration is therefore kept constant at 0.01 µg/mL and at 0.1 µg/mL in separate duplicate incubations, with and without 500-fold excess unlabeled antibody. The cell suspensions are then incubated with antibody at room temperature under constant shaking to keep the cells in suspension.

After 1.5–2 h incubation, each mixture of cells and antibody is shaken well, then 100 µL dispensed into tubes for counting and 100 µL of each mixture is layered onto 200 µL of the oil mixture in a microfuge tube and centrifuged for 5 min at 16,000g (**Fig. 2**). The tubes are then frozen in solid carbon dioxide and

For each cell concentration:

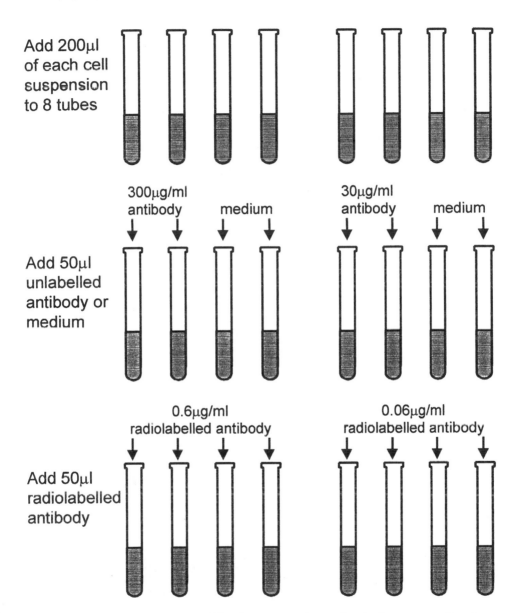

Add 200µl of each cell suspension to 8 tubes

300µg/ml antibody   medium   30µg/ml antibody   medium

Add 50µl unlabelled antibody or medium

0.6µg/ml radiolabelled antibody   0.06µg/ml radiolabelled antibody

Add 50µl radiolabelled antibody

Fig. 1. Diagram of the protocol for the assay to determine the immunoreactive fraction of a radiolabeled antibody. Two independent incubations are performed in duplicate, for two different antibody concentrations (illustrated here for final radiolabeled antibody concentrations of 0.1 µg/mL and 0.01 µg/mL), with and without unlabeled blocking antibody at a 500-fold excess.

For each incubation tube:

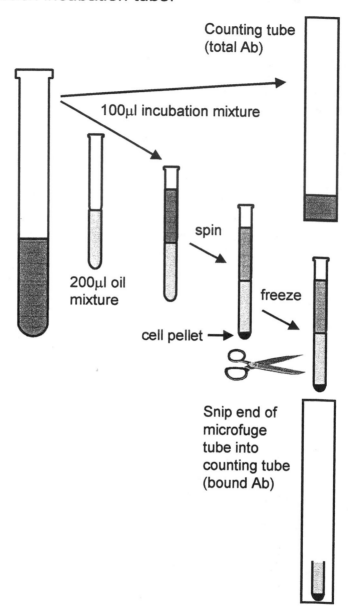

Fig. 2. Diagram of the protocol for counting the free and bound radioactive antibody after incubation with the cell suspensions. The total (bound plus free) antibody is determined by counting an aliquot of the incubation mixture. The bound antibody is determined by spinning an aliquot of the incubation mixture through oil, freezing in solid CO_2, and snipping the cell pellet into a tube for counting.

the bottom of the tube, containing the cell pellet, is snipped off into a counting tube. The most convenient way of doing this is to use a guillotine-type clipper designed for cutting dogs' claws and to cut halfway through the oil layer. The activity in the cell pellet (bound antibody) and in the 100-μl aliquot of the respective incubation mixture (total antibody) is counted in a γ-counter in the case of antibodies labeled with γ-emitting isotopes (such as ^{125}I, ^{131}I, ^{99m}Tc, or ^{111}In). The activity in antibodies labeled with β-emitting isotopes (such as ^{90}Y) is counted in a liquid scintillation counter after the addition of 4 mL scintillant to each tube. In order to account for all of the radioactivity, the top of the microfuge tube, containing the supernatant (free antibody), may also be counted, as well as an aliquot of the original radiolabeled antibody added to the cell suspensions (**Note 1**).

3.2. Binding Capacity

Cells are incubated as above, but the cell concentration is kept constant at 10^6 cells/mL, and the antibody concentration is varied between 2.5×10^{-3} and 5 μg mL. Around 20 different antibody concentrations should be used, each incubated with and without a 500-fold excess unlabeled antibody as for the immunoreactivity assay.

3.3. Calculation

The purpose of the incubation with a 500-fold excess of unlabeled antibody is to block the antigenic sites on the cells and thus prevent the radiolabeled antibody from binding. Therefore, any bound radioactivity in these incubations is the result of nonspecific protein binding to the cells. These radioactive counts are subtracted from the counts obtained without the excess unlabeled antibody to give the actual (specifically bound) antibody counts, which are then used in the following calculations (**Note 2**).

3.3.1. Immunoreactivity

In an ideal binding reaction, the equilibrium amount of antibody bound to antigen is determined by the law of mass action:

$$[B] = K_a \cdot [F] \cdot [rT - B] \tag{1}$$

where:

$[B]$ = bound antibody concentration (in the cell pellet),
K_a = association constant,
$[F]$ = concentration of free antigen,
$[T]$ = total antibody concentration (in the incubation mixture), and
r = immunoreactive antibody fraction.

therefore

$[rT - B]$ = concentration of reactive free antibody

$$[F] = N \cdot [\text{cell}] - [B] \tag{2}$$

where

N = number of binding sites per cell.

From **Eq. 1**:

$$\frac{[T]}{[B]} = \frac{1}{r \cdot K_a} \cdot \frac{1}{[F]} + \frac{1}{r}$$

$$= \frac{1}{r \cdot K_a} \cdot \frac{1}{N \cdot [\text{cell}] - [B]} + \frac{1}{r} \tag{3}$$

Extrapolating to infinite antigen excess, then as [cell] increases, the term *[B]* becomes negligible in comparison and can be ignored. The results are plotted for each antibody concentration as:

$$\frac{[T]}{[B]} \text{ v } \frac{1}{[\text{cell}]} \tag{4}$$

taking into account that the final cell concentration in the incubation mixture is only four-fifths of the initial concentration of the cell suspension, owing to dilution with the addition of the antibody. The plot will be a straight line with slope $1/(r \cdot K_a \cdot N)$. When [cell] = ∞ (i.e., 1/[cell] = 0), the intercept on the ordinate is $1/r$, the reciprocal of the immunoreactive fraction of the radiolabeled antibody (**Note 3**).

3.3.2. Binding Capacity

From **Eq. 1**, substituting for *[F]*,

$$\frac{[B]}{[rT - B]} = K_a \cdot (N \cdot [\text{cell}] - [B])$$

$$= -K_a \cdot [B] + K_a \cdot N \cdot [\text{cell}] \tag{5}$$

Scatchard analysis *(6)* is performed by using 20 different antibody concentrations and plotting:

$$\frac{[B]}{[rT - B]} \text{ v } [B] \tag{6}$$

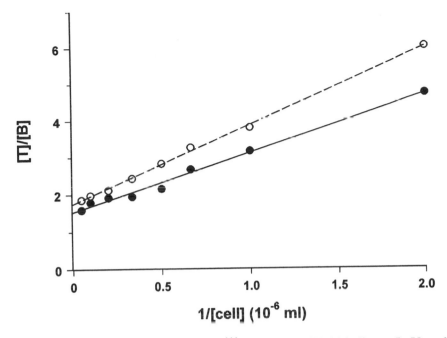

Fig. 3. Live cell radioimmunoassay of ^{111}In-labeled AUA1 binding to LoVo cells: determination of the immunoreactive fraction at 0.1 (●) and 0.01 μg/mL (○). Each point is the mean of duplicate measurements. The lines are fitted by linear regression to least squares.

The negative slope of the line, found by linear regression, gives the association constant K_a, and the intercept on the abscissa is the binding site concentration, $N \cdot [\text{cell}]$. The number of binding sites per cell can then be calculated as:

$$N = \frac{[\text{binding sites}] \cdot \text{incubation volume} \cdot N_A}{\text{number of cells}} \qquad (7)$$

where

N_A = Avogadro's constant, 6.02×10^{23}/mole (**Note 4**).

3.4. Example

Figures 3 and **4** illustrate an example of this type of analysis for ^{111}In-labeled mAb AUA1 (*7*) using the human colon carcinoma cell line LoVo (*8*) against which AUA1 was raised.

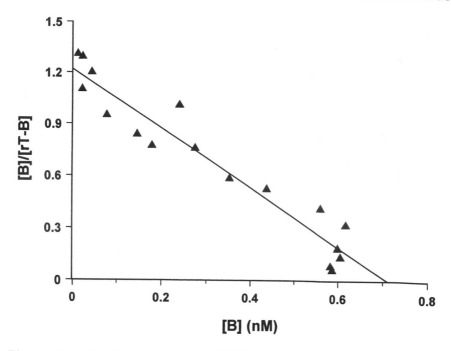

Fig. 4. Live cell radioimmunoassay of ^{111}In-labeled AUA1 binding to LoVo cells: Scatchard plot of bound/reactive free antibody against bound antibody for the determination of the number of binding sites per cell. Each point is the mean of duplicate measurements. The line is fitted by linear regression to least squares.

3.4.1. Immunoreactivity

Figure 3 is the reciprocal antigen plot for the determination of the immunoreactive fraction at two different antibody concentrations (0.1 μg/mL and 0.01 μg/mL). For these antibody concentrations, linear regression analysis gives the equations of the two lines as, respectively:

$$y = 1.60x + 1.53$$
$$y = 2.14x + 1.75 \tag{8}$$

From **Eq. 3**, the immunoreactive fraction is given by the reciprocal of the intercept on the ordinate, i.e., the value of y when x is zero. These reciprocals are 0.65 and 0.57, respectively, yielding a mean value for the immunoreactive fraction of 61%. This is a reasonable value for immunoreactivity, considering that the antibody has undergone both DTPA (metal chelate) conjugation and ^{111}In-labeling.

3.4.2. Binding Capacity

Figure 4 is the Scatchard plot of bound/reactive free antibody against bound antibody for the determination of the number of binding sites per cell. The equation of the line of best fit is:

$$y = -1.71x + 1.22 \tag{9}$$

From **Eq. 5**, this gives the affinity (K_a) directly as 1.71 nM^{-1}.

Rearranging:

$$x = \frac{1.22 - y}{1.71} \tag{10}$$

The intercept on the abscissa is the binding site concentration, i.e., the value of x when y is zero, which gives a value of 0.71 nM. The incubation volume is 300 μL and the number of cells is 3×10^5 (0.3 mL at 10^6 cells/ml) Therefore, from **Eq. 6**, the number of binding sites per cell is:

$$N = \frac{0.71 \times 10^{-9} \cdot 300 \times 10^{-6} \cdot 6.02 \times 10^{23}}{3 \times 10^5} \tag{11}$$

Note that all values are converted to moles or liters. It follows that, for the LoVo cell line used in this experiment, the number of binding sites per cell is 4.3×10^5.

4. Notes

1. If the total radioactivity in the cell suspension after incubation is significantly less than that in an equivalent aliquot of the added radiolabeled antibody, then there may be a problem with binding of the antibody to the plastic of the incubation tubes. This could be overcome by using different tubes, performing the assay in the presence of excess protein, such as bovine serum albumin, or preblocking the tubes with protein.

2. If the nonspecific binding of the antibody to the cell line is found to be low, then the blocking step with excess unlabeled antibody may be omitted.

3. Immunoreactivity: If the cell concentration is too low, i.e., at high values of 1/[cell], then the antibody may saturate the antigen, particularly at the higher antibody concentration used. In this case $[T]/[B]$ will appear too high, since there will be a component of the total antibody that cannot bind antigen, because it is already saturated. The graph will appear to curve upward at high x values. If this occurs only at 1 or 2 values, then it is valid to use the remaining linear portion of the curve for the calculation of immunoreactive fraction. If, however, a significant part of the curve is nonlinear, then the assay must be repeated using either lower antibody concentrations or more cells.

4. Binding capacity: A similar situation can occur with the Scatchard plot. As the antibody concentration increases, the antigen becomes saturated. If the antibody concentration is further increased, no more antibody can bind and so $[rT - B]$ increases, hence $[B]/[rT - B]$ decreases, and $[B]$ remains constant at the maximum amount of antibody that can bind. This results in a clustering of points at the bottom of the line at the $[B]$ value corresponding to the binding site concentration or, in fact, slightly lower, since steric hindrance will occur at a very high antibody concentration. There is some evidence of this clustering in **Fig. 4**. If the effect is greater than seen in **Fig. 4**, then the highest antibody concentrations should not be used in the analysis, if this does not exclude too much data. If too many of the data points fall into this category, then the experiment must be repeated with lower antibody concentrations or higher cell number.

References

1. Fraker, P. J. and Speck, J. C., Jr. (1978) Protein and cell membrane iodinations with a sparingly soluble chloramide, 1,3,4,6-tetrachloro-3a,6a-diphenylglycoluril. *Biochem. Biophys. Res. Commun.* **80,** 849–857.
2. Markwell, M. A. K. (1982) A new solid-state reagent to iodinate proteins. *Anal. Biochem.* **125,** 427–432.
3. Bolton, A. E. and Hunter, W. M. (1973) The labeling of proteins to high specific radioactivities by conjugation to a ^{125}I-containing acylating agent. *Biochem. J.* **133,** 529–539.
4. Lindmo, T., Boven, E., Cuttitta, F., Fedorko, J., and Bunn, P. A., Jr. (1984) Determination of the immunoreactive fraction of radiolabeled monoclonal antibodies by linear extrapolation to binding at infinite antigen excess. *J. Immunol. Methods* **72,** 77–89.
5. Segal, D. M. and Hurwitz, E. (1977) Binding of affinity cross-linked oligomers of IgG to cells bearing Fc receptors. *J. Immunol.* **118,** 1338–1347.
6. Scatchard, G. (1949) The attractions of proteins for small molecules and ions. *Ann. NY Acad. Sci.* **51,** 660–672.

7. Arklie, J. (1981) Studies of human epithelial cell surface using monoclonal antibodies. D.Phil. Thesis, Oxford University.
8. Drewinko, B., Romsdahl, M. M., Yang, L. Y., Ahearn, M. J., and Trujillo, J. M. (1976) Establishment of a human carcinoembryonic antigen-producing colon adenocarcinoma cell line. *Cancer Res.* **36,** 467–475.

29

Use of Biosensors to Measure the Kinetics of Antibody–Antigen Interactions

Andrew J. T. George

1. Introduction

The affinity and kinetics of antibody–antigen interactions are increasingly realized to be important parameters in determining the usefulness of antibodies in both in vivo and in vitro settings (*1*). As discussed in Chapter 1, the affinity of an antibody (given by the association or dissociation equilibrium constants; K_a and K_d) gives information about how much antibody will be bound to the antigen at equilibrium, or how much antibody will be required for a particular proportion of the antigen to be bound. The kinetics of the interaction (given by the association and dissociation rate constants; k_{ass} and k_{diss}) tell how rapidly the antibody–antigen complex is formed and, once formed, how rapidly it dissociates.

Until recently, most studies confined themselves to measuring the affinity of antibody–antigen interactions, because a number of methods existed to determine the affinity (*see* Chapter 28), but measuring the kinetics was more complex and tedious. However, in recent years the development of biosensors has made the determination of kinetics far simpler.

A biosensor consists of a sensing surface onto which is immobilized either the antigen or the antibody. Binding of the complementary partner to the immobilized molecules is then detected by a transducer, which sends an electronic signal that can then be analyzed to determine the degree of binding. Different biosensors vary in the type of transducer used; thus, the BIAcore series of machines (Biacore AB, Uppsala, Sweden) uses plasmon resonance to detect binding, whereas the IAsys series uses resonant mirror technology. They also vary in their configuration; the IAsys using a cuvet system and the BIAcore a flow cell (reviewed in **ref.** *1*).

From: *Methods in Molecular Medicine, Vol. 40: Diagnostic and Therapeutic Antibodies*
Edited by. A. J. T. George and C. F. Urch © Humana Press Inc., Totowa, NJ

In this chapter we will concentrate on the IAsys, because that is the system we have the most experience with. However, many of the protocols can be readily converted to other biosensors. The machine comes in different models that vary slightly in their details; for example, the size of the reaction chamber in the cuvet can be different. We will give protocols assuming a 50-μL reaction chamber, it will be necessary to scale the volumes appropriately for other chambers.

The basic configuration of the IAsys is shown in **Fig. 1**. The sensing surface is on the bottom of a cuvet that is inserted into the machine. Different surfaces can be purchased. For most applications a carboxymethylated dextran hydrogel surface, is used, which consists of a layer of dextran that extends approx 200 nm from the surface. The dextran is modified to carry carboxymethyl groups that allow for convenient covalent attachment of proteins or other molecules. Other surfaces include the "flat" amino silane surface, which lacks the hydrogel and uses amino groups for attachment. Furthermore, other surfaces are available with biotin groups already attached.

Below the sensing surface lies a resonant mirror device that acts as a transducer, monitoring the binding of material to the sensing surface. Details of how the resonant mirror work can be found elsewhere *(2,3)*; it effectively serves to measure the mass of material bound onto the surface (though it will also detect changes in the optical properties of the solution in the vicinity of the surface, as will be discussed shortly (*see* **Note 1**).

A typical experiment starts with the immobilization of one of the binding partners to the surface. We will call the immobilized molecule the ligand, and the soluble partner the ligate. We will give the main protocol used to immobilize protein onto carboxymethylated dextran hydrogel via ε amino groups. It should be noted that alternative protocols exist and are available from the manufacturer for immobilization onto "flat" surfaces or via alternative chemistries.

Following immobilization the ligate is then added (*see* **Fig. 2**). The binding is followed for a period, and then the chamber is evacuated and washed, removing all free antibody. This allows the dissociation of the antibody–antigen complex to be followed. The surface is then regenerated by adding a buffer that dissociates the immune complex, allowing the experiment to be repeated.

In this chapter we will concentrate on the use of biosensors to measure the kinetics of antibody–antigen interactions. However, they also have applications for the kinetics of interaction of other macromolecules, as well as for epitope mapping, ligand identification, and concentration determination.

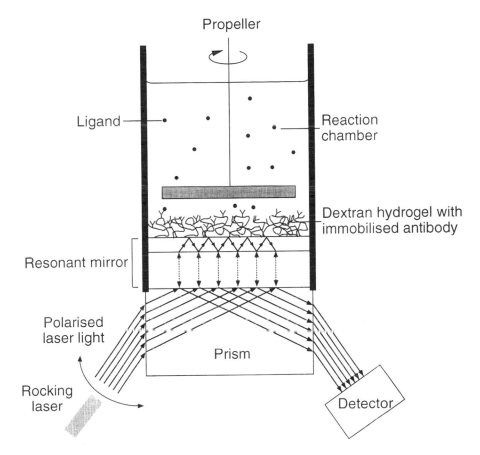

Fig. 1. Schematic representation of the IAsys resonant mirror biosensor. The sample cuvet contains a reaction chamber into which the sample is added, a dextran hydrogel surface to which the ligand is immobilized (represented in this case by Y-shaped antibodies), the resonant mirror, which is made of up to approx 100 nm high refractive index Si_3N_4 on top of 500 nm SiO_2, and a prism. Other surfaces can be used as alternatives to the dextran hydrogel. The cuvet is placed within the IAsys instrument, and the contents of the reaction chamber are efficiently stirred with a propeller or paddle. Laser light is directed at the prism at a range of angles. At one angle (the resonant angle) the light tunnels through the SiO_2 and propagates along the Si_3N_4 layer before tunneling out of the mirror. This resonant angle can be readily detected owing to a shift in the phase of the resonant light. Alterations in the amount of material bound to the dextran affect the position of the resonant angle, so the binding of the antibody to the antigen can be followed by determining the resonant angle (from **ref. *1*** with permission ©Ashley Publications).

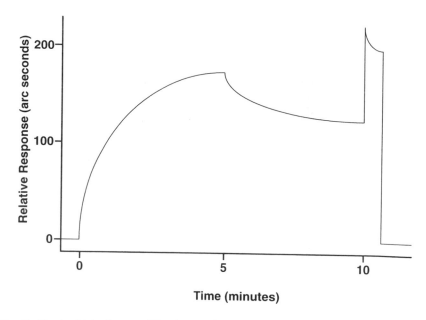

Fig. 2. Typical binding profile of experiment. This illustrates an idealized binding curve that might be obtained in an experiment. The ligand has been previously immobilized onto the sensing surface. At 0 min the ligate is added. The association of the ligate and ligand are then followed for 5 min. During this time the initially fast rate of association falls off as the reaction approaches equilibrium (at equilibrium the binding curve would reach a plateau). At this time the cuvet is washed to remove free ligate. The dissociation of the ligate from the ligand is then followed for 5 min. The regeneration buffer is then added to strip any remaining ligate off the sensing surface. Washing with PBS-Tween then returns the response to baseline. The amount of material bound to the sensing surface is given by the relative response (in arc seconds). The sudden changes in response seen when the regeneration buffer is a bulk shift caused by changes in the buffer. Similar bulk shifts can be seen when the ligate is added (or washed out) if the buffer composition of the ligate solution is different from that of the running buffer.

2. Materials

2.1. General Materials

1. IAsys machine (various models) available from Affinity Sensors (Bar Hill Cambridge, UK).
2. Carboxymethylated dextran hydrogel cuvets (appropriate for the IAsys model in use).
3. Phosphate-buffered saline containing 0.05% Tween (PBS-Tween) (*see* **Note 1**).

2.2. pH Optimization

1. Ligand to be immobilized. You will need a final concentration of 50 µg/mL in the appropriate acetate buffer.
2. 10 m*M* Acetate buffers at pH ranging from 3.0–6.0 in 0.5 unit increments (*see* **Note 2**).

2.3. Immobilization

1. EDC-coupling kit (available from Affinity Sensors). This contains 1-ethyl-3-(3-dimethylaminopropyl) carbodiimide (EDC) and *N*-hydroxysuccinimide (NHS), as well as ethanolamine. The EDC and NHS need to be aliquoted as described (*see* **Note 3**).
2. Ligand at 50 µg/mL in 10 m*M* acetate buffer of appropriate pH (determined as in **Subheading 3.1.1.**).

2.4. Kinetic Experiments

1. Ligate (typical maximum concentration of an antibody 20 µg/mL, though for lower affinity interactions may need a higher concentration).
2. Regeneration buffer (*see* **Note 4**).

3. Methods

In all experiments it is necessary to set the stirrer or vibrator of the machine at the correct speed to ensure rapid mixing of the contents of the cuvet. The setting will depend on the model of the machine, and will be recommended by the manufacturer for that model. It is also necessary to set the temperature at a constant value. The conventional setting is 25°C, though other temperatures can be used (*see* **Note 5**).

3.1. Immobilization onto Dextran Hydrogel

3.1.1. Optimization of pH

The covalent immobilization of the protein ligand onto the hydrogel relies on the electrostatic concentration of the molecule onto the negatively charged gel to obtain a sufficiently high local concentration of the molecule. The optimal pH at which this will occur will depend on the pH of the solution. If one is immobilizing a protein for the first time it is therefore necessary to optimize the pH of the reaction. This is done on a new carboxymethyl dextran surface, which can then be reused for the immobilization (**Subheading 3.1.2.**) (*see* **Note 6**).

1. Place a carboxymethyl-dextran cuvet into the IAsys. Add 50 µL PBS-Tween and allow to equilibrate for 5–10 min.
2. Make up for each of the pH values to be tested two microfuge tubes. One tube should contain 200 µL 10 m*M* acetate buffer at the appropriate pH. The other tube should contain 50 µg/mL antigen in 200 µL of the same buffer (*see* **Note 7**).

3. Replace the PBS-Tween in the cuvet with 50 μL of the 10 mM acetate buffer at the lowest pH. Wait 3 s.
4. Replace the 10 mM acetate buffer with 50 μL of the same buffer containing 50 μg/mL of the antigen. Leave for 2 min.
5. Replace the contents of the cuvet with 50 μL PBS-Tween.
6. Repeat the process from **step 3** for each of the pH values.

The expected result should be a series of binding profiles for each pH, with different maximal responses. The optimal pH is that which gives the highest profile.

3.1.2. Immobilization

This protocol has three stages: first, activation of the carboxymethyl groups on the dextran hydrogel by EDC-NHS, then immobilization of the protein onto the activated groups, and finally blocking of any remaining activated groups with ethanolamine (*see* **Note 8**).

1. Place a carboxymethylated-dextran cuvet into the machine. You can reuse the surface used for pH optimization. Add 50 μL PBS-Tween and allow to equilibrate for 5–10 min.
2. Add 25 μL NHS to 25 μL EDC and immediately replace the contents of the cuvet with this mixture. Leave for 7 min.
3. Wash the cuvet with 50 μL PBS-Tween and leave for 30 s.
4. Add your ligand at 50 μg/mL in 50 μL 10 mM acetate at the pH determined by the optimization experiment.
5. Leave for 5–15 min (*see* **Note 8**).
6. Wash the cuvet three times with 50 μL PBS-Tween and leave for 30 s.
7. Replace contents with 50 μL 1 M ethanolamine, pH 8.5. Leave for 3 min.
8. Wash three times with PBS-Tween (*see* **Note 9**).

3.2. Determination of the Kinetics of Binding

To determine the kinetics of binding, the ligate is added to the cuvet at a range of concentrations. The highest concentration depends on the affinity of the interaction. We have found, as a general rule of thumb, that for antibody (IgG) as ligate, 20 μg/mL is a good starting concentration (*see* **Note 10** for controls).

1. Regenerate the surface with appropriate regeneration buffer (*see* **Note 4**).
2. Wash the cuvet six times with 50 μL PBS-Tween and allow to equilibrate for 5–10 min.
3. Make up doubling dilutions of the antibody in PBS-Tween using a final volume of 10 μL and a top concentration 10 times greater than that which you intend to start with (i.e., for a starting concentration of 20 μg/mL make up 200 μg/mL).
4. Replace the contents of the cuvet with 45 μL PBS-Tween, and wait until the baseline is flat.

5. Add 5 μL of your starting preparation of the antibody.
6. Leave for 5 min. During this time the association of the antibody and antigen is followed.
7. Wash the surface three times in 50 μL PBS-Tween, leaving the cuvet with 50 μL PBS-Tween in it.
8. Leave for 5 min. During this time the dissociation of the antibody and antigen is followed (*see* **Note 11**).
9. Add regeneration buffer for 2 min (*see* **Note 4**).
10. Wash six times in PBS-Tween.
11. When the baseline has normalized, repeat **steps 5–10** with the next concentration of antibody.
12. Continue the process until you can no longer see a significant response.

3.3. Calculation of Results

The association and dissociation are calculated with the help of software supplied by the manufacturer of the machine (*4*). Because this is updated on a continual basis there is no point in describing in detail how to use it to calculate the association and dissociation. In this section I will indicate the overall strategy in calculating the rate constants and equilibrium constants. It should be remembered, however, that there are several alternative methods to calculate the affinity and rate constants, each of which may have advantages in particular settings. It should also be remembered that the accuracy of your analysis depends on the amount of effort spent on both experimentation and analysis. For highly accurate values to be obtained it is necessary to perform many experiments using different experimental conditions and compare the resulting analyses. However, for simple comparison or order of magnitude type studies, in which the results are reasonably accurate, simpler protocols are sufficient. In many cases highly accurate results are not needed (*see* **Note 12**).

3.3.1. Calculation of Association Rate Constants

1. Select using FASTfit software the baseline regions of the binding curve and the association regions.
2. Select the appropriate equations to fit the curve (either monophasic or biphasic depending on whether you believe there are one or two types of interaction occurring).
3. Fit the data to the equation.
4. This will give a value termed k_{obs} or k_{on} (I prefer the term k_{obs} because it avoids confusion with the association rate constant). Repeat this process for every concentration of ligate used.
5. Plot k_{obs} against the concentration of ligate. The relationship between k_{obs} and k_{ass} is given by:

$$k_{obs} = k_{ass}[L] + k_{diss} \tag{1}$$

Thus, the slope of the curve gives k_{ass}.

3.3.2. Calculation of Dissociation Rate Constant

The dissociation rate constant is calculated directly from the dissociation part of the curve. Although the intercept of the plot used in **Subheading 3.3.1.** can give the k_{diss}, this tends to be an inaccurate approach.

1. Select regions of the curves corresponding the baseline and dissociation curves (this can be done at the same time as fitting the association curves).
2. Select the appropriate equation(s) to fit the dissociation to (*see* **Note 13**).
3. Fit the data to the equations.

3.3.3. Calculation of the Equilibrium Constants

The equilibrium constants are simply given by:

$$K_a = \frac{1}{K_d} = \frac{k_{ass}}{k_{diss}} \qquad (2)$$

4. Notes

1. The experiments can be carried out in any buffer. We tend to use PBS-Tween. However, it should be noted that changes in the buffer cause changes in the optical properties at the surface. This leads to changes in the resonant angle, seen as sudden "bulk shifts" in the response (i.e., instantaneous changes in the response). Although these are often unavoidable, it is a good idea to minimize them during kinetic experiments by ensuring that the ligand is diluted in the same buffer as is being used in the experiment.
2. The acetate buffers are used at 10 mM. However, it is more sensible to make the stock acetate buffers as 100 mM buffers at the appropriate pH and then dilute them in distilled water when needed to make 10 mM acetate buffers.
3. Dissolve separately the EDC (1.15 g) and NHS provided (0.2 g) in 15 mL water each. Aliquot in 100 µL volumes and freeze immediately. These reagents are relatively unstable and they should only be thawed once you are ready to use them. Any unused reagents should be thrown away and not refrozen.
4. The regeneration buffer is used to strip any ligate from the sensing surface, allowing it to be reused for another experiment. The regeneration buffer must be able to remove all the ligate without damaging the covalently coupled ligand. On the whole the cuvet is capable of withstanding any sensible regeneration buffer that you might want to use; it is the immobilized ligand that will be destroyed. For every ligand it is therefore necessary to find a regeneration buffer that works. The simplest way to do this is to repeat cycles of binding-dissociation-regeneration and observe the responses, checking that all the ligate is removed by the buffer and that the same concentration of ligate shows the same binding response on subsequent cycles. It should be noted that when the surface is used for the first time you may see a higher response than on subsequent times, because of ligand that is weakly bound to the surface. However, after one regeneration cycle all the responses should be the same.

A number of regeneration buffers can be tried. 20 m*M* glycine, pH 2.2, is commonly used. More recently we have found that "Gentle Elution" buffer sold by Pierce works for many ligands. When choosing a regeneration buffer consider any features that you know about the ligand that will give you a clue regarding a suitable buffer: Is the molecule unstable in acid/basic conditions? Is there a buffer that you can use during affinity purification of the molecule?

It is important to apply the regeneration buffer to the surface for the minimum time possible to minimize damage to the ligand. Typically regeneration cycles of 2 min are used, followed by extensive washing with PBS-Tween.

5. The temperature alters the optical properties of the surface, and changes in temperature cause changes in the response seen. Therefore, ensure that all buffers are warmed to the same temperature before use, and if the ligate is stored on ice for the experiment, warm the dilutions immediately before adding to the sensing surface.

6. If your ligand is very expensive or difficult to obtain it may be unnecessary to do a pH optimization. You can try immobilizing at pH 4.5 and hope that you get good enough immobilization. However, you run the risk of it not working and having to repeat the immobilization on a fresh surface at a different pH. You should also note that if your ligand is very impure then the pH optimization may be telling you the best pH to immobilize the contaminants—not the ligand!

7. If your ligand is very expensive or difficult to obtain (or is at a very low concentration) then you can try using just 10 μg/mL and immobilizing for longer. The volume could also be reduced to 30 μL.

8. The amount of material that you need to immobilize onto the surface depends on what experiments you want to do. If you are interested in concentration determination, it is important to immobilize as much ligand as possible. On the other hand, for kinetic determination the lower the concentration of ligand (consistent with seeing good binding with the ligate) the better. As a rule of thumb for kinetic experiments you should immobilize <1000 arc s of ligand (for large molecules this may need to be scaled up).

9. The manufacturers recommend regenerating the surface before proceeding. This is the correct thing to do if you are using a ligand regeneration buffer combination that you have used before. However, we recommend that if this is the first time you have immobilized a ligand you should first check that the ligate binds, then regenerate the surface, and then check that the ligate still binds. This allows you to confirm whether any failure to see binding is caused by loss of ligand (or its structure) during immobilization, or whether it is the result of using too harsh regeneration conditions (see **Note 4**).

10. It is important to carry out appropriate controls when using the biosensor. The negative controls would be similar to those used in other assays and in most cases will involve using a control ligate or possibly a control ligand. You should run the controls not only at the start of the experiment, but should also check that repetitive cycles of regeneration have not damaged the ligand, rendering it nonspecifically "sticky," by repeating the controls at the end of a run. It is also

useful to run a positive control at intervals, to check that the response seen is the same throughout the experiment.

11. We have outlined a useful starting point for kinetic experiments. However, this can be modified as needed. For example, it can be useful when obtaining accurate values for the dissociation phase to add high concentrations of the ligate, allow the association to occur for a short time (90 s), and then carry out the dissociation.

12. When designing experiments, remember the effects of avidity. Multivalent binding has a higher functional affinity than univalent binding. Therefore, if you are using a monovalent antigen as the ligand, and a bivalent IgG antibody as the ligate, the affinity will be higher than if the antibody is the immobilized ligand and the antigen the ligate. In addition, the increase in functional affinity caused by multivalent binding will depend on such parameters as the concentration of immobilized ligand.

13. The k_{diss} can be calculated using equations that either extrapolate the dissociation to baseline (i.e., assume that eventually all the ligate will dissociate from the ligand) or else produce the best fit, making no assumptions regarding the amount of dissociation seen. The first type of fitting is clearly what should theoretically occur, and we have tended to find that this type of equation gives the most useful data. However, because some of the ligate can be trapped within the hydrogel (especially at high-ligand concentrations), this can cause inaccuracies.

References

1. George, A. J. T., Rashid, M., and Gallop, J. L. (1997) Kinetics of biomolecular interactions. *Expert Opin. Ther. Patents* **7,** 947–963.
2. Buckle, P. E., Davies, R. J., Kinning, T., Yeung, D., Edwards, P. R., Pollard-Knight, D., and Lowe, C. R. (1993) The resonant mirror: a novel optical biosensor for direct sensing of biomolecular interactions part II: applications. *Biosensors Biolectr.* **8,** 355–368.
3. Cush, R., Cronin, J. M., Stewart, W. J., Maule, C. H., Molloy, J., and Goddard, N. J. (1993) The resonant mirror: a novel optical biosensor for direct sensing of biomolecular interactions part I: principles of operation and associated instrumentation. *Biosensors Biolectr.* **8,** 347–353.
4. George, A. J. T., French, R. R., and Glennie, M. J. (1995) Measurement of kinetic binding constants of a panel of anti-saporin antibodies using a resonant mirror biosensor. *J. Immunol. Methods* **183,** 51–63.

VI

APPLICATION OF ANTIBODIES IN VITRO

30

How to Set Up an ELISA

Bill Jordan

1. Introduction

The enzyme-linked immunosorbent assay (ELISA) represents a simple and sensitive technique for specific quantitative detection of molecules to which an antibody is available *(1,2)*. Although there are a huge number of variations based on the original ELISA principle, this chapter will focus on the two perhaps most useful and routinely performed: the indirect sandwich ELISA, providing high sensitivity and specificity; and the basic direct ELISA, useful when only one antibody to the sample antigen is available.

During the indirect sandwich ELISA (**Fig. 1A**), an antibody specific for the substance to be measured is first coated onto a high capacity protein-binding microtiter plate. Any vacant binding sites on the plate are then blocked with the use of an irrelevant protein, such as fetal calf serum (FCS) or bovine serum albumin (BSA). The samples, standards, and controls are then incubated on the plate, binding to the capture antibody. The bound sample can be detected using a secondary antibody recognizing a different epitope on the sample molecule, thus creating the "sandwich." The detection antibody is commonly directly conjugated to biotin, allowing an amplification procedure to be carried out with the use of streptavidin bound to the enzyme horse-radish peroxidase (HRP). Because streptavidin is a tetrameric protein, binding four biotin molecules, the threshold of detection is greatly enhanced. The addition of a suitable substrate, such as 3,3',5,5;-tetramethylbenzidine (TMB), allows a colormetric reaction to occur in the presence of the HRP that can be read on a spectrophotometer, with the resulting optical density (OD) relating directly to the amount of antigen present within the sample.

In some cases, however, only one specific antibody may be available, and in such a small quantity that directly conjugating it to biotin would be impracti-

From: *Methods in Molecular Medicine, Vol. 40: Diagnostic and Therapeutic Antibodies*
Edited by: A. J. T. George and C. E. Urch © Humana Press Inc., Totowa, NJ

A

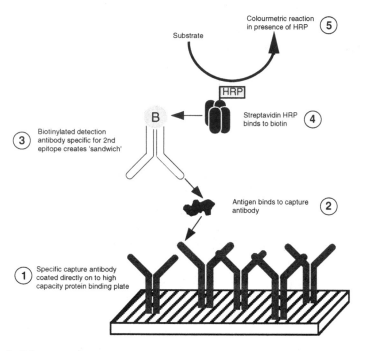

Fig. 1. Diagramatic representation of **(A)** the indirect sandwich ELISA, and **(B)** *[facing page]* the basic direct ELISA.

cal. In this situation a direct ELISA should be used. During the direct ELISA the sample itself is coated directly onto the microtiter plate and is then detected using the specific antibody. If this antibody is biotinylated, the procedure can proceed as in the indirect ELISA; if not, then a secondary biotinylated antibody directed against the species of the detecting antibody itself can be used. **Figure 1B** demonstrates this technique.

To set up a reliable and durable ELISA it is essential to first optimize a number of the parameters mentioned above. The level of optimization will, of course, depend on exactly what is required from the assay. In some cases a simple "yes or no" answer is desired and a simple standard procedure may be sufficient. If, however, high sensitivity is the aim with accurate quantatation of the molecule in question, then carefully setting up the optimal conditions in advance will pay dividends and save a great deal of time in the long term.

B

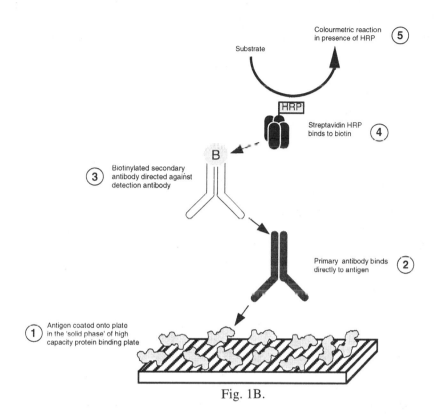

Fig. 1B.

2. Materials

1. Antibodies: For the indirect ELISA, antibody pairs can often be bought commercially and consist of a capture antibody and a biotinylated detection antibody. Both antibodies are specific for the molecule in question, with the detection antibody being directly biotinylated and able to recognize the sample molecule when it is bound to the capture antibody on the plate. For the direct ELISA, one specific detection antibody is required, preferably biotinylated, but if not a secondary biotinylated antibody specific for the detection antibody is also needed. Aliquot and freeze at $-20°C$ or lower in small, usable quantities with a carrier protein, at such as 10% FCS or 1% BSA (*see* **Note 1**).

2. Blocking buffer: Phosphate-buffered saline (PBS), pH 7.4, supplemented with either 1% fatty-acid-free BSA or filtered 10% FCS. If measuring in tissue culture samples, use protein representing that within the culture conditions, i.e., 10% FCS; in effect the sample will have been preabsorbed with this protein during culture and thus any nonspecific binding to the blocking buffer is avoided.

3. Carbonate coating buffer: 8.41g Na_2HCO_3 in 1 L freshly made PBS. Dissolve and adjust to desired pH with HCl or NaOH. Store for no more than 1 mo at 4°C (*see* **Note 2**).

4. High-capacity protein-binding 96-well microtiter plates: There are a large number of suitable makes including Maxisorp (Nunc, Roskilde, Denmark), Immunoware (Pierce, Chester, UK), Immunlon II (Dynex, Middlesex, UK), and Costar (*see* **Note 3**).

5. PBS/Tween/10% FCS: Add 0.05 mL Tween 20 to 90 mL PBS, pH 7.4, and 10 mL filtered FCS. Make up fresh as required.

6. Plate sealers or plastic wrap.

7. Plate-washing apparatus: Adequate washing is a vital element of achieving a successful ELISA. Although a number of automatic plate washers are available, they are expensive and the use of a wash bottle with good pressure is perfectly suitable, though a little more time consuming.

8. Samples/standards: Standards of known amounts are required for positive controls, and for estimation of levels within samples (via comparison to a titration of known amounts). All standards should be diluted in medium as near as, or identical to, that of the sample solution. Standards are best obtained from a reliable commercial source that has already mass calibrated them and should be frozen in small, concentrated aliquots at –20°C or lower. Repeated freeze–thaw cycles must be avoided.

9. Spectrophotometer: Any suitable microplate reader able to measure absorbance at the appropriate wavelength.

10. Stop solution: 0.5 *M* H_2SO_4.

11. Streptavidin HRP: Use in accordance with the manufacturer's instructions. Sources of TMB include Sigma (St. Louis, MO), Pierce, and Zymed.

12. Substrate: One-step TMB (Zymed). Although many other substrates are available for HRP, TMB has high sensitivity with a quick development time. OD can be monitored at 650 nm while the color develops, then at 450 nm when the reaction is stopped with H_2SO_4. TMB may also be obtained in a lyophilized state and made up fresh with hydrogen peroxidase, however, the pre-prepared solution is quick, easy, and, more importantly, extremely consistent (*see* **Note 4**).

13. Washing buffer: Add 0.5 mL Tween-20 to 1 L PBS, pH 7.4. Make up fresh as required.

3. Methods

3.1. Basic Sandwich ELISA Protocol

1. Dilute the capture antibody to 1 µg/mL in coating buffer, pH 9.5. Add 100 µL to each well of a high-capacity protein-binding 96-well microtiter plate.

2. Seal the plate to avoid evaporation and incubate overnight (12–18 h) at 2–8°C.

3. Wash plate: Discard unbound antibody by inverting and flicking the plate over a sink. Fill each well with 300 µL washing buffer and leave for at least 10 s before discarding once more. Ensure all liquid has been removed between each wash by repeatedly tapping the plate onto clean paper towels. Repeat three times.

4. Add 200 µL blocking buffer to each well. Seal the plate and incubate for at least 2 h at room temperature.
5. Discard blocking buffer. Wash the plate three times as in **step 3**.
6. Prepare a titration series of known standards (for example, in 1.5 mL Eppendorf tubes) diluted in a matrix representing that of the samples (e.g., culture medium or human serum). Include a negative control (i.e., culture medium only). Transfer samples and antigen standards to the ELISA plate in duplicate at 100 µL per well. Seal the plate and incubate at room temperature for at least 2 h, or overnight at 4°C for increased sensitivity.
7. Wash plate three times as in **step 3**.
8. Dilute biotinylated detection antibody to 1 µg/mL in PBS, pH 7.4. Add 50 µL per well. Incubate at room temperature for 2 h. If problems with nonspecific binding of the biotinylated antibody to the plate occur, dilute the antibody in PBS/Tween/10% FCS rather than just PBS (*see* **Note 5**).
9. Wash plate three times as in **step 3**.
10. Dilute streptavidin HRP according to the manufacturer's instructions. Add 100 µL/well. Incubate at room temperature for 30 min.
11. Wash plate four times as in **step 3**.
12. Add 100 µL/well of "one step" TMB. Allow color to develop for 10–60 min (20 min is usually sufficient). OD may be monitored at this stage at 630 nm as the color develops (*see* **Note 6**).
13. Add 100 µL 0.5 M H_2SO_4 to each well to stop the reaction. Read OD at 450 nm.
14. Estimate the amount of antigen within the samples by comparing ODs to those of known standards.

3.2. Direct ELISA Protocol

1. Make serial dilutions of samples from neat to 1:16 in coating buffer, pH 9.5. Add 100 µL to each well of a high-capacity protein-binding microtiter plate. Also set up wells with antigen standards and a negative control diluted in the same coating buffer.
2. Seal the plate with an acetate plate sealer or cling film wrap to avoid evaporation and incubate overnight (12–18 h) at 2–8°C.
3. Wash plate: Discard unbound antibody by inverting and flicking the plate over a sink. Fill each well with 300 µL washing buffer, leave for at least 10 s, and discard once more. Ensure all liquid has been removed between each wash by repeatedly tapping the plate onto clean paper towels. Repeat three times.
4. Add 200 µL blocking buffer to each well. Seal the plate and incubate for at least 2 h at room temperature.
5. Discard blocking buffer. Wash plate three times as in **step 3**.
6. Dilute detection antibody to 2 µg/mL in PBS. Add 50 µL/well. Incubate at room temperature for 2 h. If the antibody is biotinylated proceed to **step 9**.
7. Wash plate three times as in **step 3**.
8. Add secondary antibody (100 µL, 2 µg/µL) specific for the detection antibody (i.e., if the detection antibody is mouse, use biotinylated rabbit antimouse Ig) (*see* **Note 5**).

9. Wash plate three times as in **step 3**.
10. Dilute streptavidin HRP according to the manufacturer's instructions. Add 100 μL/well. Incubate at room temperature for 30 min.
11. Wash plate four times as in **step 3**.
12. Add 100 μL per well of "one step" TMB. Allow color to develop for 10–60 min (20 min is usually sufficient). OD may be monitored at this stage at 650 nm as the color develops.
13. Add 100 μL 0.5 M H_2SO_4 to each well to stop the reaction. Read OD at 450 nm.
14. Estimate amount of antigen within samples by comparing ODs to those of known standards of sample.

3.3. Optimization of ELISA

At this stage the ELISA may be more than adequate, although optimization of the following parameters is usually required (*see* **Note 7**):

1. pH of carbonate coating buffer (pH 7.0–10.0). Also try PBS at pH 7.4.
2. Concentration of capture antibody (0.5–10.0 μg/mL).
3. Concentration of secondary antibody (indirect ELISA, 0.5–4.0 μg/mL).
4. Concentration of biotinylated detection antibody (0.1–2.0 μg/mL).
5. Concentration of streptavidin-HRP conjugate (usually between 1:1000 and 1:10,000).

4. Notes

1. The quality of the antibodies used is perhaps the most important aspect in setting up a good ELISA. Antibodies need to have a high affinity for the sample to be measured, reducing the chance of being "washed off" during the assay. The indirect ELISA relies on two specific antibodies and thus the increased specificity increases sensitivity of the assay by reducing background.
2. The pH of the coating buffer can have a huge effect on the amount of antibody that will bind to the plate and thus to the ELISA as a whole. Basically, a higher pH will result in more antibody binding but may have a detremental effect on its immunoreactivity. Thus, a pH must be found that is suitable for the antibody in question; this can vary dramatically. When beginning optimization of the assay, test a range of carbonate buffers from pH 7.0 to 10.0 as well as PBS, pH 7.4. We usually find a carbonate buffer pH of 9.5 gives good results. In some cases we have found commercially available coating antibodies recommended by the manufacturer to be adsorbed onto the plate at pH 7.4 to be far more effective at higher pHs, improving the lower detection limit of sensitivity by up to 1000%, and thus allowing the coating concentration to be vastly reduced and creating an extremely cost-effective assay.
3. There can be a significant difference in the protein binding capabilities of different makes, and even batches of microtiter plates. Some appear to be extremely good for binding antibodies, whereas others more useful for other proteins. The only real way to choose a suitable plate is by trial and error, or using a recommended make known to be good for the protein you intend to coat.

4. Although the HRP/TMB system represents a good, reliable, and sensitive combination, HRP has a number of alternative substrates that can be used, such as *o*-phenylene diamine (OPD). Enzymes other than HRP can also be used, such as alkaline phosphatase (AP), which can be used in combination with the substrate *p*-nitrophenyl phosphate (p-NPP). The choice of enzyme–substrate system depends on a number of factors, including price, sensitivity, and whether a filter is available for the substrate-specific wavelength to be measured.

5. The use of biotinylated secondary antibodies (or detection antibody in the indirect sandwich ELISA) in conjunction with enzyme-conjugated streptavidin (or avidin, extravidin, and so forth) both increases sensitivity and saves time in that a further step is eliminated from the assay and therefore another step of optimization is not required.

6. If the major aim of the ELISA is to obtain quantitation of substances present in extremely low concentrations, a number of adaptations to the technique can be used. Such techniques often use alkaline phosphatase enzyme systems that can be used, for example, to lock into a circular redox cycle, producing an end product, such as red formazan, that is hugely amplified in comparison to standard amplification methods *(3)*. Chemiluminescent amplified ELISA principles have also been shown to give very high sensitivity *(4)* and can be optimized to measure as little as 1 zeptomole (about 350 molecules!) of alkaline phosphatase *(5)*. Although extremely sensitive, such techniques are extremely time-consuming to set up and optimize, and are far more expensive than the simple colormetric ELISAs described in this chapter.

7. In some cases, molecules present in a sample are masked by the solution they are in. This problem can sometimes be solved by diluting the samples in PBS/Tween/ 10% FCS. If this is performed, remember to make similar adjustments to the solution used for the standards. Possible interference molecules within samples, such as soluble receptors for the antigen, can also cause a problem. Commercially available matched antibody pairs for molecules should have been pretested and guaranteed against being affected by such problems.

References

1. Kemeny, D. M. and Challacombe, S. J. (1988) *ELISA and Other Solid Phase Imunoassays. Theory and Practical Aspects,* Wiley, Chichester, UK.
2. Kemeny, D. M. (1991) *A Practical Guide to ELISA*. Permagon, Oxford, UK.
3. Self, C. H. (1985) Enzyme amplification—a general method applied to provide an immunoassisted assay for placental alkaline phosphatase. *J. Immunol. Methods* **76,** 389–393.
4. Bronstein, I., et al. (1993) Chemiluminescent assay of alkaline phosphatase applied in an ultrasensitive enzyme immunoassay of thyrotropin. *Clin. Chem.* **35,** 1441–1446.
5. Cook, D. B. and Self, C. H. (1993) Determination of one-thousandth of an attomole (1 zeptomole) of alkaline phosphatase: application in an immunoassay of proinsulin. *Clin. Chem.* **39,** 965–971.

31

Measurement of HAMA
and Anti-Idiotypic Antibodies

Steve Nicholson

1. Introduction

Murine monoclonal antibodies (mAbs) when administered to patients are perceived much as any other foreign antigen: an immune response is usually mounted against them, the result of which is the generation of human antimouse antibodies (HAMA). Even in the absence of such immunization some patients may possess HAMA activity because of polyclonal IgM rheumatoid factors that crossreact with Fc epitopes on both human and mouse IgG (1).

If mAbs are administered for diagnostic purposes the resulting HAMA is an undesirable byproduct. The investigation may not be repeatable and immunoassay results may be spuriously elevated as a result of the crosslinking of "catcher" and "tracer" antibodies in the absence of the antigen being assayed (2,3).

Where mAbs are administered for therapeutic purposes, HAMA may be a mixed blessing. The use of mAbs as a targeted delivery system, e.g., in the radioimmunotherapy of B-cell non-Hodgkin's lymphoma (4), may be restricted by the sequestration of the therapeutic mAb in the circulation caused by HAMA binding. Where the mAb is itself the therapeutic agent, in so-called idiotypic/anti-idiotypic vaccination schedules (5), the generation of HAMA is both an indication of antigenicity and part of the goal. HAMA generated in these regimens remains principally anti-Fc; this can be used as a measurement of successful vaccination. The more specific anti-idiotypic (Ab2) component, although slightly harder to quantify, may be a more rewarding subject for study.

From: *Methods in Molecular Medicine, Vol. 40: Diagnostic and Therapeutic Antibodies*
Edited by: A. J. T. George and C. E. Urch © Humana Press Inc., Totowa, NJ

2. Materials

Phosphate-buffered saline/0.05% Tween 20 is used as wash buffer throughout unless otherwise stated. Blocking buffer is wash buffer + 1% bovine serum albumin unless otherwise stated.

2.1. Measuring HAMA

1. Wash buffer and blocking buffer.
2. Immunizing mAb or mouse IgG.
3. Enzyme-labeled antihuman immunoglobulins or any enzyme-labeled mouse immunoglobulin (*see* **Note 1**).
4. Chromogenic substrate (*see* **Note 1**).
5. "HAMA ELISA" (medac, Hamburg, Germany).
6. "ImmuSTRIP HAMA IgG" (Immunomedics, Morris Plains, NJ).

2.2. Eliminating HAMA Interference in Immunoassays

1. Mouse serum.
2. Murine IgG.
3. Immunoglobulin Inhibiting Reagent® (IIR) (Bioreclamation Inc., East Meadow, NY).

2.3. Measuring Anti-Idiotypic Antibodies

1. Wash buffer and blocking buffer.
2. Administered mAb and isotype-matched control mAb.
3. "Labcoat" carbohydrate-binding ELISA plates (Costar, Cambridge, MA).
4. Fetal bovine serum.
5. Secondary antibody: enzyme-conjugated antihuman Ig (*see* **Note 1**).
6. Chromogenic substrate (*see* **Note 1**).

2.4. IAsys™

1. Carboxymethyl dextran IAsys cuvets (Affinity Sensors, Cambridge, UK).
2. Administered mAb.
3. Wash buffer.
4. 10 mM sodium acetate, pH 5.0.
5. 1 M ethanolamine hydrochloride, pH 8.5.
6. Gentle elution buffer (Pierce Warriner, Rockford, IL).

3. Methods

3.1. Measuring HAMA

Refer to Chapter 30 for further information.

3.1.1. General Protocol

The choice of coating antibody will depend on availability and whether the investigator is interested in measuring combined HAMA and anti-idiotypic antibodies or HAMA alone: the immunizing antibody should be used for the former whereas any mouse immunoglobulin (or mixture thereof) should suffice for measuring HAMA alone.

1. Coat all wells of a 96-flat well microtiter plate with murine IgG diluted in wash buffer. A concentration of 2 ng/100 µL/well should be sufficient. Incubate for at least 1 h at room temperature.
2. Wash plate and block with blocking buffer for at least 1 h at room temperature. Wash plate repeatedly.
3. Prepare serial dilutions of serum samples in wash buffer. Reference serum, if available, should be similarly diluted.
4. Add duplicates of sample dilutions and standards to wells. Incubate for 1 h at room temperature. Aspirate all wells (*see* **Note 2**) and wash three times.
5. Add "tracer," which may be either enzyme-labeled antihuman or any labeled mouse immunoglobulin. This step may be coincubated with **step 4**, particularly if using nonspecific labeled mouse immunoglobulin as tracer. Incubate for 30–45 min. Aspirate all wells and wash at least three times.
6. Add chromogenic substrate and measure signal.

3.1.2. HAMA ELISA and Immustrip HAMA IgG

The HAMA ELISA (medac) and Immunstrip HAMA IgG (Immunomedics) are one-step enzyme immunoassays that measure HAMA quantitatively, standardized against antimouse IgG. Results are expressed as HAMA in ng/mL. The microtiter plate or strip is supplied precoated with mouse IgG, the tracer is HRPO-conjugated mouse IgG, and the substrate is tetramethylbenzidine (TMB) for the medac kit or *o*-phenylenediamine (OPD) for the Immunomedics kit.

1. Dilute serum samples in wash buffer.
2. Add samples and standards to duplicate wells of the preblocked assay plates (100 µL/well) together with 100 µL/well of the HRPO/mouse IgG tracer.
3. Incubate the plate at 37°C for 30 min.
4. Aspirate all wells and wash four times with wash buffer.
5. Add chromogenic substrate to each well.
6. Incubate the plate for 15 min at room temperature.
7. Stop the reaction by the addition of 100 µL/well of 0.5 M H_2SO_4.
8. Read absorbance at 450 nm. The curve is linear in the range 1–160 ng/mL for the medac assay, whereas the Immunomedic assay measures HAMA equivalents up to 220 ng/mL. I have found that further dilution of serum samples is often required for samples that are strongly positive for HAMA.

See **Subheading 3.4.** for measuring HAMA using IAsys™.

3.2. Methods for Eliminating HAMA Interference in Immunoassays

3.2.1. Small-Scale and Noncommercial Methods

These approaches are most useful when preliminary immunoassays have raised the possibility of HAMA being present, but the assay itself is not optimized, or when the serum sample is routinely assayed after dilution.

1. Prepare dilution buffer:
   a. Wash buffer containing 1–10% mouse serum.
   b. Wash buffer containing 10–1000 μg/mL mouse IgG. Ideally this should be of the same isotype as the mAb to which the patient has been exposed (*see* **Note 3**).
2. Prepare the sample over a range of dilutions using dilution buffer. Incubate for 1 h at room temperature.
3. Proceed with immunoassay as usual.

Results from a preliminary experiment along these lines will allow the investigator to choose an appropriate buffer and sample dilution. An example of such an optimizing experiment is shown in **Fig. 1**.

3.2.2. Immunoglobulin Inhibiting Reagent

This commercially available reagent (Bioreclamation Inc., New York) is especially useful when batched immunoassays are being performed using an automated or semiautomated procedure. IIR, a mixture of multiple isotypes from a variety of species, is supplied lyophilized in Eppendorf tubes.

1. Add up to 500 μL of serum to tubes.
2. Invert the tube to mix and incubate at room temperature for at least 1 h.

The assay (or assays) is then run as usual. We have validated IIR in eliminating HAMA interference in the Roche Cobbas Core second-generation CA125 assay, which is run in an automated process at the tumor marker laboratory in the department of medical oncology, Charing Cross Hospital (*6*). We found no perturbation in HAMA-free samples or standards. Spurious elevations were corrected as efficiently as can be achieved by adding mouse serum, but without the need for volume adjustment calculations (*see* **Note 4**).

3.3. Measuring Anti-Idiotypic Antibodies

The aim here is to measure the anti-idiotypic element of a polyclonal HAMA response without the confounding effect of the anti-Fc component drowning the much smaller Ab2 signal. The first protocol has been used by numerous investigators (*7,8*) with a variety of modifications to suit their reagents. The second protocol is my preferred system. Both methods outlined below have

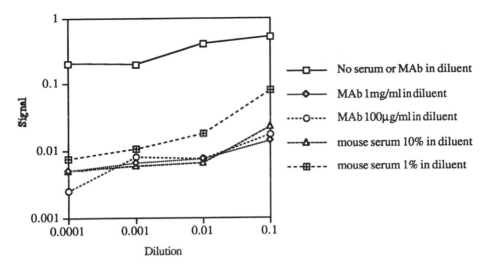

Fig. 1. Serum from a patient who had completed an idiotypic vaccination regimen with the murine IgG1 HMFG1. Serial dilutions of serum were assayed in ELISA against a microtiter plate coated with murine IgG. This experiment shows that at a 1:100 dilution, diluent containing 10% mouse serum, MAb 1 mg/mL, or 100 μg/mL are equally successful at absorbing HAMA, whereas diluent containing 1% mouse serum is inadequate. This patient had a grossly elevated result on the CA125 tumor marker immunoassay in the absence of any evidence of recurrent tumor as a result of HAMA interfering with the assay.

been applied to the measurement of Ab2 generated in the clinical trial setting. The choice will depend on the investigator's access to relevant antibodies and microtiter plates. Both protocols will benefit from a purified, quantitated positive control. The third protocol may be applicable in some settings and is mentioned for completeness.

3.3.1. Assay Using the Immunizing Antibody as Both "Catcher" and "Tracer"

The precise methodology will vary depending on the availability of labeling procedures or humanized versions of the immunizing mAb. Some variants and modifications are included, but investigators will need to adapt the protocol to their own needs.

1. Coat the wells of a microtiter plate with "catcher" mAb (*see* **Note 5**) in the range 1 ng–1 μg/well in 50–100 μL wash buffer. Allow to incubate for at least 1 h at room temperature, or overnight at 4°C. Individual polystyrene tubes may be preferred if a radioimmunoassay is intended.

2. Aspirate wells and wash repeatedly. Block with blocking buffer for at least 1 h at room temperature.

3. Dilute serum sample in buffer containing mouse serum or immunoglobulin to absorb non-Ab2 HAMA (*see* **Subheading 3.2.1.**) and incubate for 1 h at room temperature (*see* **Note 6**).

4. The "tracer" may be added concurrently with the sample or after a further incubation and series of washes. "Tracer" is most often the immunizing mAb that has been labeled with ^{125}I for radioimmunoassay (*see* Chapter 27) enzyme (peroxidase, alkaline phosphatase), or biotin for ELISA (Chapter 30). Alternatively, labeled antihuman immunoglobulin or antihuman isotype antibodies may be used, in which case these should ideally be from a species other than mice. The optimal dilution of "tracer" will vary from protocol to protocol.

5. Incubate for 45 min at room temperature, aspirate wells, and wash repeatedly.

6. Add chromogenic substrate for ELISA and read in a spectrophotometer or divide the plate into single wells and count for RIA.

3.3.2. Assay Using Site-Orientated Binding of the Immunizing Antibody

This method uses the "Labcoat" carbohydrate-binding plate manufactured by Costar. The carbohydrate moieties on the mAb Fc region are oxidized by reaction with sodium periodate to form dialdehydes, which form covalent bonds with the hydrazide coating on the ELISA plate. The aim is to immobilize mAb on the ELISA plate in a less random manner than occurs with passive adsorption of proteins onto plastic. The antigen-binding site is thus presented for interaction with its anti-idiotype, whereas the Fc region is relatively less accessible, reducing signal caused by non-Ab2 HAMA (*see* **Note 7**).

1. Dilute immunizing mAb and isotype-matched control mAb to 1 mg/mL in distilled water.

2. To 2 mL mAb samples add 3.2 mL 15 m*M* sodium periodate in 0.1 *M* sodium acetate buffer, pH 5.5. Stir for 30 min at room temperature.

3. Add 200 μL 1:100 ethylene glycol in water to stop the reaction.

4. Buffer-exchange the mAb samples into 0.1 *M* sodium acetate buffer, pH 5.5, diluted to 1–10 μg/mL (*see* **Note 8**).

5. Add samples to alternate halves of a "Labcoat" plate, 100 μL/well. Incubate for 1 h at room temperature.

6. Aspirate away sample and wash all wells three times with wash buffer.

7. Add blocking buffer to all wells and incubate for at least 30 min.

8. Dilute all serum samples in dilution buffer (*see* **Subheading 3.2.1.**) containing 10% FBS (*see* **Note 9**). A typical protocol will use 1:100 dilution in buffer containing 100 μg/mL of isotype-matched mouse mAb. Incubate for 1 h at room temperature.

9. Aspirate blocking buffer. Do not wash wells.

10. Add serum samples to duplicate wells coated with immunizing mAb and duplicate wells coated with control mAb. Incubate for 1 h at room temperature.
11. Aspirate individual wells (*see* **Note 2**) and wash four times.
12. Add "tracer" secondary antibody. Include 10% FBS in diluent (*see* **Note 8**). Incubate for 45 min. Wash at least four times.
13. Add chromogenic substrate and read absorbance on the spectrophotometer.

This assay allows one to measure the success with which HAMA has been excluded from the final signal, giving anti-isotype binding as a background signal for each sample (*see* **Note 10**).

3.3.3. Measuring Anti-Idiotypic Antibodies Using FACS

McIntyre and Higgins described this interesting assay *(9)*, which hinges on the observation that OKT3 binding to CD3 is inhibited only by IgG anti-idiotypic antibodies. The ability of patients' serum, neat and in dilution, to inhibit the binding of OKT3, to a CD3-expressing cell line (Jurkat) is measured by mixing serum samples with FITC-conjugated OKT3, then adding the cell line and measuring fluorescence. The major advantage of this system is its rapidity (about 45 min). Full details of FACS protocols are given in Chapter 33.

1. Prepare dilution of serum samples. Add 20 μL of each sample dilution to Falcon 2052 tubes. The Ab2-negative control will consist of diluent alone.
2. Add 20 μL FITC-labeled immunizing antibody (OKT3) diluted in PBS + 0.1% bovine serum albumin + 0.1% sodium azide. Incubate for 10 min at 4°C.
3. Prepare cell line (Jurkat). Harvest cells and wash/resuspend three times in PBS + 0.1% bovine serum albumin + 0.1% sodium azide. Add 50 μL cells at a concentration of 10^7/mL. Incubate for 10 min at 4°C.
4. Wash/resuspend cells three times and analyze for fluorescence intensity.

See **Subheading 3.4.** for measuring anti-idiotypic antibodies using IAsys.

3.4. Using the IAsys Resonant Mirror Biosensor to Measure HAMA and Anti-Idiotypic Antibodies

The IAsys resonant mirror biosensor measures antigen–antibody binding in a nonisotopic, nonenzymatic system where the interaction between fixed antigen and antibody in the sample causes changes in the refractive index at the detection surface. Resonance changes are detected using polarized laser light, which is reflected back to a detector/transducer. This system enables the kinetics of antigen–antibody interactions to be studied in real time. The system is discussed in greater detail in Chapter 29.

The resonant mirror biosensor has been used to study HAMA and the anti-idiotypic antibody response in serum samples from patients with epithelial ovarian cancer who received the murine IgG1 monoclonal antibody HMFG1 (anti-MUC1) in a phase I clinical trial *(10)*. Changes in both quantity and affinity can be measured; to measure absolute levels reference standards are required, but to demonstrate maturation of the Ab2 response, e.g., in idiotypic vaccination protocols, relative changes compared to pretreatment levels may be sufficient.

The key parameters for these purposes are the initial slope of the association curve, which depends on quantity of HAMA or Ab2 in the sample, and the dissociation rate constant "k_{off}" which is inversely proportional to affinity *(11,12)*.

1. Dilute administered antibody to a concentration of 50 µg/mL in 10 mM sodium acetate, pH 5.0 (*see* **Note 11**).
2. Add 200 µL to an IAsys cuvet (Affinity Sensors) whose carboxymethyl dextran surface has been activated. Incubate for 10 min.
3. Wash the binding surface three times then block remaining binding sites with 1 M ethanolamine hydrochloride, pH 8.5, for 2 min. Wash three times.
4. Dilute samples 1:20 in wash buffer (to measure HAMA) or HAMA-elimination buffer (**Subheading 3.2.1.**) if measuring Ab2 (isotype-matched mouse IgG).
5. Allow the machine readout to achieve a flat baseline, aspirate, and add diluted sample. Follow the association curve (5 min is usually sufficient).
6. Wash twice rapidly. Follow dissociation curve (5 min is usually sufficient).
7. Regenerate the surface with 200 µL of gentle elution buffer for 2 min. Perform three rapid washes and allow the readout to return to flat baseline. Proceed to the next sample.

Figure 2 shows an IAsys experiment demonstrating both affinity maturation and increasing quantity of anti-idiotypic antibodies in one patient as she progresses through an idiotypic vaccination regimen.

4. Notes

1. Horseradish peroxidase-conjugated tracer antibody should be used with *o*-phenylenediamine as the chromogenic substrate and read at an absorbance of 450 nm. Alkaline phosphatase-conjugated tracer should be used with *p*-dinitrophenyl phosphate as the substrate and the color reaction is read at 405 nm.
2. Aspirating samples from individual wells is time-consuming and tedious, but the results speak for themselves. There is much less risk of crosscontamination between wells. It is often best to add the first wash well-by-well and aspirate this also. Subsequent washes can use the "rinse and flick" method. Do not immerse the plate in a sandwich box filled with wash buffer—you are asking for a high background.
3. It should be remembered that if the administered antibody is used this will absorb anti-idiotypic atibodies as well as HAMA—not wise if you are planning to mea-

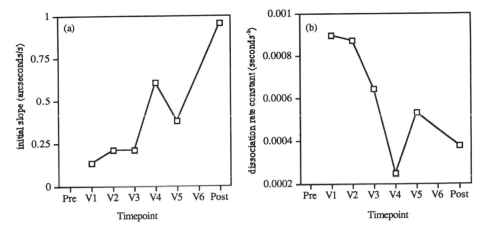

Fig. 2. Anti-idiotypic antibody results for a single patient analyzed by IAsys™ resonant mirror biosensor. An ovarian cancer patient underwent idiotypic vaccination with the murine MAb HMFG1. An initial dose was given on commencement ("Pre") followed by six intradermal booster doses (V1–V6) given at monthly intervals. Serum was also collected 1 mo after completion of the regimen ("Post"). Pretreatment serum showed an erratic and uninterpretable initial slope with a dissociation rate constant too high to be measured accurately. As the patient progressed through the vaccination protocol the quantity of anti-idiotypic antibody rises (**a**), but its mean dissociation rate constant falls (**b**), indicating affinity maturation.

    sure the former after treating your sample. Similarly, if the blocking antibody used is either the "catcher" or the "tracer" from your immunoassay the antigen of interest will be bound at the blocking stage rather than in the assay.

4. A similar reagent, Scantibodies Laboratory HBT (Heterophilic Blocking Tube), is available from Bionostics Limited, Bedfordshire, UK; I have no experience of this particular product.

5. If in possession of a humanized or chimeric version of the immunizing murine mAb, this should be used, in preference, as the "catcher" (*13*).

6. Where humanized or chimeric antibody is the "catcher" it may prove possible to dilute in wash buffer alone without compromising the result.

7. Plates coated with Protein A and Protein G are also commercially available and the same protocol may be modified to use these to immobilize mAbs via their Fc region. Normal ELISA plates may suffice for qualitative purposes and have been used in similar protocols.

8. Traditionally, buffer should be exchanged by dialyzing against 0.1 *M* sodium acetate buffer, pH 5.5. I prefer to use Centricon centrifuge concentrator tubes, concentrating then rediluting my mAb sample twice in buffer.

9. This is the recommendation of the manufacturer to reduce background signal. If using 10% mouse serum as the HAMA-eliminating buffer the addition of further

serum should be unnecessary. I have had excellent results using dilution buffer containing 100 μg/mL isotype-matched mAb with no FBS, but allowing the plate to block for longer (2–4 h) in **step 7**.

10. Where an individual serum sample still shows a high anti-isotype signal the concentration of the blocking buffer may need increasing. Consider also the possibility that the patient may have genuine Ab2 against that antibody; an alternative isotype-matched control may correct for this.

11. Binding conditions may vary between pH 4.0 and 5.0.

References

1. Courtenay-Luck, N., Epenetos, A. A., Winearls, C. G., and Ritter, M. A. (1987) Preexisting human anti-murine immunoglobulin reactivity due to polyclonal rheumatoid factors. *Cancer Res.* **47,** 4520–4525.

2. Boscato, L. and Stuart, M. (1988) Heterophilic antibodies: a problem for all immunoassays. *Clin. Chem.* **34,** 27–33.

3. Boerman, O., Segers, M. F., Poels, L. G., et al. (1990) Heterophilic antibodies in human sera causing falsely increased results in the CA125 immunofluorometric assay. *Clin. Chem.* **36,** 888–891.

4. Kaminski, M. S., Zasadny, K. R., Francis, J. R., et al. (1996) Iodine-131-anti-B1 radioimmunotherapy for B-cell lymphoma. *J. Clin. Oncol.* **14,** 1974–1981.

5. Herlyn, D., Wettendorff, M., Schmoll, E., et al. (1987) Anti-idiotype immunization of cancer patients: modulation of the immune response. *Proc. Nat. Acad. Sci. USA* **84,** 8055–8059.

6. Nicholson, S., Fox, M., Epenetos, A., and Rustin, G. (1996) Immunoglobulin inhibiting reagent: evaluation of a new method for eliminating spurious elevations in CA125 caused by HAMA. *Int. J. Biol. Markers* **11,** 46–49.

7. Cheung, N.-K., et al. (1994) Antibody response to murine anti-GD2 monoclonal antibodies: correlation with patient survival. *Cancer Res.* **54,** 2228–2233.

8. Tibben, J., Thomas, C. M., Massuger, L. F., et al. (1995) Humoral anti-OV-TL-3 response after the intravenous administration of radiolabelled Fab′ or F(ab′)$_2$ fragments in ovarian cancer patients. *Nucl. Med. Commun.* **16,** 853–859.

9. McIntyre, J. and Higgins, N. (1995) A novel and rapid assay to detect anti-idiotypic anti-OKT3 antibodies. *Transplantation* **59,** 1507–1508.

10. Nicholson, S., Gallop, J. L., Law, P., et al. (1999) Monitoring antibody responses to cancer vaccination with a resonant mirror biosensor. *Lancet* **353,** 808.

11. George, A., Danga, R., and Gooden, C. (1995) Quantitative and qualitative detection of serum antibodies using a resonant mirror biosensor. *Tumor Target.* **1,** 245–250.

12. George, A., Gallop, J., and Rashid, M. (1997) Kinetics of biomolecular interactions. *Expert Opin. Ther. Patents* **7,** 947–963.

13. Madiyalakan, R., Sykes, T. R., Dharampaul, S., et al. (1995) Anti-idiotype induction therapy: evidence for the induction of immune response through the idiotype network in patients with ovarian cancer after administration of anti-CA125 murine monoclonal antibody B43.13. *Hybridoma* **14,** 199–203.

32

SDS-PAGE and Western Blotting

Abdulhamid A. Al-Tubuly

1. Introduction

Proteins can be separated according to their molecular sizes and charges, since these factors will determine the speed at which they will travel through a gel. The SDS-PAGE method involves the denaturation of proteins with the detergent sodium dodecyl sulfate (SDS) and the use of an electric current to pull them through a polyacrylamide gel, a process termed polyacrylamide gel electrophoresis (PAGE). SDS binds strongly to proteins, with approximately one detergent molecule binding to two amino acids when SDS is present at 0.1% *(1,2)*. When boiled with SDS, proteins gain a negative charge in proportion to their molecular size, and thus travel in the acrylamide gel according to their molecular sizes. The smaller the size of the running protein, the faster it travels through the pores of the gel (**Fig. 1**).

The polyacrylamide gel is formed by polymerization of monomers of acrylamide with monomers of an appropriate crosslinking substance. The most commonly used crosslinking agent is *N,N'*-methylene-*bis*-acrylamide (usually abbreviated bisacrylamide, or BIS). Gel polymerization is usually initiated with ammonium persulfate (APS), and the reaction is accelerated by addition of the catalyst *N,N,N',N'*-tetramethylenediamine (TEMED). A three-dimensional network is then formed by the crosslinking of randomly growing polyacrylamide chains. The concentrations of acrylamide and the crosslinking agent used will determine the length of the polymers and the extent of the crosslinking, which in turn will affect the physical properties of the gel, such as density, elasticity, fragility, and, most importantly, pore size *(3,4)*. Careful consideration must, therefore, be given to the choice of acrylamide concentration for the optimal separation of different proteins. Gels with large pore size allow faster running of large size proteins, whereas gels with high density (i.e.,

From: *Methods in Molecular Medicine, Vol. 40: Diagnostic and Therapeutic Antibodies*
Edited by: A. J. T. George and C. E. Urch © Humana Press Inc., Totowa, NJ

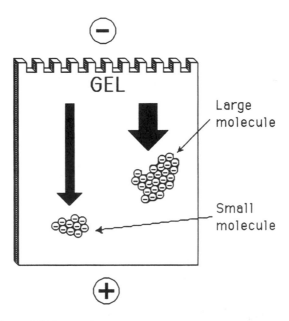

Fig. 1. Migration of different size proteins in a vertical flat slab gel. The smaller the molecular size of the protein, the smaller the charge conferred to it. Migration through the gel is determined by the pore size of the gel, with smaller molecules moving faster.

smaller pore size) would slow large proteins down, permitting better separation of smaller molecules (**Table 1**). The best way to analyze a novel protein with no prior information about its size range is to adopt a method of trial and error, in which gels of different concentrations are tested.

The two main approaches for SDS treatment of proteins are the reducing and nonreducing methods. In the former approach, by adding a reducing thiol agent, such as urea, 2-mercaptoethanol, or dithiothreitol (DTT), to the sample buffer, the proteins will totally unfold and a separation according to their molecular weight is possible (*see* **Note 1**). In the latter (nonreducing) method, the proteins are not fully unfolded, and thus sensitive proteins are not destroyed (*see* **Note 1**). Furthermore, the cleavage of disulfide bonds is prevented *(5,6)*. Two types of gels can be made for the SDS-PAGE method: the cylindrical rod gel or the flat slab gel. The latter is more commonly used and can be applied either horizontally or vertically. The vertical flat gel is currently the method of choice, particularly the small format (7 × 7 cm) minigel, because of its easy use, reduced procedure time, and the effectiveness of electrophoretic transfer (i.e., Western blotting) of proteins from the gel onto a membrane. Only the vertical SDS-PAGE minigel method, based on that outlined by Laemmli *(1)*, will be summarized in this chapter.

Table 1
Separation Ranges of Gels
with Different Acrylamide Concentrations

Gel concentration, %	Molecular weight range, kDa
<5	>200
5–12	20–200
10–15	10–100
>15	<15

2. Materials
2.1. Preparation of Tissue Lysates

1. Eppendorf microfuge tubes (Hamburg, Germany). Keep on ice.
2. Lysis buffer (**Table 2**). Prepare and keep at 4°C (*see* **Note 2**).
3. Sample buffer (**Table 2**). Prepare and keep at room temperature.
4. If reduction of samples is required; 2-mercaptoethanol or dithiothreitol (*see* **Note 1**). To every 1 mL of sample buffer add 20 μL of 2-mercaptoethanol or 31 μg dithiothreitol
5. Hot water bath for boiling samples with SDS.
6. Tissue sample, frozen in liquid nitrogen as for preparing tissue section (*7*) (*see* Chapter 34).
7. Cryostat.
8. Microfuge.

2.2. SDS-PAGE

1. Vertical mini-gel (7 × 7 cm) apparatus (available from many commercial suppliers, such as Hoefer Scientific Instruments, San Francisco, CA; Bio-Rad Laboratories, Richmond, CA; and Integrated Separation Systems, Hyde Park, MA). An illustration of a minigel apparatus (made by Hoefer Scientific Instruments) is shown in **Fig. 2**.
2. Acrylamide (30% in H_2O) (*see* **Note 3**).
3. 1 *M* Tris-HCl, pH 8.8.
4. 1 *M* Tris-HCl, pH 6.8.
5. 10% SDS.
6. Ammonium persulfate.
7. TEMED, *N,N,N',N'*-tetramethylethylendiamine.
8. 70% ethanol. Keep at room temperature.
9. Distilled water. Keep at room temperature.
10. Electrophoresis buffer (*see* **Table 2**). Keep at 4°C.
11. Molecular weight markers (MWM), which are prestained proteins with known molecular size. These can be purchased ready made from commercial suppliers (e.g., Sigma, Poole, UK).
12. Hamilton syringe (Hamilton, Reno, NV).

Table 2
Buffers and Solutions for (Minigel) SDS-PAGE and Western Blotting

Buffers	Volume or weight used
Lysis buffer (500 mL, pH 7.2)	
10 mM Tris-HCl	0.606 g
150 mM NaCl	4.383 g
0.5% Nonidet-P40	2.5 mL
1 mM PMSF	10 µL/mL
Sample buffer (5 mL, pH 6.8)	
10% SDS	500 µL
Glycerol	500 µL
1 M Tris-HCl	400 µL
0.1% bromophenol blue	500 µL
Distilled H$_2$O	3.1 mL
Electrophoresis buffer (1 L, pH 8.3)	
0.025 M Tris-HCl	3 g
0.192 M glycine	14.42 g
0.1% SDS	1 g
Distilled H$_2$O	Add to 1 L
Transfer buffer (1 L, pH 8.3)	
0.025 M Tris-HCl	3 g
0.192 M Glycine	14.42 g
20% Methanol	200 mL
Distilled H$_2$O	Add to 1 L

13. Glass pipets for overlaying ethanol/water.
14. Powerpack.
15. Staining solution: 2:5:5 acetic acid:methanol:distilled water containing 0.25% Coomassie Blue.
16. Destaining solution: 2:5:5 acetic acid:methanol:distilled water.
17. 7% acetic acid.
18. Gel dryer.

2.3. Western Blotting

1. Vertical transferring tank. An illustration of a minitank (7 × 7 cm) with buffer cooling system (made by Hoefer Scientific Instruments) is shown in **Fig. 3**.
2. Nylon membranes (Imobilon-polyvinylidene difluoride, PVDF; Millipore, Bedford, UK).
3. Transfer buffer (*see* **Table 2**). Keep at 4°C.
4. Filter papers (cut to 7 × 7 cm).
5. Large tray.
6. Powerpack.
7. PBS containing 0.02% sodium azide.

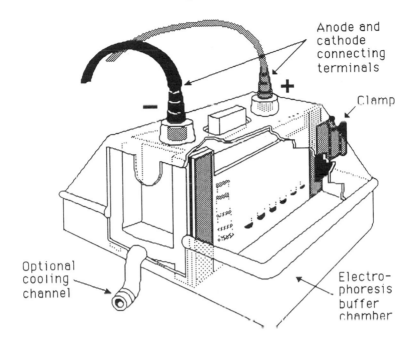

Fig. 2. Miniaturized (7 × 7 cm) vertical flat gel electrophoresis apparatus.

2.4. Materials for Visualization of Proteins

1. Blocking buffer: 2.5% dried milk powder in PBS.
2. Washing solution: 0.5% dried milk powder in PBS.
3. Primary antibody (approx 10 µg/mL in washing solution).
4. Rotator or shaker.
5. Small plastic tray to hold membrane (or 15 mL conical tubes if cut into strips).
6. Appropriate secondary antibody (e.g., peroxidase-conjugated rabbit antimouse immunoglobulin).
7. 0.1% Nonidet P40 (Tween) in PBS.
8. DAB substrate: 30 mg diaminobenzidine, 50 mL PBS, 15 µL 30% H_2O_2.
9. ECL kit (available from Amersham International, Little Chalfont, UK).
10. X-ray films (Hyperfilm MP; Amersham).

3. Methods

There are several methods for preparing samples for SDS-PAGE. If the sample is available in solution, then simply go to **Subheading 3.1., step 3** of the protocol below. However, we have found it useful to prepare lysates from frozen tissue blocks to analyze the antigen recognized by a variety of antibodies.

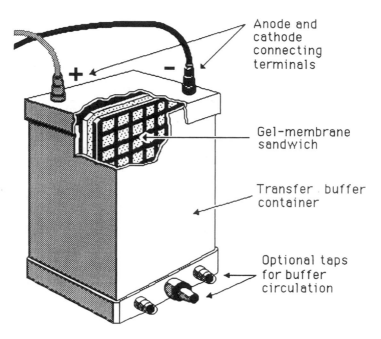

Anode and
cathode
connecting
terminals

Gel-membrane
sandwich

Transfer buffer
container

Optional taps
for buffer
circulation

Fig. 3. Small format (7 × 7 cm) Western blotting transfer tank with optional buffer cooling channels. It is recommended that the buffer be cooled and recirculated, if longer transfer periods are required.

3.1. Preparation of Lysates from Frozen Tissue Blocks

1. Cut several (approx 50) 15 μm thick sections (at –30°C) using a cryostat and place in prechilled (on ice) Eppendorf microfuge tubes containing 110 μL lysis buffer (*see* **Table 2**) for 15 min. Phenyl methyl sulfonyl fluoride (PMSF), a protease inhibitor, can be included in the lysis buffer to prevent the degradation of protease-sensitive molecules (*see* **Note 2**).
2. Centrifuge in a microfuge at 4°C for 5 min.
3. Collect the resulting cell/debris-free supernatant, mix with an equal volume of sample buffer (*see* **Table 2**), and boil for 2–5 min at 100°C. If you want the sample to be reduced add 2-mercaptoethanol (1 μL) or DTT.
4. Allow the sample to cool (5–10 min), aliquot, and either analyze immediately or store at –20°C until required.

SDS-PAGE and Western blotting of lysates made from frozen tissue samples are of great significance. For example, the comparison of the expression of a certain protein (analyzed by immunohistochemistry of tissue sections) with the size of bands from a Western blot analysis of lysates made from the same tissue can give valuable information regarding the amount of protein present in that tissue *(7,8)*.

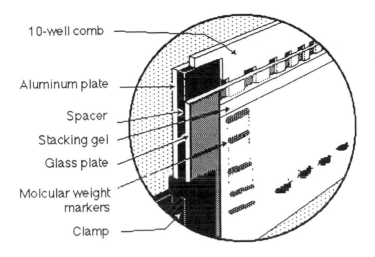

10-well comb

Aluminum plate

Spacer

Stacking gel

Glass plate

Molcular weight markers

Clamp

Fig. 4. Polyacrylamide gel cassette assembly.

3.2. SDS-PAGE

1. Clean carefully all parts of the minigel apparatus with 70% ethanol (particularly the two aluminum plates, two glass plates, two spacers, and the comb).
2. Assemble the apparatus as in **Figs. 2** and **4**, ready to prepare, and add the stacking and separation gel molds.
3. Prepare part "A" of the separation gel first (**Table 3**) (*see* **Note 3**), then immediately prepare the sealing gel (**Table 4**) to seal the lower edge of the cassette (*see* **Notes 3–8**). The sealing gel will set (i.e., polymerize) very quickly (*see* **Note 4**); therefore, immediately apply the gel mold to the lower edge of the cassette using a Pasteur pipet, allowing the gel to be sucked in by capillary action. Apply some sealing gel also to the sides of the cassette (between the spacers and the plates).
4. Leave to stand for approx 5 min to allow the sealing gel to polymerize. For possible causes of delayed polymerization, *see* **Table 5**.
5. Select a suitable comb that is available in several shapes (e.g., uniwell comb or multiwell comb) and mark on the glass plate the level to which to fill the separating gel (**Fig. 4**). It is recommended to mark 0.5 cm lower than the comb.
6. Pour the running gel (after mixing parts "A" and "B"; *see* **Table 3**) in the space between the two plates (*see* **Note 4**).
7. Overlay with 0.5 mL distilled water (or 10% ethanol), and allow to stand for approx 60 min (*see* **Notes 5** and **6**).
8. Pour off the overlaying water, fit the comb in its place, then prepare the stacking gel (*see* **Table 4**) and pour on top of the running gel, covering the teeth of the comb. Let stand for 30–40 min to ensure that the gels are completely set (*see* **Notes 7** and **8**).

Table 3
Separating Gel Solutions for Selected Acrylamide Percentages
(Designed for a Minigel Apparatus)

Running gel[a]	7.5% Acrylamide (20–200 kDa range)	12.5% Acrylamide (10–100 kDa range)
Part A		
Acrylamide (30%)	3.75 mL	6.25 mL
1 M Tris-HCl, pH 8.8	5.6 mL	5.6 mL
Distilled H_2O	5.6 mL	3.1 mL
10% SDS	150 μL	150 μL
Part B		
10% APS	50 μL	50 μL
TEMED	10 μL	10 μL

[a]Parts A and B should be mixed immediately before use to prevent untimely polymerization.

9. Fill the apparatus reservoir with electrophoresis buffer (*see* **Table 2**).
10. Load the samples (15 μL/well) along with the MWM using a Hamilton syringe. The MWM are run alongside the samples to help in estimating the molecular weight of proteins analyzed.
11. Cover the apparatus with the lid, connect to the main power, and begin the electrophoresis (for 90 min) starting at 50–60 V and increase to 100 V when the dye front has reached the running gel.

When proteins have been separated by electric current they can be visualized within the gel by incubating the gel in a 2:5:5 solution of acetic acid, methanol, and distilled water containing "Coomassie blue," which stains proteins blue. Gels can either be stored in 7% acetic acid or dried using a gel dryer (follow instructions appropriate to the make of gel dryer). The polyacrylamide gels are difficult to handle (break easily), so instead of staining the proteins inside the gel they are first transferred onto a membrane to which they bind and are immobilized (i.e., Western blotting). The membranes are much easier to work with than the gels and they can be stained with different antibodies, allowing specific detection of particular proteins. Gels destined for Western blotting should not be stained with Coomassie blue (though it can be useful to stain the gels after the transfer procedure described below to check that transfer is successful). In addition, the lane containing the molecular weight markers can be cut off and stained using Coomassie to aid in determination of molecular weight if prestained markers are not used.

3.3. Western Blotting

1. Remove the gel cassette from the minigel apparatus and pull out the two spacers.

Table 4
Sealing and Stacking Gel Solutions
(Designed for a Minigel Apparatus)

Gel Solution	Volume used
Sealing gel[a]	
Part A	
From part A of the separation gel (*see* **Table 3**)	1.5 mL
Part B	
10% APS	25 μL
TEMED	5 μL
Stacking gel (5%)[a]	
Part A	
Acrylamide (30%)	1 mL
1 *M* Tris-HCl, pH 6.8	750 μL
Distilled H$_2$O	3.76 mL
10% SDS	60 μL
Part B	
10% APS	30 μL
TEMED	6 μL

[a]Parts A and B should be mixed immediately before use, to prevent untimely polymerization.

2. Carefully lever off the glass plate without breaking the gel and transfer the aluminum plate (with the gel still on top) into a tray containing transfer buffer (**Table 2**).
3. Prewet a (7 × 7 cm) piece of nylon membrane with methanol and slide it between the gel and the aluminum plate (still in the transfer buffer tray).
4. Cover the gel-membrane with transfer buffer-soaked (7 × 7 cm) filter papers and sponges and place in the transfer cassette, thus forming the transfer sandwich (**Fig. 5**).
5. Place the cassette in the transferring tank containing transfer buffer (as in **Fig. 3**) (*see* **Note 9**).
6. Connect to the main power and run an electric current of 300 mA for approx 60 min to transfer the proteins from the gel onto the membrane. At this stage membranes can be stored at 4°C in PBS containing 0.02% sodium azide (*see* **Notes 10 and 11**).

3.4. Immunostaining of Western Blot Membrane

1. Incubate the membrane overnight at 4°C (or 2 h at room temperature) with a blocking buffer (2.5% milk powder in PBS) to block any unoccupied charges that may lead to nonspecific binding of proteins to the membrane. This can be conveniently done in a small plastic tray.

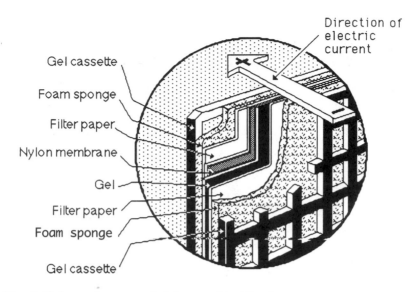

Fig. 5. Gel-membrane sandwich assembly. The foam sponges and filter papers are used to ensure close contact of the gel on the membrane. Proteins transfer from the cathode to the anode side (arrow).

2. Rinse several times in a washing solution (0.5% milk powder in PBS). The membrane can either be cut into several strips to be stained with different antibodies (which can be placed in 15-mL conical tubes), or stained as a whole membrane with only one antibody (in a tray).

3. Incubate with the primary antibody (diluted in 0.5% milk powder in PBS) for 1–2 h at room temperature, either in a tube on a rotator (if small strips) or in a tray on a shaker (if whole membrane).

4. Wash the membrane thoroughly (three times for 5 min each wash) in washing solution.

5. Incubate for 1 h at room temperature with a peroxidase-conjugated antibody specific for the primary antibody you are using (e.g., rabbit antimouse, or sheep antirabbit). The antibody should be diluted according to the manufacturer's instructions or titration by previous experiments to give the best staining with no background.

6. Wash several times as before, then incubate with diaminobenzidine (DAB) substrate for approx 10 min (or until brown bands appear) at room temperature.

7. Wash the stained membrane in tap water (for 5 min) then allow to air dry.

8. Alternatively, in order to get a higher sensitivity, bands can be visualized using the enhanced chemiluminescence (ECL) method. In this method, the peroxidase-conjugated secondary antibody reacts with the substrate plus a

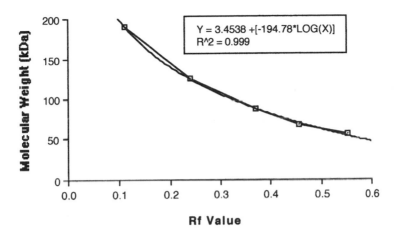

Fig. 6. A typical curve for calculating molecular weights.

luminescent compound (such as luminol). This results in emission of light, which can be detected using a photosensitive film, with short exposure times (seconds–minutes).

3.5. Enhanced Chemiluminescence

1. Wash the membrane with 0.5% milk powder in PBS three times for 5 min each wash.
2. Wash further with 0.1% Tween in PBS (three times for 5 min). At this stage membranes can be stored overnight in 0.1% Tween/PBS at 4°C.
3. Drain the membrane briefly, then apply the ECL reagents for 1 min (following the manufacturer's instructions).
4. Drain the membrane, wrap with cling film, put in an X-ray cassette, and expose to X-ray films for 10 s–10 min.

3.6. Calculation of the Molecular Weight of a Protein

In order to determine the molecular weight of a protein, the relative distance (R_f) for each molecular weight marker and experimental proteins had to be determined. R_f is calculated by measuring the distance each of the molecular markers and experimental proteins had traveled within the gel and dividing that number by the distance the dye front had traveled within the gel. A curve can be constructed from the molecular weight markers, with R_f on the x-axis and molecular weight (in kDa) on the y-axis (**Fig. 6**). A logarithmic curve fit can then be made that will provide an equation from which the molecular weight (in kDa) of the stained proteins could be calculated by using their R_f values (*see* **Fig. 6**).

Table 5
SDS-PAGE and Western Blotting: Troubleshooting

Problem	Cause	Remedy
SDS-PAGE		
Leakage of gel molds	Incorrect assembly of apparatus	Reassemble the apparatus carefully using a hydrophobic ointment (e.g., Vaseline) for sealing
	Broken/cracked glass plate	Use unbroken glass plates
	Dirty glass plates	Clean the plates with 70% alcohol/water before and after use
Delayed/no polymerization	Presence of air in the gel mold	Tilt apparatus to let air escape. Cover gel molds with water or 10% ethanol/water to prevent air being absorbed into the gel
	Old reagents/buffers	Always use fresh reagents (especially ASP) Use proper concentrations for catalysts and accelerators
	Incorrect concentrations of TEMED/APS	Make sure that buffers and reagents have reached room temperature (polymerization occurs best at 20–30°C)
	Low temperature	
White/cloudy gel	High concentration of BIS	Lower BIS concentration
	Precipitation of SDS	Check temperature (should be 20–30°C)
No electric current	No main power	Check the main, leads, and tank lid. Clean all wirings with 70% alcohol, and dry before use
	Faulty leads	
	Loose tank lid	
	Dirt plugs (no contact)	
	Insufficient buffer in tank	
Reversed migration of dye	Incorrect electrical polarity	Remember that negatively charged proteins will migrate toward the anode (i.e., the positive side)

Problem	Cause	Solution
Distorted/wavy migration of dye	Uneven pore size Air bubbles present in gel Poor quality gel	Mix gel mold quickly and properly Avoid air bubbles formation (*see above*) Use fresh reagents and buffers
Western blotting and immunostaining		
No transfer	Incorrect assembly of apparatus Incorrect polarity of electric current (proteins lost in transfer buffer) Insufficient transfer time	Assemble the apparatus properly Check polarity of lid plugs (remember proteins transfer from gel to membrane, i.e., cathode to anode direction) Allow enough time for transfer (1–2 h for minigel apparatus)
No proteins (bands) in certain areas	Air bubbles in gel Uneven contact between gel and membrane	Prevent air bubbles formation; *see above* Roll a glass pipet on the gel-membrane sandwich to expel any trapped air bubbles
High background staining	Excess antibodies used Severe degradation of proteins Prolonged exposure to substrates in enzyme-based staining procedures	Titrate all antibodies and dilute in PBS as required Use protease inhibitors (e.g., PMSF) Use sufficient amounts of washing solutions and adequate washing times
Incorrect/unexpected MWM values	Samples diffused into gel because of delayed running samples Larger sample volumes than the wells	Start running the samples immediately after loading Use equal and sufficient amounts of protein samples

4. Notes

1. The use of the reducing agent DTT is preferred over 2-mercaptoethanol or urea because of the following advantages: DTT is less volatile, and hence, produces less smell; and when both reducing and nonreducing samples are to be separated in the same gel, the reducing action of DTT can be blocked with iodoacetamide, thus preventing DTT from diffusing into the lanes of the nonreducing proteins.
2. If needed, use 10 µL of PMSF/1 mL lysis buffer. This should be done in a fume cupboard and preferably on ice. PMSF is neurotoxic and should not be inhaled or touched. Always wear protective gloves, a face mask, and a safety goggles.
3. Acrylamide is an accumulative neurotoxin (and a possible carcinogen). Handling of the powder form can easily produce airborne particles that can be inhaled. Always wear protective gloves, a face mask, and safety goggles, and dispense in a fume cupboard. Gloves should be worn also when handling acrylamide solutions.
4. APS and TEMED will quickly initiate gel polymerization. Always keep the addition of APS/TEMED to the last moment.
5. Dissolved oxygen may inhibit the process of gel polymerization. It is essential to cover the running gel with 0.5 mL distilled H_2O or 10% ethanol. The overlying of water or ethanol will also ensure a straight running/stacking gel interface.
6. Extreme temperatures can affect the process of gel polymerization and should be avoided. The optimum temperatures are in the range of 20–30°C.
7. When applying the sealing gel, make sure that the level of the gel is even to prevent distortion of the separation. If the gel has formed a concave or convex line, try to slightly tilt the apparatus to one side.
8. The stacking gel is of a lower acrylamide concentration (5%, **Table 4**) than the running gel (7.5 or 12.5%, **Table 3**) and is buffered at lower pH. The passage of proteins from the lower acrylamide concentration and pH to the higher acrylamide concentration and pH at the stacking/running gel interface has the effect of concentrating the proteins into narrow bands.
9. Make sure that the transfer sandwich is tightly held to avoid air bubble accumulation.
10. When removing the membrane from the transfer sandwich, remember to mark with a pencil the side on which the proteins were transferred.
11. For safety reasons it is essential to switch off the mains when checking the leads or polarity.

References

1. Laemmli, U. K. (1970) Cleavage of structural proteins during the assembly of the head of bacteriophage T4. *Nature* **227,** 680–685.
2. Reynolds, J. A. and Tanford, C. (1970) Binding of dodecyl sulfate to proteins at high binding ratios. Possible implications for the state of proteins in biological membranes. *Proc. Natl. Acad. Sci. USA* **66,** 1002–1007.

3. Andrews, A. T. (1986) *Electrophoresis: Theory, Techniques and Biochemical and Clinical Applications.* Oxford University Press, Oxford, UK.

4. Dunn, M. J. (1993) *Electrophoresis: Proteins.* BIOS Scientific Publishers, Oxford, UK.

5. Dunbar, B. S. (ed.) (1994) *Protein Blotting: A Practical Approach.* Oxford University Press, Oxford, UK.

6. Cann, J. R. (1996) The theory and practice of gel electrophoresis of interacting macromolecules. *Anal. Biochem.* **237,** 1–16.

7. Al-Tubuly, A. A., Luqmani, Y. A., Shousha, S., Melcher, D., and Ritter, M. A. (1996) Differential expression of gp200-MR6 molecule in benign hyperplasia and down-regulation in invasive carcinoma of the breast. *Br. J. Cancer* **74,** 1005–1011.

8. Al-Tubuly, A. A. (1997) The role of IL-4 receptor complex in normal and transformed epithelial cells: structural and functional analysis. PhD thesis, University of London.

Further Readings

Beynon, R. J. and Easterby, J. S. (1996) *Buffer Solutions: The Basics.* Oxford University Press, Oxford, UK.

Hawcroft, D. M. (1997) *Electrophoresis: The Basics.* Oxford University Press, Oxford, UK.

Westermeier, R. (1997) *Electrophoresis in Practice: A Guide to Methods and Applications of DNA and Protein Separations.* VCH–Wiley, Oxford, UK.

33

Flow Cytometric Analysis

Paul F. McKay

1. Introduction

Flow cytometry, as the name suggests, is the analysis of cells (which carry one or more fluorescent labels) moving in a fluid flow *(1,2)*. This technique has become widely used because of the enormous increase in the number and range of specificities of antibodies to cell determinants. Monoclonal and polyclonal antibodies to both murine and human antigens, indeed antibodies that have a fluorochrome covalently attached (and which have already been tested in various assay systems), are readily commercially available.

Flow cytometry has been used clinically in a number of ways, including:

1. The determination of the number and proportion of CD4+ve T cells in the whole blood of HIV+ve patients;
2. Identification of neoplastic cells in the blood and determination of their cell lineage origin using dual or triple fluorochrome labeling; or
3. The matching of major and minor histocompatibility antigens for the purpose of organ transplantation.

It is most important when using this technique to have a suspension of single cells in an isotonic medium. Having single cells growing in suspension in vitro provides perhaps the simplest starting material, but adherent cells in culture, whole blood, solid tissue, and even whole organs can be used to provide the cells for analysis.

When the single cell passes through the laser beam the light is scattered. Forward scatter is an indirect measure of the size of the cell; the larger the cell, the more scatter in the forward direction. Side scatter is a measure of the "granularity" of the cell. Denser areas within the cell deflect more light and so cause greater side scatter *(3)*. Forward scatter and side scatter are two further

From: *Methods in Molecular Medicine, Vol. 40: Diagnostic and Therapeutic Antibodies*
Edited by: A. J. T. George and C. E. Urch © Humana Press Inc., Totowa, NJ

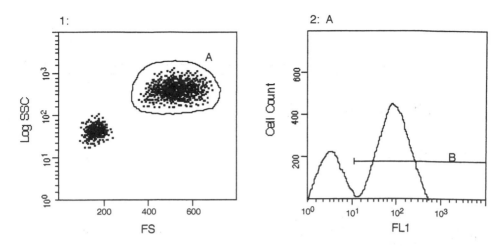

Fig. 1. One-color flow cytometric analysis, showing positive population of the A region. The position of line B is defined by the negative control and is used to determine the positive population.

parameters (as well as the fluorochromes that label the cell antigens of interest) that are used to identify and categorise cell subpopulations of interest.

For example, in **Fig. 1**, which shows a one-color analysis, the forward scatter (FS) and the log of the side scatter (log SSC) distinguish two populations of cells. In this case it may be active and resting cells. The population being analyzed is the large and slightly more granular cells that have been surround by an analysis region named A (This is called "gating" the cells of interest.). The relative position of the cells in the histograms can be altered by changing the voltage "gain," which can be convenient if one of the cell populations being analyzed falls outside the histogram window. When the "gated" cells are analyzed for their emitted fluorescence when stimulated by the laser they are shown to be positive for the fluorochrome of interest and therefore must have the antibody with the attached fluorochrome on their cell surface. The positivity is decided by the line named B and is shown on the axis labeled FL1 (fluorescence log 1). This is set (for each experiment) by using the negative isotype-matched control antibody. This isotype-matched antibody controls for nonspecific binding of the test antibody and should have a histogram profile similar to that shown in **Fig. 2**.

The B region is set so that about 1% of the cell counts are to the right of the start of region B and the rest (99%) are to the left. The cell population can be moved up and down the FL axis by increasing or decreasing the voltage "gain." By having a discrete negative cell population (as above) even a small population shift can be seen and the analysis will be clearer.

2: A

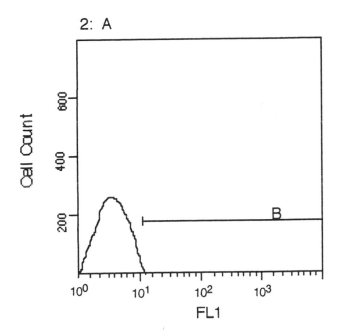

Fig. 2. An example of a negative staining profile.

In two-color immunofluorescence the principles are the same but the "gating" is done in a slightly different way. The histograms in **Fig. 3** show the percent positivity of the cells for each fluorochrome (FL1 [fluoroscein isothiocyanate; FITC] and FL2 [phycoerythrin; PE]). Each region C and D has been set with reference to the relevant isotype-matched negative control. The fourth histogram is a visual representation of the cells using both the FL1 and FL2. We can see that some of those cells that are FL1-positive are also FL2-positive (R2), whereas some cells are positive for one or the other fluorochrome (R1 and R3) and some are negative for both (R4). The percentage of cells in each of these regions can be informative. A problem that does arise in two- and three color analysis is the spillover of the emission spectrum of one fluorophore into the emission spectrum of the other fluorophore. This happens commonly with FITC- and PE-conjugated antibodies. FITC has an emission maximum at 525 nm but the emission ranges from 495 to 600 nm. Likewise, PE has an emission maximum at 578 nm but ranges over 545–640 nm. Obviously, the two fluorochrome emission spectra overlap at 545–600 nm *(4,5)*. If no action is taken the FL1 detector will read some fluorescence coming from the FL2 fluorophore and vise-versa. A procedure termed "compensation" is undertaken that basically ensures that the FL1 detector (FITC) does not read wavelengths above 545 mm and the FL2 (PE) detector does not read any fluorescent wavelength below 600 nm *(6)*.

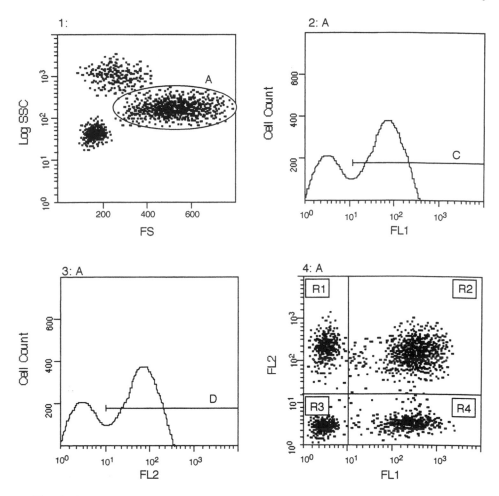

Fig. 3. Two-color analysis showing the two positive populations in FL1 and FL2 and the "double positive" population in R2.

In three-color immunofluorescence it is possible to draw a further "gate" around the cells in each of these regions and analyze the population for a third fluorochrome. This technique is quite advanced and is outside the remit of this chapter, but for those interested in the benefits of this technique there are textbooks and a cytometry journal available in most university libraries.

2. Materials

1. Phosphate-buffered saline (PBS): 0.138 M NaCl, 2.7 mM KCl, pH 7.4.
2. Ficoll-Histopaque 1077 or 1083.
3. Nylon cell strainer (70 μm).

4. Hemocytometer.
5. 21 Gage needles.
6. Scalpel.
7. Paraformaldehyde.
8. Primary antibody.
9. Secondary fluorochrome-labeled antibody.

3. Methods

3.1. Preparation of a Single-Cell Suspension for Analysis

3 1 1 From Cells in Culture

1. Remove cells and growth medium from the culture flask (for adherent cells *see* **Note 1**).
2. Spin cells in an appropriate tube at 300g for 10 min at 4°C.
3. Discard growth medium.
4. Resuspend cells in residual medium, then add 1 mL PBS.
5. Count cells using a hemocytometer.
6. Adjust cell concentration to 1×10^7 cells/mL.

3 1 2 From Whole Blood

1. Use whole heparinized blood from a human or animal source.
2. Layer blood over Ficoll-Histopaque (*see* **Note 2**).
3. Centrifuge at 750g for 20 min at room temperature.
4. Remove the yellowish layer at the interface and place in a 50 mL tube.
5. Top up to 50 mL with PBS.
6. Spin at 300g for 10 min at 4°C.
7. Discard PBS and resuspend cells in residual fluid.
8. Add 50 mL PBS.
9. Spin at 300g for 10 min at 4°C.
10. Discard PBS and resuspend cells in residual fluid.
11. Resuspend cells in residual medium, then add 1 mL PBS.
12. Count cells using a hemocytometer.
13. Adjust cell concentration to 1×10^7 cells/mL.

3.1.2. From Tissue/Organs

1. Chop tissue or organ into 1 cm^3 pieces.
2. Use two needles to "tease" out the cells from the tissue matrix (**Note 3**).
3. Harvest the lacerated tissue/cell suspension from the Petri dish.
4. Sieve the mixture through a 70 μm cell strainer (**Note 3**).
5. Centrifuge the strained cells at 300g for 10 min at 4°C.
6. Discard PBS and resuspend cells in residual fluid.
7. Add 1 mL PBS.
8. Count cells using a hemocytometer.
9. Adjust cell concentration to 1×10^7 cells/mL.

3.2. One-Color Immunofluorescence

The cell sample can be stained with the fluorochrome in either a "FACS" tube or, if a large number of samples are to be processed, in a 96-well V-bottomed plate. One-color analysis is the most basic staining procedure and is used to identify positive populations; for example, a cell line that has been transfected with a gene encoding an antigen to which there is an antibody. Those cells that are positive can be identified using the antibody against the newly expressed antigen and then a second layer FITC-anti-Ig polyclonal antibody as described below (always include a sample stained only with an isotype-matched primary antibody as a negative control). All steps should be carried out on ice and all reagents/centrifuges should be chilled to 4°C before starting the procedure

1. Use 100 µL of a single-cell preparation (as above) (1×10^6 cells).
2. Add 100 µL of primary antibody dilution (**Note 4**).
3. Incubate at 4°C for 30–60 min with occasional agitation.
4. Centrifuge at 300*g* for 10 min.
5. Discard supernatant.
6. Resuspend the cell pellet in residual medium.
7. Add 200 µL PBS (4°C) to the wash.
8. Repeat **steps 4–7** a further two times.
9. Centrifuge at 300*g* for 10 min.
10. Discard supernatant.
11. Resuspend the cell pellet in residual medium.
12. Add 100 µL secondary antibody (4°C) (**Note 5**).
13. Incubate at 4°C for 30–60 min with occasional agitation.
14. Repeat **steps 4–7** three times.
15. Centrifuge at 300*g* for 10 min.
16. Discard supernatant.
17. Resuspend the cell pellet in residual medium.
18. Add 200 µL 1% paraformaldehyde.
19. Analyze the stained cells in a flow cytometer.

3.3. Two-Color Immunofluorescence

The two-color immunofluorescence technique uses two directly labeled antibodies for staining. The fluorochromes most often used are FITC and PE because they are both stimulated to fluoresce using a laser emitting light at 488 nm. The antibodies can be added to the cells at the same time and because they are directly conjugated there is no need for a second-layer antibody (**Note 6**). It is always useful to stain a cell sample with isotype-matched antibodies as the a negative control; if both primary antibodies are of the same isotype it will only be necessary to add that isotype but if they are different add both isotypes at the same time. For the purposes of clarity the example shown is the procedure for staining with CD4-FITC and CD8-PE, which are both markers for blood T cells. The mature T cells in the peripheral blood generally fall into one of two types, CD4 or CD8, and it is sometimes useful to measure the relative proportions of these cells. All steps should be carried out on ice and all reagents/centrifuges should be chilled to 4°C before starting the procedure

1. Use 100 μL of a single-cell preparation (as above) (1×10^6 cells)
2. Add 50 μL primary antibody CD4-FITC and 50 μL primary antibody CD8-PE (**Note 7**).
3. Incubate at 4°C for 1 h.
4. Centrifuge at 300 g for 10 min.
5. Discard supernatant.
6. Resuspend the cell pellet in residual medium.
7. Add 200 μL PBS (4°C) to wash.
8. Repeat **steps 4–7** a further three times.
9. Centrifuge at 300g for 10 min.
10. Discard supernatant.
11. Resuspend cell pellet in residual medium.
12. Add 200 μL 1% paraformaldehyde.
13. Analyze the stained cells in the flow cytometer.

4. Notes

1. For adherent cells first discard the growth medium, then incubate the cells with an appropriate volume of nonenzymatic cell dissociation medium (Sigma, Poole, UK; cat. no. c5914; 5 mL/75 cm^3 cell-culture flask). The cells should be incubated at 37°C until most are in suspension and any large clumps have dissipated (any remaining small clumps will be forced into single-cell suspension by the shear forces when taken up by the pipet).
2. When using human blood, layer over Ficoll-Histopaque 1077 (Sigma; cat. no. 1077-1), which has a density of 1.077 g/mL. When separating murine white blood cells Ficoll-Histopaque 1083 (density 1.083 g/mL; Sigma; cat. no. 1083-1) is used because murine cells are slightly more dense.
3. For teasing out the cells from an organ or tissue matrix it is quite convenient to use two 21-gauge needles. One of the needles can be used to "hold" the tissue firmly on the base of a Petri dish containing about 10 mL PBS. The other needle is used to lacerate the tissue and liberate the cells from the connective tissue. The cell/tissue mixture is then strained through a 70 μm nylon mesh, which allows single cells to pass through but retains the connective tissue (cell strainer; Becton Dickinson, Franklin Lakes, NJ; cat. no. 2350).
4. The primary antibody used for the staining can either be undiluted hybridoma supernatant or a dilution of a commercial antibody. (Optimum dilution varies but it is best to start with a range of dilutions from approx 1–50 μg/mL, and to use 100 μL/analysis, i.e., 0.1–5 μg/analysis.) For any cell antigen this will be in excess.

5. The secondary antibody will be a fluorochrome-labeled anti-Ig. The fluorochrome used is usually FITC, simply because antibodies are most commonly labeled with this fluorochrome, but PE, tetramethyl-rhodamine, and Texas Red can also be used. The optimum dilution varies, but generally 10–20 µg/mL works well. The Ig species type to be used is dictated by the primary antibody.

6. In the example given, using CD4-FITC and CD8-PE can both be added to the sample together to double-stain the cell sample and because they have a direct label (i.e., the fluorochrome is attached directly to the primary antibody) there is no need for the second-layer antibody. However, when the cell expresses very low cell-surface levels of the antigen of interest, it may be necessary to use a second-layer antibody in order to "amplify" the signal. In such a case it would be necessary to carefully select the species Ig of the primary antibodies so that you do not get crossreactivity.

7. Each of the antibodies used should be tested to ascertain the best dilution to be used. Usually, each antibody should be used at 0.1–5 µg/analysis but, as always, different antibodies will have different staining efficiencies and for this technique the antibody is almost always used in excess.

References

1. Hercher, M., Mueller, W., and Shapiro, H. M. (1979) Detection and discrimination of individual viruses by flow cytometry. *J. Histochem. Cytochem.* **27,** 350–352.

2. Shapiro, H. M. (1977) Fluorescent dyes for differential counts by flow cytometry: does histochemistry tell us much more than cell geometry? *J. Histochem. Cytochem.* **25,** 976–989.

3. Cairo, M. S., Vandeven, C., Toy, C., Tischler, D., and Sender, L. (1988) Fluorescent cytometric analysis of polymorphonuclear leukocytes in Chediak-Higashi syndrome: diminished C3bi receptor expression (OKM1) with normal granular cell density. *Pediatr. Res.* **24,** 673–676.

4. Corver, W. E., Cornelisse, C. J., and Fleuren, G. J. (1994) Simultaneous measurement of two cellular antigens and DNA using fluorescein-isothiocyanate, R-phycoerythrin, and propidium iodide on a standard FACScan. *Cytometry* **15,** 117–128.

5. Gruber, R., Reiter, C., and Riethmuller, G. (1993) Triple immunofluorescence flow cytometry, using whole blood, of CD4+ and CD8+ lymphocytes expressing CD45RO and CD45RA. *J. Immunol. Methods* **163,** 173–179.

6. Weyde, J., Wassermann, K., and Schell-Frederick, E. (1997) Analysis of single and double-stained alveolar macrophages by flow cytometry. *J. Immunol. Methods* **207,** 115–123.

Further Reading

Shapiro, H. M. (1988) *Practial Flow Cytometry*, 3rd ed., Wiley-Liss Inc., New York.

The Cytometry Journal.

34

Immunocytochemistry

Susan Van Noorden

1. Introduction

Immunocytochemistry provides an accurate way of localizing antigens *in situ* in tissue sections or cell preparations using antibodies combined with a label that can be identified microscopically. The most frequently used labels are fluorescent compounds that can be excited by light of specific wavelength, enzymes that can act on a specific substrate with a chromogen to give a colored end-product, and colloidal gold (for electron microscopy). Antibodies are applied to tissue preparations, often in a series of layers, one applied antibody acting as an antigen for the next (antispecies) antibody to build up the amount of label at the original site of reaction.

1.1. Conditions

For any antigen localization, the antigen and the tissue must be fixed so that the antigen is insoluble and the tissue components are immobilized and protected from osmotic damage. Unfortunately, the "best" fixation for histology uses formalin, which crosslinks protein groups, followed by processing to paraffin sections; this fixation can sometimes damage antigenicity by altering the epitopes to which the antibody binds. For some antigens it is still necessary, therefore, to use fresh-frozen sections or cell preparations, postfixed in a precipitant fixative, such as acetone or alcohol. However, standard histological fixatives, such as formalin in its various combinations, can now usually be used in diagnostic histopathology, provided that antibodies have been selected during testing to react with fixed antigens, and with heat-mediated antigen retrieval methods an increasingly wide range of antibodies can be used on paraffin sections.

From: *Methods in Molecular Medicine, Vol. 40: Diagnostic and Therapeutic Antibodies*
Edited by: A. J. T. George and C. E. Urch © Humana Press Inc., Totowa, NJ

1.2. Diagnostic Applications

Immunocytochemistry is now a routinely used diagnostic test for tumor type and innumerable other conditions in histo- and cytopathology, as well as in immunology, microbiology, and hematology. Immunocytochemistry is most useful in differential diagnosis, where a panel of antibodies to relevant antigens is used to distinguish among various options on material that cannot be diagnosed satisfactorily on standard histological preparations. Because this is a relatively expensive test, a blanket approach is not usually justified. Clinical history and preliminary examination of the histological preparations are important in selecting the panel to be used. The antibodies should have been extensively tested for specificity, sensitive methods should be used, and the appropriate negative and positive controls must always be carried out at the same time as the tests to ensure that the technique is in good working order and that the result is not caused by nonspecific reactions.

1.2.1. Antibody Screening

During production of monoclonal antibodies (mAbs), rapid screening is required (Chapter 17). If the antibodies are to be used for immunocytochemistry, the screening test should be carried out on tissue containing an abundance of the antigen in question, in its known localization, prepared in the same way as for the final use of the antibodies, i.e., if the antibodies are to be used for histological diagnosis they should be screened on paraffin sections of formalin-fixed tissue, using the standard method of the laboratory. Polyclonal antibodies are screened in the same way, but with less need for hurry. If the antibodies are to be used as therapeutic reagents, different conditions may apply (*see* **Subheading 1.3.**). When antibodies are being produced to identify an antigen that has not yet been identified in tissue, possibly in an unknown localization, the matter is more complicated and tissue prepared with different fixatives and types of section may be required to establish the correct conditions. An additional control in this case will require the antibody to be adsorbed with pure antigen to test positive-appearing staining for specificity.

1.3. Therapeutic Applications

An antibody for use as a therapeutic agent will generally be monoclonal. It must be shown to target its antigen accurately and solely if it is to be used as a toxin carrier or "magic bullet." For testing such antibodies, in the first instance, the tissue should be in as natural a state as possible to be comparable with in-body conditions. The nearest we can get to this is to use fresh-frozen tissue sections or fresh cell preparations, but usually light fixation (alcohol or acetone) will be necessary to prevent the antigen from dissolving and the tissue from disintegrating during immunostaining. A simple method, such as the indirect two-layer technique, should be used. Once it has been shown that the antibody reacts well with its antigen in this type of preparation, it can be tested on formalin-fixed paraffin sections. If this test is positive and specific, a wide variety of normal and pathological material will be available in the archives for further testing. It is unlikely that there will be a sufficiently varied tissue bank of frozen material and it is much easier to produce paraffin sections than frozen ones from numerous cases. On frozen sections or cell preparations, it may be necessary to use Fab fractions of antibodies to avoid possible binding to Fc receptors in immunocytochemical testing, as in therapy.

Many different types of imunocytochemical reactions using a variety of labels are in use today. Only the most commonly used will be detailed here. Further reading on practical *(1,2)*, diagnostic *(3)*, and theoretical *(4,5)* aspects of immunocytochemistry is detailed in the reference list.

1.4. Labels

1.4.1. Fluorescent Labels

The most popular fluorescent labels are still fluorescein isothiocyanate (FITC), which fluoresces bright apple green at excitation wavelength 495 nm, and tetrarhodamine isothiocyanate (TRITC) or Texas red, both of which fluoresce red at excitation wavelength 530 nm. For double immunofluorescence using fluorescein- and rhodamine-conjugated antibodies to visualize two antigens in the same preparation, the microscope must be provided with two narrow-band filters so that the two labels can be excited alternately. There are also yellow- and blue-fluorescing compounds and, most recently developed, a group of cyanine dyes with long-lasting fluorescence in various bright colors. Appropriate filters must be available.

Immunofluorescence provides a rapid test but has the disadvantages that a special microscope is required and the final product is not permanent. The ability of the label to fluoresce will fade over time, and particularly during exposure to the exciting light; it is difficult to photograph, requiring a fast film. On the other hand, it is very suitable for lightly fixed frozen sections, where the poor preservation of the background tissue structure will not be noticed. In addition, the eye is very sensitive to fluorescence and can discern small quantities easily. If living cells are to be immunostained, e.g., for cell sorting and flow cytometry, fluorescent labels would be the correct choice because they do not kill the cells. Formalin-fixed tissue tends to have greenish background fluorescence, which can be confusing if FITC is the label, but may have to be accepted if the antigen requires crosslinking fixation, as many small peptides do, to make them insoluble. The answer here would be to use an alternative fluorescent label.

1.4.2. Enzyme Labels

Enzyme labels were brought in to provide permanent preparations that could be viewed in an ordinary light microscope and are suitable for either frozen or paraffin sections. At the end of the series of antigen–antibody reactions finishing with an enzyme-labeled reagent, a "histochemical" reaction is carried out to reveal the site of enzyme activity. The criteria for a useful enzyme are that it can be conjugated to an antibody and that it can split an applied substrate so that one of the products will react with a suitable chromogen to precipitate at the site of reaction an intensely colored product that is insoluble and microscopically visible.

The first enzyme label to be introduced was horseradish peroxidase, followed by calf intestinal alkaline phosphatase. Any endogenous enzyme activity in the tissue preparation, such as myeloperoxidase, the peroxidase-like enzyme in red blood cells, or the alkaline phosphatase in vascular endothelium, must be blocked so that it cannot take part in the reaction. For peroxidase, this is usually done with an excess of its substrate, hydrogen peroxide, often at the beginning of the technique but at any stage before the application of the peroxidase-labeled reagent. Alkaline phosphatase exists in several tissue-specific isoforms (bone, liver, endothelial, intestinal). All except the intestinal isoform are inhibited by levamisole, which is added to the final incubating solution. Alkaline phosphatase is an unsuitable label for immunoreactions on intestinal tissue. Other enzymes (glucose oxidase, β-D-galactosidase) are also used as labels, but will not be discussed here.

The color of the endproduct of reaction depends on the substrate and chromogen. The reaction of peroxidase with hydrogen peroxide and 3-3'-diaminobenzidine (DAB) is dark brown and can be made black by addition of heavy metal salts to the incubation medium, or by depositing them on the DAB precipitate in a postreaction. If 3-amino-9-ethylcarbazole (AEC) is used instead of DAB, the endproduct is red. Alkaline phosphatase splits naphthol phosphate, and the released naphthol couples with a diazonium salt, such as Fast Red TR, to give an azo dye, in this case a bright red color. Blue and other colors are also available, depending on the substrate and chromogen. The pH of the buffer, its molarity and temperature, and the concentration of the substrate and chromogen are important in achieving optimal results from the enzyme reaction.

1.4.3. Colloidal Gold

Colloidal gold was introduced as a label for electron microscopic immunocytochemistry (Chapter 35) because it is electron-dense, but it can also be used

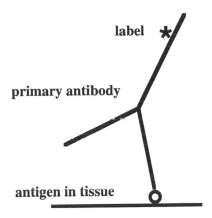

Fig. 1. Direct one-step method.

at light microscopic level. It has intrinsic color (magenta) but needs to be used in high concentration for this to be usefully visible. However, enhancement of the colloidal gold by deposition of metallic silver from a silver salt solution increases the sensitivity by giving an intensely black, stable product, which allows the use of very dilute antibodies and can be useful when little antigen is present.

1.4.4. Biotin

Biotin itself cannot be made visible, but binds very strongly to a much larger molecule, avidin (or streptavidin), which can be heavily labeled with a fluorescent marker, enzyme, or colloidal gold. Antibodies can carry many molecules of biotin, which is a very small molecule, so further binding of many labeled avidin molecules provides a large amount of label, again producing a very sensitive method, able to mark intensely a very small quantity of antigen.

1.5. Overview of Staining Methodologies

1.5.1. Direct (One-Step) Method

The simplest method is the single-layer application of a labeled antibody, the "direct" method, but this is relatively insensitive and requires the labeling of individual antibodies. Therefore, it is little used diagnostically (with the exception of Dako's EPOS [extended polymer one-step] antibodies that are heavily labeled with peroxidase) (**Fig. 1**).

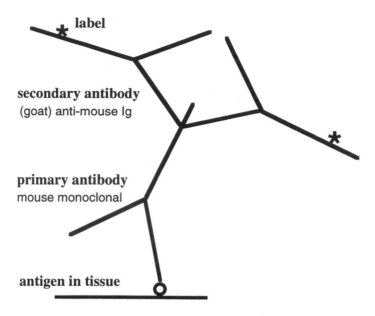

Fig. 2. Indirect two-step method.

1.5.2. Indirect (Two-Step) Method

More useful, particularly where mAbs are concerned, since the dilution factor is of less importance than for polyclonal antibodies, is the two-layer, "indirect" method. This is usually the method used when testing mAbs during production because it can be done more rapidly than the even more sensitive, three-layer techniques, and if a fluorescent label is used, the extra steps associated with enzyme-linked reactions are not required. The primary antibody is unlabeled and is identified by a labeled antibody raised to the immunoglobulin of the species providing the primary antibody (**Fig. 2**).

1.5.3. Indirect (Three-Step) Methods

1.5.3.1. Enzyme Antienzyme Methods

Enzyme antienzyme methods, such as peroxidase antiperoxidase (PAP) or alkaline phosphatase-antialkaline phosphatase (APAAP), increase the sensitivity considerably in terms of dilution of the primary antibody, because the three-layered technique results in a build-up of label on the site of reaction. The high dilution of the primary antibody that is possible with this method is a particular advantage when it is a polyclonal antibody since unwanted contaminating antibodies, in much lower concentration in the antiserum than the antibodies to the immunogen, are diluted out, resulting in a cleaner preparation. The primary antibody is unlabeled. The second, antiprimary species antibody

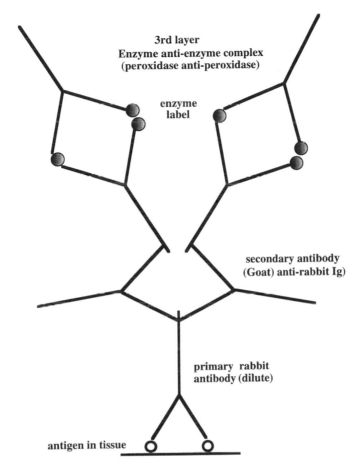

3rd layer
Enzyme anti-enzyme complex
(peroxidase anti-peroxidase)

enzyme
label

secondary antibody
(Goat) anti-rabbit Ig)

primary rabbit
antibody (dilute)

antigen in tissue

Fig. 3. Three-step PAP method.

is concentrated with respect to the primary, so that only one antigen-binding site of each antiprimary immunoglobulin is occupied. The third layer consists of a complex of enzyme label bound to an antienzyme immunoglobulin raised in the same species as the primary antibody. This complex will therefore bind to the free antigen-binding sites of the second layer antibody. The peroxidase antiperoxidase complex is a stable, cyclic structure composed of two antiperoxidase molecules with one antigen-binding site of each sharing a peroxidase molecule and the other bound to an unshared molecule. Thus, the maximum amount of peroxidase is associated with each primary antibody molecule bound to its tissue antigen (**Fig. 3**). The APAAP complex is employed in a similar way but is not cyclic and is composed of two AP molecules per anti-AP.

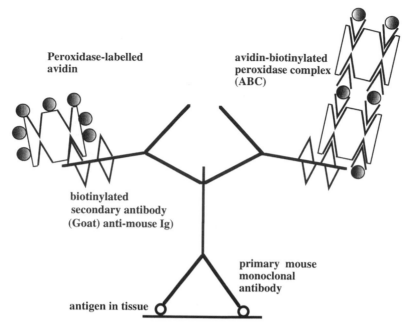

Fig. 4. Three-step avidin–biotin methods.

1.5.3.2. AVIDIN–BIOTIN METHODS

The remaining methods of routine importance are based on the strong attraction between a small vitamin, biotin, and a large glycoprotein, avidin (or protein, streptavidin). Antibodies can be labeled with large numbers of biotin molecules. Avidin (or streptavidin) has four binding sites for biotin, which has one binding site for avidin. Both avidin and biotin can be labeled with enzymes, colloidal gold, or fluorescent dyes. In the simplest system, labeled avidin is bound to a biotinylated second-layer antibody, producing a large amount of label on the site of reaction. A more complicated system, said to be more sensitive, is to combine biotinylated label and unlabeled avidin prior to use. A complex of avidin and labeled biotin is formed, since biotin molecules can share molecules of label. The components must be mixed in the proportions specified by the manufacturer so that enough unfilled biotin-binding sites are left on the avidin for the complex to bind to the biotinylated second antibody (**Fig. 4**).

1.6. Nonspecific and Unwanted Binding

One of the problems in all immunocytochemical methods is non-specific or unwanted binding of antibodies or other reagents to the tissue substrate. For further discussion and remedies *see* **Notes 7–12**.

1.6.1. Fc Receptors

Antibodies can bind via their Fc portions to Fc receptors in frozen or fresh tissue, and then be identified with the subsequent labeled antibody system. If they cannot be blocked with normal serum (**Note 8**) it may be necessary to use Fab fractions of antibodies. In paraffin sections, Fc receptors are destroyed, so this is not a problem.

1.6.2. Nonspecific Binding

Even in paraffin sections antibodies may bind through physical forces to hydrophobic or charged sites in the tissue, and these will be picked up in the staining reaction.

1.6.3. Specific Unwanted Binding

Specific unwanted binding can also take place. For example, in unpurified polyclonal antisera there may be populations of antibodies in addition to the ones resulting from immunization that could by chance find their own or similar antigens in the tissue and both polyclonal and monoclonal antibodies are candidates for crossreaction with molecules that have amino acid sequences or configurations similar to their own antigens.

1.7. Fixation

The type of fixation depends on the nature of the antigen to be localized. Large proteins are adequately denatured by precipitant fixatives, such as alcohol or acetone, or a combination fixative, such as Carnoy's or Methacarn, which contain reagents to prevent shrinkage of the tissues. These fixatives are suitable for postfixing fresh frozen sections or cell preparations and some of them (not acetone, except in freeze-substitution) can be used to fix small blocks of tissue prior to further dehydration and embedding in paraffin. However, in frozen sections of unfixed tissue these small peptides can dissolve and diffuse away during the brief thaw associated with the act of cutting the section so postfixation, even in formalin, may be unsuitable. Peptides generally require crosslinking fixation with formaldehyde or glutaraldehyde to make them insoluble before freezing the tissue block or processing it through graded alcohols and embedding in paraffin. The crosslinking fixatives will also fix the larger proteins and are best for tissue preservation in general, sometimes combined with a precipitant fixative, such as picric acid (Bouin's fixative). This type of fixation is used routinely for histopathologic specimens but there is a danger of overfixation of antigens so that the required epitopes are concealed. This can be a particular problem with tissues that have been fixed for a long period (more than 24 h) but, fortunately, there are now methods for retrieving these antigenic sites by treating sections with heat or protease digestion (*see* **Subheading 3.6.**). In tissue that has been fixed for a long time one of the more sensitive immunocytochemical techniques, such as the PAP or avidin–biotin complex (ABC) methods, is recommended.

2. Materials

2.1. Preparation of Frozen Blocks

1. Iso-pentane in a beaker precooled in liquid nitrogen to the solid state.
2. OCT compound (Bayer).
3. Cork disks or other nonconducting material (e.g., cardboard) to support block.
4. Hollow aluminum foil mold, made by wrapping a double thickness of foil around a suitably shaped, flat-bottomed object. The object is then removed.
5. Ball-point pen for labeling supporting structure on the back.
6. Storage container for frozen blocks, e.g., aluminum screw-top cylinder (Delapak Ltd.), that can be filed in a deep-freeze at –70°C or suitable cryogenic vials for long-term storage in a liquid nitrogen tank.
7. Cryostat (–20°C) with microtome.
8. Slides, suitably coated (*see* **Subheading 3.4.**) or multiwell slides.

2.2. Coating Slides with Poly-ʟ-Lysine

1. Clean, dry slides.
2. Poly-ʟ-lysine hydrobromide of high molecular weight (> 150,000) (Sigma P 1399), 0.1% solution in distilled water. Store aliquots frozen at –20°C and thaw completely before use. Replace in freezer after use. Ready-to-use solutions are commercially available (e.g., Sigma [St. Louis, MO] P 8920).

2.3. Coating Slides with APES

1. 3-Aminopropyltriethoxysilane (APES) (Sigma A3648).
2. Acetone.

2.4. Blocking Endogenous Peroxidase

2.4.1. Frozen Sections and Cell Preparations

1. Hydrogen peroxide (e.g., 30%).
2. 70% methanol in PBS, stored at room temperature. Methanol alone may be used. It is itself a partial inhibitor of peroxidase activity.

2.4.2. Paraffin Sections

1. Freshly prepared 0.3% hydrogen peroxide in tap water, distilled water, phosphate-buffered saline (PBS), or methanol.

2.5. Antibody Diluent (Not for Enzyme-Labeled Reagents)

1. 0.01 *M* phosphate-buffered 0.9% NaCl, pH 7.0–7.4, containing 0.1% bovine serum albumin (BSA) and 0.1% sodium azide (*see* **Note 4**).

2.6. Antigen Retrieval by Trypsin Treatment

1. Trypsin (crude porcine pancreatic, e.g., ICN 150213).
2. Distilled water or buffer (e.g. 0.001 M Tris-HCl buffer, pH 7.6) containing 0.1% calcium chloride, kept at 37°C.
3. pH meter and 0.1 M NaOH.

2.7. Antigen Retrieval by Microwaving in Citrate Buffer

1. Microwave oven with revolving plate and variable wattage.
2. Plastic slide carrier.
3. Plastic container with lid, for about 500 mL (e.g., sandwich box).
4. 0.01 M sodium citrate/citric acid buffer, pH 6.0 (adjusted with 0.2 M NaOH). This solution can be stored at room temperature for a few days.
5. Distilled water for topping up.

2.8. Indirect Immunofluorescence

1. Frozen sections or cell preparations appropriately fixed.
2. Humid incubation chamber, e.g., large Petri dish containing a rack made from glass rods or wooden applicator sticks to support slides off the bottom, and paper tissue wads well dampened with distilled water.
3. Slide rack and container or Coplin jar for rinsing slides.
4. PAP pen, available from most immunoreagent-supplying companies.
5. Buffer: 0.01 M 0.9% PBS, pH 7.0–7.4 (*see* **Note 1**).
6. Normal serum from species providing second antibody at 1/20 dilution in PBS antibody diluent (*see* **Subheading 2.5.**) for blocking nonspecific binding (e.g., normal goat serum).
7. Primary antibody at predetermined optimal dilution in PBS antibody diluent (e.g., mouse mAb).
8. Fluorescein- or rhodamine-labeled second antibody against species of primary antibody (e.g., goat-antimouse immunoglobulin) at predetermined optimal dilution in antibody diluent.
9. Pasteur pipets or pipet with disposable tips.
10. Paper tissues.

2.9. Indirect Immunoperoxidase

1. Sections or cell preparations on slides, endogenous peroxidase blocked and antigen retrieval done as above if appropriate.
2. Racks, buffer, and humid chamber as for immunofluorescence.
3. PAP pen.
4. PBS buffer.
5. Normal serum as for immunofluorescence.
6. Primary antibody as for immunofluorescence.
7. Second antibody, peroxidase labeled, at its predetermined optimal dilution in PBS/TBS without azide or in Protexidase (ICN).

8. DAB, H_2O_2, and PBS for developing the peroxidase.
9. Hematoxylin for counterstaining.
10. Alcohols, solvent, mountant.

2.10. Three-Step PAP Method

1. **Items 1–6** from **Subheading 2.9.**
2. Unconjugated second antibody at predetermined optimal dilution in PBS diluent.
3. PAP complex, same species as primary antibody, at predetermined optimal concentration in PBS without azide or in Protexidase.
4. Other reagents as in **Subheading 2.9.**

2.11. Three-Step Peroxidase-Labeled Avidin–Biotin Method

1. **Items 1–6** from **Subheading 2.9.**
2. Biotin-conjugated second antibody at predetermined optimal dilution in PBS antibody diluent.
3. Peroxidase-labeled avidin or streptavidin (labeled avidin method) at optimal dilution in PBS without azide or in Protexidase, or biotinylated peroxidase and unlabeled avidin or streptavidin (ABC method).
4. Other reagents as in **Subheading 2.9.**

2.12. Development of Peroxidase with Diaminobenzidine

1. Diaminobenzidine tetrahydrochloride, $2H_2O$ (e.g., Sigma D 5637).
2. Hydrogen peroxide solution.
3. PBS.

2.13. Development of Alkaline Phosphatase to Give a Red Color

1. 0.1 *M* Tris-HCl buffer, pH 8.2.
2. Levamisole hydrochloride (Sigma L 9756) (inhibitor of endogenous nonintestinal alkaline phosphatase isoforms).
3. Fast Red TR salt (chromogen) (Sigma F 8764).
4. Naphthol AS-MX phosphate, sodium salt (Sigma N 5000).
5. *N,N*-Dimethyl formamide.
6. Mayer's hematoxylin (nuclear counterstain).
7. Aquaperm (Immunon, Life Sciences 484975) or other aqueous mountant.

3. Methods

3.1. Paraffin Sections

After fixation, dehydration through graded alcohols, and embedding in a paraffin wax block, thin sections (2–5 μm) are cut, floated on a warm water bath, picked up on glass microscope slides and dried for several hours or overnight at 37–45°C. Brief drying in a 60°C oven will not harm most antigens and may help to keep the sections on the slides, but heating the sections on a hotplate is not advised. The slides must be precoated with a section adhesive, such as poly-L-lysine (*see* **Subheading 3.4.1.**) or, for methods requiring heat-mediated antigen retrieval, APES (*see* **Subheading 3.4.2.**). Suitable pretreated slides, such as Vectabond or Polysine slides, are commercially available. Once dried, paraffin sections may be stored for months or years at room temperature without apparent damage to antigenicity. Paraffin blocks are suitable for recutting after many years of storage.

To prepare paraffin sections for immunostaining, remove the paraffin in two or three changes of xylene or other solvent, and hydrate through several changes of 100, 90, and 70% alcohol to water. Block endogenous peroxidase (*see* **Subheading 3.5.**), carry out any antigen-retrieval methods required (*see* **Subheading 3.6.**), and place the slides in phosphate-buffered or Tris-buffered saline (PBS or TBS).

3.2. Preparation of Frozen Sections

Correct rapid freezing technique is essential for the preparation of sections with good structure. Liquid nitrogen is the coldest available freezing medium but is a poor conductor, so a layer of gaseous nitrogen is formed around a warm tissue block immersed in it, preventing conduction and resulting in slow freezing and the formation of ice crystals in the tissue, which distort the structure. Isopentane is a good conductor and the rapidity of freezing compensates for the slightly higher temperature of liquid isopentane. It is used at its melting point that is the lowest possible temperature compatible with the liquid state.

It is helpful to freeze the block on a supporting structure that can be labeled and, after cutting, removed from the object holder for storage at low temperature. Once tissue has been snap-frozen it is important not to let it thaw, because this will result in movement of molecules within the tissue and ice crystal formation if it is refrozen. Frozen blocks may be stored at –20°C for a few hours, or at –40° to –70°C for long-term storage. In all cases, seal the blocks in plastic bags or other containers, excluding as much air as possible to prevent the tissue from drying out.

Arrange the block so that the cutting surface contains the parts of the tissue required in the correct orientation.

1. Place tissue block (not more than 5 mm thick) either with the cutting surface up on a drop of OCT on a cork or cardboard disk that can be labeled on the back with a ballpoint pen, directly on the object holder on a drop of OCT, or in a hollow aluminum foil mold with the cutting surface down. Fill the mold with OCT and place a labeled cork on top. After freezing, remove the foil and you will have a frozen, even-sided, flat-surfaced block of OCT containing the tissue on a labeled base.

2. Remove the beaker of isopentane from liquid nitrogen and allow it to stand at room temperature until the isopentane is partly melted.
3. Holding the cork disk, the object holder, or the foil mold with forceps, immerse the block in melting isopentane for a few seconds until frozen.
4. Place the cork/cardboard disk carrying the frozen block on a drop of OCT on a precooled object holder in the cryostat until it is frozen on.
5. Cut sections (5 μm) and pick up on poly-L-lysine-coated slides.
6. Dry sections at room temperature for at least 1 h; several hours or overnight may improve adhesion.
7. Fix in acetone or alcohol for 10 min.
8. Allow evaporation of the fixative. If desired, draw round sections with a hydrophobic pen to create an antibody chamber (*see* **Subheading 3.7.**). If sections are not to be used within a day, store them at –20°C, wrapped back-to-back in "cling-film" or foil, sealed in a plastic bag containing some silica gel or other dehydrating agent. Before use remove the entire bag from the deep-freeze and allow it to warm to room temperature before opening, This allows any water from condensation to be taken up by the silica gel and not to condense on cold sections, which might damage the tissue structure, particularly if the sections are stored without fixation.
9. Block endogenous peroxidase if necessary.
10. Place slides in PBS or TBS (*see* **Note 2**).

3.3. Preparation of Cells

These may be made on poly-L-lysine-coated slides and treated in the same way as frozen sections. Cell cultures on coverslips can also be used but are more difficult to handle. Excess medium should be rinsed off before the cells are fixed.

Cell preparations for formalin fixation should be fixed immediately after the cells have settled on the slide without drying, and should then be transferred to buffer for storage until used. After alcohol fixation, cell preparations can be left in the alcohol (store at 4°C) or air-dried.

3.4. Slide Coating

3.4.1. Coating Slides with Poly-L-Lysine

This procedure can be used for paraffin sections or prefixed frozen sections. Many slides may be coated at one time and stored indefinitely at room temperature.

Place a small amount (about 10 μL) of poly-L-lysine (0.1%) at one end of a slide. Using another slide, rock the end of the slide in the drop to spread the solution then, holding the applicator slide at an angle of about 30°, push the solution along the slide to form an even film over the surface. Interference colors should be seen, indicating that the film is suitably thin. If droplets of solution form on the slide, the surface is not clean enough, and the slide should be discarded. The film dries immediately. Mark the coated side, because it is otherwise indistinguishable from the uncoated slide.

For unfixed frozen sections or cell preparations the above method is satisfactory, but an alternative for preparations that will not require antigen retrieval is to use poly-L-lysine of lower molecular weight (30,000), dip racks of slides into the solution, and allow them to dry.

3.4.2. Coating Slides with APES

1. Rinse racks of slides in acetone for 5 min.
2. Immerse in 2% APES in acetone for 2 min.
3. Rinse in two changes of acetone, 5 min each.
4. Allow to dry and store indefinitely at room temperature.

3.5. Blocking Endogenous Peroxidase

3.5.1. Frozen Sections and Cell Preparations

1. Just before use, add hydrogen peroxide to 70% methanol in PBS to a final concentration of 0.3%.
2. Incubate fixed preparations taken from the dry state or from alcohol or PBS for 30 min, then rinse in PBS and leave in PBS until the next step. Do not let the preparations dry from this stage on.

For an alternative method, see **ref. 8**.

3.5.2. Paraffin Sections

1. Incubate sections for 30 min at room temperature in 0.3% hydrogen peroxide solution. Alternatively, use 0.6% hydrogen peroxide for 15 min.
2. Rinse in water and transfer sections to PBS.

3.6. Antigen Retrieval

It is now well established that some antigen molecules, particularly large proteins, become excessively crosslinked internally during formaldehyde fixation, obscuring the antigenic sites and preventing binding of the primary antibody. Two main strategies for overcoming this problem have been developed. The first is to "digest" the fixed tissue sections with a protease, such as trypsin or protease XXIV. The second, more recently discovered *(9,10)*, is to apply intense heat by microwaving or pressure cooking in a calcium-chelating solution. The time of treatment must be determined by experiment (usually within the range of 2–20 min). If the initial immunostaining test is unsuccessful, it is advisable to try with antigen retrieval techniques before abandoning hope. The two most common methods are given here. Antigen retrieval applies only to aldehyde-fixed preparations, after bringing to water, and can be done before or after peroxidase blocking. The time determined for antigen retrieval varies with the antigen and may have to be increased if the preparation has been fixed for an abnormally long time. It is very important that the method for antigen retrieval be standardized in each laboratory so that preparations are always treated under the same conditions.

3.6.1. Antigen Retrieval by Trypsin Treatment

1. Weigh appropriate amount of trypsin for 0.1% final concentration.
2. Dissolve it in appropriate amount of warm buffer/water with calcium chloride.
3. Quickly adjust the pH to 7.8 with NaOH.
4. Immerse sections at 4°C for the predetermined time.
5. Rinse in running water and proceed with the immunostaining method.

Enzyme solutions can be applied in drops on the preparations, but a more uniform and reproducible effect is achieved by immersion in a large volume of solution. For more expensive enzymes, such as protease XXIV, which may be more useful for some antigens, the drop method is preferred.

3.6.2. Antigen Retrieval by Microwaving in Citrate Buffer

1. In the microwave oven place 500 mL of buffer in the plastic dish with the lid on loosely and a separate plastic beaker containing 200 mL of distilled water.
2. Heat at 750 W for 2 min (about 60°C).
3. Remove the beaker of water, centralize the buffer container on the revolving plate, and immerse the sections in the plastic slide carrier. Replace the lid loosely. If no lid is available, cover the dish with cling-film.
4. Heat at 750 W for 5 min (solution will boil).
5. Check the level of the liquid in the dish and if necessary top-up to the 500 mL mark with the warm distilled water.
6. Repeat **steps 4** and **5** for the predetermined heating time.
7. Cool the preparations by running cold water into the dish of slides. Do not remove slides from the hot solution or the buffer will crystallize on the preparations and drying artifacts will be introduced. Continue with the immunostaining method. If preparations with different optimal heating times are being treated at the same time, begin with the slides that need the longest incubation time, then add the others at the appropriate time. Thus, you can avoid removing hot slides from the solution. Other calcium chelating solutions that have been used in this method include urea and ethylenediaminetetraacetic acid (EDTA).

3.7. Isolating Sections with Water-Repellent Pen

Encircle sections on the slide with a water-repellent PAP pen to contain the drops of antibody over the section and reduce the care needed when drying around the sections before applying antibody. This also allows several sections on the same slide to be immunostained with different concentrations of antibody or with different antibodies without danger of the solutions mixing. The same effect can be obtained by mounting sections on multiwell slides that are already compartmentalized with Teflon, but these may not be coated with poly-L-lysine, risking detachment of sections.

3.8. Finding the "Correct" Antibody Dilution (see Note 3)

1. Select a tissue known to contain a large quantity of antigen.
2. Immunostain with doubling dilutions of primary antibody, using the conditions that you intend to use in your experiments.
3. Choose the dilution that gives a good positive stain with minimal background, at the stage in the series before the positive staining begins to be reduced. This dilution can then act as standard for subsequent work, and it should not be necessary to alter it unless you change your method.

This test assumes that the dilution of the second/third layer reagents has already been standardized in another system. It is not usually necessary to adjust them for different primary antibodies.

3.9. Immunostaining Methods

It is important in all staining to include appropriate positive and negative controls (see **Notes 5** and **6**). As discussed in **Subheading 1.**, nonspecific binding can cause false positives. For methods to overcome this *see* **Notes 7–12**.

3.9.1. Indirect Immunofluorescence

Treat slides one at a time until you become proficient. It is important that the preparations do not dry.

1. Remove the slide from the buffer. With a paper tissue, dry around the section or cells, making sure the section stays damp but that there is either a dry PAP pen circle around it or a well dried area of slide to create surface tension between the drop of antibody on the section and the glass around it.
2. Place the slide in the humid chamber and apply a drop of normal serum. When all preparations have been treated, cover the dish and leave for 10 min (or longer).
3. Drain the serum onto a paper tissue, but do not rinse the slide; the preparation should stay moist with serum. Make sure the area around the preparation is dry.
4. Apply a drop of primary antibody or negative or positive control solution to cover the preparation (*see* **Note 4**). Repeat for the remaining slides, cover the dish, and leave for the appointed time at room temperature or at 4°C, according to the method you are using.
5. Drain off the antibody and rinse the preparations in three changes of PBS for 5 min each.
6. Dry around the preparations as before and apply a drop of fluorescent second antibody. Cover the dish and leave for 30 min to 1 h at room temperature, according to your method.
7. Drain off the antibody and rinse in three changes of PBS as in **step 5**.
8. Mount in a water-based, fluorescence-free mountant containing a fluorescence preserver (e.g., Permafluor, Immunon, Life Sciences 434980).
9. View in a fluorescence microscope with appropriate filters.

3.9.2. Indirect Immunoperoxidase

Tissue is prepared as in **Subheading 2.9.1.**

1. Follow **Subheading 3.9.1.** for indirect immunofluorescence up to **step 5**.
2. Dry the slides as before and apply a drop of peroxidase-labeled second antibody. Cover the dish and leave for 30 min to 1 h at room temperature.
3. Rinse in three changes of PBS.
4. Develop peroxidase (*see* **Subheading 3.9.5.**).
5. Rinse in water, counterstain lightly in hematoxylin, differentiate in acid alcohol, Blue in Scott's or tap water, dehydrate through graded alcohols, clear in solvent, and mount in permanent mountant.

3.9.3. Three-Step PAP Method

1. Follow **steps 1–5** in **Subheading 3.9.1.**
2. Apply unconjugated second antibody. Leave for 30 min.
3. Rinse in three changes of PBS.
4. Apply PAP complex. Leave for 30 min.
5. Rinse in three changes of PBS.
6. Develop enzyme and finish as in **Subheading 3.9.2.**

3.9.4. Three-Step Peroxidase-Labeled Avidin-Biotin Method

1. Follow **steps 1–5** in **Subheading 3.9.1.**
2. Apply biotinylated second antibody. Leave for 30 min at room temperature. At this stage, if the ABC method is being used, mix the biotinylated peroxidase and avidin or streptavidin as recommended by the manufacturer and allow them to react for at least 30 min.
3. Rinse in three changes of PBS, 5 min each.
4. Apply the ABC or labeled avidin. Leave for 30 min at room temperature.
5. Rinse in three changes of PBS, 5 min each.
6. Develop peroxidase and finish as for **Subheading 3.9.2.**

3.9.5. Development of Peroxidase with Diaminobenzidine

The incubating solution should be fresh, but remains functional for at least 1 h after being made.

1. Make a 0.05% solution of DAB in PBS in sufficient volume to immerse a rack of slides.
2. Add hydrogen peroxide to 0.01% final concentration.
3. Immerse the preparations for 10 min.
4. Remove the preparations to a container of PBS and check the staining under a microscope. A dark brown reaction product should be seen. If the reaction is weak, redevelop for a further 5 min. Beyond this time, little improvement can be expected.

5. Rinse in tap water, counterstain lightly with hematoxylin, differentiate in acid alcohol, and "blue" in Scott's alkaline tap water substitute if desired or in running tap water. Dehydrate through graded alcohols, clear in solvent, and mount in synthetic mountant.

See safety **Note 13.**

3.9.6. Alkaline Phosphatase-Labeled Methods

Methods using alkaline phosphatase as the label are the same as the peroxidase methods, but the endogenous peroxide blocking step is omitted. Many alkaline phosphatase endproducts of reaction are alcohol-soluble so the preparations must be mounted in a water-based mountant. The latest type are applied without coverslip and dry as a film on the preparation. Their refractive index is the same as that of glass and a drop of synthetic mountant and coverslip can be applied after the film is dry if desired.

3.9.6.1. DEVELOPMENT OF ALKALINE PHOSPHATASE TO GIVE A RED COLOR

1. Make stock solution of naphthol AS-MX phosphate (substrate). Weigh 20 mg naphthol AS-MX phosphate. Place in a beaker and (in a fume hood) dissolve in 2 mL dimethyl formamide. Add quickly, with stirring, 18 mL 0.1 M Tris-HCl buffer, pH 8.2. Divide into 1 mL aliquots, each containing 1 mg naphthol AS-MX phosphate, and store frozen.
2. Thaw one aliquot of substrate and mix it with 4 mL of Tris-HCl buffer, pH 8.2, containing 1.2 mg Levamisole (final concentration 1 mM).
3. In this dissolve 5 mg Fast Red TR salt, shake well, and filter onto the preparations in a damp chamber. Cover and incubate at room temperature or 37°C for 5–10 min (possibly longer).
4. Examine preparations microscopically for a red reaction product.
5. Rinse in water and counterstain nuclei lightly with Mayer's hematoxylin.
6. Do not differentiate in acid-alcohol (reaction product is alcohol-soluble). Blue in tap water or Scott's solution. Rinse in water and mount in aqueous mountant.

4. Notes

1. The buffer used for diluting the antibodies and for rinsing the preparations is 0.01 M 0.9% PBS, pH 7.0–7.4. Alternatively, TBS may be used throughout. Methods given here use PBS, but TBS could be substituted.
2. Once frozen sections have become wet with an aqueous solution it is very important not to let them dry at all. Drying produces structural artifacts.
3. The aim in immunostaining is to use an antibody concentration that is in excess of any expected amount of antigen in the tissue, to ensure that all antigenic sites are occupied by detecting antibody. Provided that the antibody is tested on a tissue that contains a large amount of antigen, the selected concentration will be

adequate for a tissue that contains less antigen, provided that the same method is used. Optimal concentrations using a very sensitive three-layer method will be lower than for a less sensitive two-layer method. The time of incubation with the primary antibody is also important, particularly for polyclonal antibodies, which may contain a variety of antibodies to different epitopes of the antigen. In a short incubation (i.e., 1 h at room temperature) only the most avid of the antibody populations will bind. Given a longer incubation, such as 4 h at room temperature or overnight at 4°C, the less avid antibodies have a chance to find their targets, so a higher dilution is possible. For reasons of economy and to avoid as much background binding as possible, it is sensible not to use a higher concentration of antibody than necessary. A "correct" dilution for a polyclonal antiserum is usually in the region of 1/100–1/5000 or higher. If the immunoglobulin fraction is being used, rather than the whole serum, different values may be found. The supplier may give some guidelines in the data-sheet, but it is as well to test the antibody in your own system.

Monoclonal antibodies should be tested similarly. Because it is possible to arrive at a known concentration for a mAb, the procedure is easier. A concentration of 1–10 µg/mL is usually "correct" for a mAb, depending on its avidity and the sensitivity of the method used.

4. For immediate use, concentrated antibodies can be diluted in PBS. For storage of antibody solutions at their working dilution at 4°C, use PBS containing 0.1% BSA, a high concentration of an "inert" protein, which protects the antibody molecules from attaching to protein-binding sites on the walls of the storage vessel, and 0.1% sodium azide, to prevent microbial and fungal growth. Many antibodies can be stored conveniently for months at their working dilution, but some are better stored more concentrated, snap-frozen rapidly by immersion in liquid nitrogen, in aliquots that can be diluted to a convenient volume when required. Repeated thawing and freezing is not recommended for any mAb. Polyclonal antibodies are more robust but, if kept frozen, should be diluted not more than 1/10–1/100 in PBS to maintain a high protein concentration. Antibodies can be kept at –20°C diluted 1:1 with glycerine, which will prevent freezing. Storage preferences should be checked before committing a large volume of antibody to any option.

Enzyme-labeled reagents should not be stored in azide-containing solutions, since azide is an enzyme inhibitor. Peroxidase-linked reagents can be kept ready diluted at 4°C in one of the proprietary solutions (e.g. Protexidase, ICN 980631).

5. It is essential to carry through a positive control with every immunostaining run. The control consists of known positive tissue prepared in the same way as the test tissue, and will show that all reagents are in working order. Failure of the control staining means that a negative result on the test cannot be trusted.

6. Negative controls consist of the test tissue immunostained in the absence of the primary antibody (substitute buffer) or using an inappropriate primary antibody (to an antigen that is absent from the test tissue or in a different location). This will show the level of background staining that may be expected in the test reaction from the second (and third) layer reagents and will highlight problems, such

as pigment, endogenous enzyme or biotin, immunoglobulin receptors, or damaged cells that take up antibodies indiscriminately. If an inappropriate mAb is used, ensure that it is of the same immunoglobulin subclass as the test antibody.

If an "unknown" antibody is being tested, with antigen in an unknown localization, it will be necessary to test any perceived positive staining for specificity by absorption of the antibody with pure antigen *(2,7)*. Additional evidence of specificity can be achieved by using the test antibody on inappropriate tissue that does not contain the antigen; this should give a negative result.

7. With avidin–biotin methods, it may be necessary to block endogenous biotin, particularly in liver and kidney. This is simply done by prior application of unlabeled avidin (1 mg/mL for 20 min) followed, after rinsing, by unlabeled biotin (0.1 mg/mL for 20 min) *(6)*.

8. Binding to Fc receptors or nonspecific tissue sites can be reduced before application of the primary antibody by applying nonimmune serum or immunoglobulins from the species providing the second antibody. This will occupy the binding sites and prevent binding by the primary antibody. Since the blocking immunoglobulin is of the same species as the second antibody, no binding of this layer can occur, and neither PAP (or APAAP) nor labeled avidin can bind to it.

    Nonspecific binding reactions are weak compared with specific ones, and can be reduced by including detergent in the rinsing buffer (e.g. 0.05% Tween 20) or by raising the salt content of the antibody diluent from 0.9 to 2.5%.

9. Unwanted antibody populations binding to their antigens in the tissue can best be eliminated by diluting the primary (polyclonal) antibody as far as possible, thus reducing the concentration of unwanted antibodies, and by using a sensitive method to identify the wanted antigen. Optimal dilutions for both polyclonal and monoclonal antibodies must be established (*see* **Note 3**).

10. An area for vigilance is the crossreaction (specific) of a second layer immunoglobulin, i.e., a goat antimouse immunoglobulin, with the immunoglobulin of the host tissue species. If human tissue is being stained, unpurified antimouse immunoglobulin may contain some crossreacting antibodies to human immunoglobulin, simply because of the general resemblances among immunoglobulins of different species. With antibodies to mouse immunoglobulins applied to rat tissue the danger of crossreactivity of the antimouse immunoglobulin with rat immunoglobulin in the tissue is even greater because of the close relation between the species. The answer is to buy species-specific second antibodies that have been absorbed with immunoglobulins from the host tissue species or, in the laboratory, simply add 1% of the host species serum to the diluted second antibody and allow it to react for at least 30 min before using it. The stock diluted solution can be absorbed in bulk. Test the effectiveness of the absorption by applying the absorbed antibody to frozen sections of spleen or tonsil from the host species. If no immunoglobulin-containing plasma cells are immunostained, the absorption has been successful. It may be necessary to increase the standard working concentration of the second antibody after this treatment because some of the previously reacting antibody population has been made inactive.

11. Crossreactivity of the wanted primary antibody with related molecules is relatively rare. It occurs when the antigen is part of a family of structurally related molecules present in the same tissue, e.g., gastrin and cholecystokinin in the small intestine. It is difficult to eliminate and impossible with mAbs that, by definition, react with one epitope only. The best remedy is to be aware of the possibility of crossreaction, to absorb the antibody with different fragments of the antigen molecule, if available, to identify the crossreacting epitopes, and to try different antibodies to the same antigen, in the hope of finding one that is noncrossreactive.

12. Other common hazards to be aware of are pigment in the tissue that could be construed as a positive immunoperoxidase reaction (look at an unstained section) or incompletely blocked endogenous enzyme (develop a section that has not been subjected to the immunostaining reagents). For further discussion of problems see **ref. 7**.

13. DAB is a potential carcinogen. Work in a fumehood to avoid aerosol inhalation. Wear gloves. Dispose of the used solution by oxidizing it with sodium hypochlorite (a few drops of household bleach). The solution will become black. It can then be poured down the drain with plenty of water. Rinse the container well with water to avoid traces of bleach contaminating the next DAB solution to be used in it.

    A safe way of using DAB *(11)* is to buy a preweighed amount and dissolve it in water to give a 50 mg/mL solution. Store aliquots of the solution at –20°C and use as required. A 1-mL aliquot will give 100 mL 0.05% DAB incubating solution. As for the protease digestion, enzyme development can be done in drops on the preparations but the risk of contacting the carcinogen is greater and a uniform development time for all the preparations in a run is harder to achieve than if the preparations are put in a slide carrier and immersed in a large volume of solution.

    DAB can be bought in tablet or liquid form, which is convenient, but the expense of this dictates the drops-on-slides method of development.

References

1. Beesley, J. (ed.) (1993) *Immunocytochemistry, A Practical Approach,* Oxford University Press, Oxford, UK.
2. Polak, J. M. and Van Noorden, S. (1997) *Introduction to Immunocytochemistry,* 2nd ed., Bios Scientific Publishers, Oxford, UK.
3. Leong, A. S.-Y. (1993) *Applied Immunocytochemistry for the Surgical Pathologist,* Edward Arnold, Melbourne, Australia.
4. Sternberger, L. A. (1986) *Immunocytochemistry,* 3rd ed., Wiley, New York.
5. Larsson, L.-I. (1988) *Immunocytochemistry, Theory and Practice,* CRC, Boca Raton, FL.
6. Wood, G. S. and Warnke, R. (1981) Suppression of endogenous avidin-binding activity in tissues and its relevance to biotin-avidin detection systems. *J. Histochem. Cytochem.* **34,** 1196–1204.
7. Van Noorden, S. (1993) Problems and solutions, in *Immunocytochemistry, A Practical Approach* (Beesley, J., ed.), Oxford University Press, Oxford, UK, pp. 207–239.

8. Andrew, S. and Jasani, B. (1987) An improved method for the inhibition of endogenous peroxidase non-deleterious to lymphocyte surface markers. Application to immunoperoxidase studies on eosinophil-rich tissue preparations. *Histochem. J.* **19,** 426–430.

9. Cattoretti, G., Pileri, S., Parravicini, C., et al. (1993) Antigen unmasking on formalin-fixed, paraffin-embedded tissue sections. *J. Pathol.* **171,** 83–98.

10. Morgan, J. M., Jasani, B., and Navabi, H. (1997) A mechanism for high temperature antigen retrieval involving calcium complexes produced by formalin fixation. *J. Cell. Pathol.* **2,** 89–92.

11. Pelliniemi, L. J., Dym, M., and Karnovsky, M. J. (1980) Peroxidase histochemistry using diaminobenzidine tetrahydrochloride stored as a frozen solution. *J. Histochem. Cytochem.* **28,** 191,192.

35

Immunolabeling for Electron Microscopy

Catherine E. Sarraf

1. Introduction

The protocols in this chapter concern postembedding immunolabeling for transmission electron microscopy; other schedules, such as pre-embedding methods, frozen tissue processes, and procedures for scanning electron microscopy, can be found elsewhere (1). In principle, immunolabeling at the electron microscope (EM) level follows the same precepts as immunolabeling at the light microscope level; in tissues or cells, the location of an antigen of interest is identified by a specific antibody, and must be visualized appropriately for investigation. Electron microscopy permits us to distinguish subcellular organelles, and therefore ultrastructural localization of antigen position. At the EM level, however, the "visualizing step" needs to be provided by an electron-dense entity, most often a heavy metal, which reflects incident electrons; this is in contrast to the final step of light microscope level techniques, in which the final reaction product is sought to be colored (and where there is an element of choice of which color to use). Tissue processing for EM is considerably more severe than that for light microscopy, and thus maintenance of antigenicity in tissue is more taxing. Before immunolabeling for electron microscopy can be fruitful, the first step is to ensure that the antigen of interest is present (or is still present) in the tissue; this is done by performing a thorough procedure at the light microscope level on wax-embedded sections. Once a positive result has been obtained, studies can progress to the ultrastructural level. If the presence of an antigen *cannot* be demonstrated in a wax-embedded block, it *will not* be demonstrable in a resin-embedded EM block of the same tissue. In such a case, pre-embedding and frozen tissue techniques can be of use at both light and electron microscope levels.

From: *Methods in Molecular Medicine, Vol. 40: Diagnostic and Therapeutic Antibodies*
Edited by: A. J. T. George and C. E. Urch © Humana Press Inc., Totowa, NJ

EM postembedding immunolabeling requires tissue sections to be cut at a thickness of approx 100 nm, and collected on nickel grids (<0.5 cm in diameter). For this procedure, the tissue must be fixed (chemically preserved), possibly treated with osmium, dehydrated, and embedded by impregnation with liquid resin, which is then polymerized into a solid block from which the sections are sliced. Each step is accompanied by a reduction in antigenicity in the specimen; to obtain optimal immunolabeling a balance must be reached between retention of antigenicity and provision of good morphology.

1.1. Fixation

The most commonly used fixatives before EM immunolabeling are glutaraldehyde and paraformaldehyde. The former is a bifunctional reagent and crosslinks proteins well, but it does not penetrate tissue very quickly; paraformaldehyde penetrates rapidly but because it is only unifunctional, preservation of morphology is less precise. Mixtures are frequently used to combine the favorable characteristics of each. In general, paraformaldehyde fixation is kinder to tissue that is to be immunolabeled, because the crosslinking property of glutaraldehyde can deform the tertiary structure of many antigens. Organs or, indeed, whole animals can be perfused with fixative, or else small tissue blocks (<1 mm^3) are immersed in the solution for at least 1 h. Overexposure to glutaraldehyde hardens tissue, so after the fixation period blocks are removed and held in phosphate buffer solution until the next step is to be performed; when blocks are fixed in paraformaldehyde the tissue can be left in it until required.

1.2. Preosmication

Osmium is a metal of high atomic number, and as such its compounds are highly electron dense. They also have crosslinking properties, so in electron microscopy they have the dual purpose of providing visual contrast in tissues and adding a further level of fixation. This procedure is frequently omitted when immunolabeling is to be performed, although this is not a total necessity as antigenicity can be partially restored when grid-mounted sections are immersed in sodium metaperiodate. As ever, retention of both antigenicity and ultrastructural integrity have to be weighed against each other.

1.3. Dehydration

Water is immiscible with resin, and it has to be removed from tissue blocks before they can be impregnated by the liquid monomer. Progression through graded alcohols can reduce antigenicity, but even this is preferable to dehydration by such reagents as 2,4,6 tri(dimethylaminomethyl) phenol (DMP).

1.4. Embedding

Broadly, two types of resin are commonly used for electron microscopy, the hydrophilic acrylic resins and the hydrophobic epoxies. In general, the resin of choice is frequently Araldite (epoxy) Araldite TAAB® Laboratories, Aldermaston, UK); it allows penetration of antibodies, particularly if mildly etched with hydrogen peroxide, and is totally electron-beam stable. However, there are many advantages to be gained from using acrylic resins, such as Lowicryl (Agar Scientific, Stanstead, UK); because these are hydrophilic severe dehydration can be avoided and tissue can be embedded directly from 70% alcohol. In addition, the acrylic resins polymerize at lower temperatures than the epoxies, eliminating the possibility of heat denaturation of antigens.

Postembedding immunolabeling has many advantages and results are easily reproducible; it is always the strategy of first choice. Subcellular localization of antigens is much more specific than by pre-embedding techniques, where the tissue components are still labile. In postembedding methods there is no reduction in labeling from diffusion variables because antibodies are applied directly to ultrathin sections after they have been cut from the block. This leaves the block unlabeled, so an immense number of serial sections is potentially available that can be called into use as controls, for quantitation comparisons, to identify different antigens on different occasions, and for simultaneous multiple labeling. The disadvantages, however, have to be borne in mind; there is the inevitable reduction in antigenicity, so sensitivity of the procedures is incontrovertibly lower than with pre-embedding or frozen-tissue methods. The only other drawback is when the antigen of interest is sparingly and heterogeneously distributed through a tissue. EM blocks are very small, and it may be that antigen-expressing cells are not present in all samples. In routine electron microscopy, sections 1 μm thick are always cut from EM blocks and are examined at the light microscope level first to determine that the structure/ cell type of interest is present in the block. When EM immunolabeling is to be undertaken, this stage is even more rigorously important, and it might be necessary to first perform immunolabeling at the light microscope level on 1 μm sections from the EM blocks.

Whichever method of tissue preparation has been selected, the objective is to label the antigen and render it visible on the electron microscope. The most sensitive techniques employ indirect immunolabeling, and in the simplest case a primary antibody is directed against the antigen of interest, and a secondary antibody, conjugated to an electron dense moiety, is directed against immunoglobulin (IgG) of the species in which the primary antibody was raised. For example, when a certain human antigen is to be detected, the primary incubation might be rabbit antihuman antigen; the secondary incubation would be labeled goat antirabbit IgG.

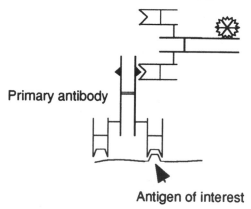

Fig. 1. Diagrammatic representation of indirect immunolabeling using an immunogold technique. Although the amplification of the antibody/antigen signal is only 2× (one primary antibody can bind two secondary antibodies + gold grain), the electron density of gold is so high that it is easily discernible.

As in light microscopy, to eliminate nonspecific background staining and to increase sensitivity of the method, further steps can be incorporated. Monoclonal or polyclonal primary antibodies are available commercially or directly from their source, but final layer polyclonal antibodies are commercially available and fall into one of two groups: particulate or enzymatic conjugates.

Particulate conjugates are high-atomic-number metal particles noncovalently bound to the final (secondary in this case) antibody. Ferritin and iron/dextran complexes have been used in the past, but these are now largely obsolete. In general, since the introduction of immunogold conjugates by Faulk and Taylor in 1971 *(2)*, gold is virtually always the particulate marker of choice (**Fig. 1**). Anti-immunoglobulin antibodies are adsorbed on to the surface of colloidal gold, so when the conjugate locates the primary antibody, gold grains are specifically bound to the appropriate organelle at the site of the antigen of interest (**Fig. 2**). This method can also be used to label the site of uptake of synthetic antigenic precursors *(3)*.

Commercially produced immunogold colloids have grains of regular ovoid or spherical shape and various standard sizes are produced determined by the method in which gold chloride is reduced: yellow or white phosphorous results in grains of 3–5 nm diameter, sodium ascorbate results in grains of 5–15 nm diameter, by sodium citrate results in the largest diameter grains, depending on the quantity of citrate present. For transmission electron microscopy the largest gold particles routinely used are 40 nm in diameter, but larger grains may

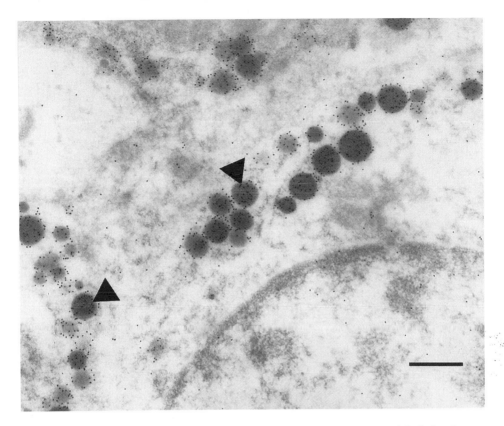

Fig. 2. High-power electron micrograph of rat pituitary immunolabeled using an immunogold technique: the gold grains demonstrate the presence of growth hormone on the granules of somatotrophs (arrows) (bar = 0.4 μm).

be desired for scanning electron microscopy. The advantages of using smaller sized particles are the lower cost, higher efficiency, and lower steric hindrance between them; the advantages of larger particles are generally related to their ease of detection. Choice of gold particle size clearly depends on the use to which it is to be put, but in general, smaller particle sizes can be advantageous on nonosmicated sections, or on tissue that is not highly counterstained, whereas larger sizes are preferable to label comparatively large or electron dense organelles.

Enzymatic conjugates are detectable because the final layer, antibody/ enzyme conjugate, is provided with the enzyme's substrate; the reaction between the two is visualized to an electron-dense final reaction product (FRP) at the site of the immunolabel. Historically, several enzyme systems have been used in this way, including the cytochromes, glucose oxidase, and acid phos-

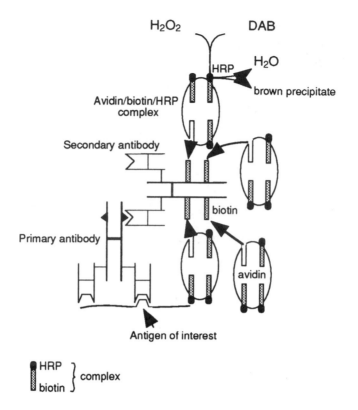

Fig. 3. Diagrammatic representation of indirect immunolabeling using an avidin/biotin/HRP complex technique. This amplifies the antibody/antigen signal by as much as 32 times, because one primary antibody can bind two secondary antibodies, thus 2 × 16 peroxidase molecules.

phatase; however, the most commonly used enzyme today is horseradish peroxidase (HRP, substrate: hydrogen peroxide). It can be used in simple indirect techniques, peroxidase antiperoxidase, and avidin/biotin complex (ABC) techniques. Diaminobenzidene (DAB) is provided, which is oxidized by an oxygen radical after enzymatic fission of hydrogen peroxide (**Fig. 3**). The familiar dark brown FRP is produced, which is then amenable to osmication. At the EM level HRP techniques are most useful for labeling membranous structures, such as Golgi-associated peptides *(4,5)* (**Fig. 4**), but on organelles that have inherent electron density, such as nuclei, endocrine granules, or even whole red blood cells, this final reaction product is less easily distinguishable from the morphology of the organelle. At low magnification, however, demonstration of highly expressed antigen can be dramatic with this method (**Fig. 5**).

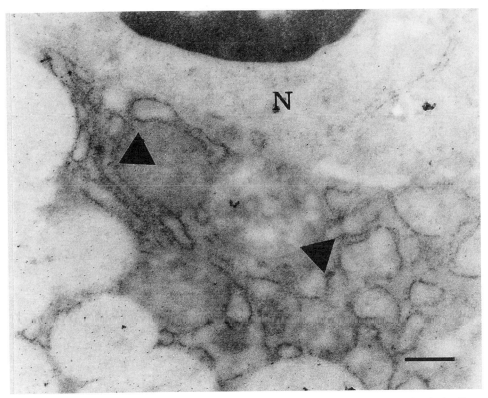

Fig. 4. Golgi apparatus from a human small intestine epithelial cell in Crohn's disease. Cells of an ulcer-associated cell lineage produce trefoil factors (concerned with healing and mucus production), and here pS2 (trefoil factor, TFF 1) has been labeled with an ABC method (arrows). The FRP is an electron-dense deposit evenly distributed on the antigenic membranes. N is a neighboring cell that has no pS2 and thus provides an excellent integral negative control (bar = 0.4 μm).

Optimal immunostaining is achieved when there is maximum preservation of antigen, when antigen/antibody binding is highly specific, when it is highly efficient, and when the final preparation is clearly visible on the electron microscope.

2. Materials

All incubations are carried out in multiwell microtest "Terasaki" plates; washing is done in drops of solution on pieces of fresh dental wax.

Primary antibodies may be mono- or polyclonal. For immunogold techniques the secondary antibody is an immunogold conjugate, whereas for the ABC immunoperoxidase technique the second layer is biotinylated and the third layer is an avidin/biotin/peroxidase conjugate. In both cases the normal

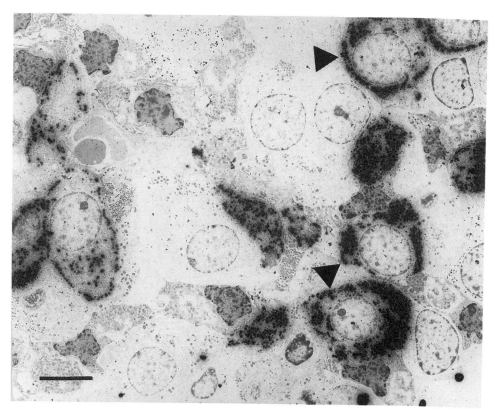

Fig. 5. Low-power electron micrograph of rat pituitary immunolabeled using an ABC technique to demonstrate the presence of growth hormone in the granules of somatotrophs (arrows); no counterstain has been applied, so other cell types are scarcely visible. When compared with **Fig. 2** it can be seen that the ABC technique shows immunoreactivity at a magnification too low to resolve 15 nm gold particles, whereas the gold technique labels granules specifically without obliterating their morphology (bar = 5 μm).

serum for the "blocking" stage is derived from the species that provides the second layer antibody.

1. Antiserum diluent: 0.01 *M* standard phosphate buffer, pH 7.4, 0.15 *M* NaCl, 0.1% globulin-free bovine serum albumin, 0.01% sodium azide.
2. Standard Tris buffer: Tris is the name for solid hydroxymethyl methylamine; the standard buffer is made from the following solutions:
   a. Stock A: dilute stock 0.2 *M* Tris (2.42 g Tris in 100 mL dH$_2$O) to 0.05 *M* with distilled water.
   b. Stock B: dilute stock 0.2 *M* Tris (2.42 g Tris and 1.7 mL HCL to 100 mL dH$_2$O) to 0.05 *M* with distilled water.

3. Tris I: 25 mL stock A + 20.7 ml stock B made up to 100 mL with dH$_2$O.
4. Tris II: 25 mL stock A + 20.7 mL stock B made up to 100 mL with dH$_2$O + 0.1% bovine serum albumin (BSA).
5. Tris III: 25 mL stock A + 11 mL stock B made up to 100 mL with dH$_2$O + 1.0% BSA.
6. Peroxidase substrate/DAB solution: 0.025–0.05%, 3'3-diaminobenzidine tetra HCl (DAB), 50 mM phosphate-buffered saline (PBS) buffer, pH 7.0–7.2, plus H$_2$O$_2$ to a final concentration of 0.01–0.03%.

3. Methods

To fulfill optimal conditions, always process approx six grids simultaneously (*see* **Note 1**), one acting as a positive control, one as a negative control (*see* **Note 2**) and four different test categories, varying only one parameter (e.g., etching time or antibody concentration) at a time.

3.1. Indirect Immunogold Method
for Single Labeling Applications

1. Etch grid-mounted ultrathin sections to permeabilize the resin (nonosmicated tissue: 10% H$_2$O$_2$ *or* osmicated tissue: saturated sodium metaperiodate) for 10–30 min at room temperature (*see* **Note 3**).
2. Wash thoroughly in microfiltered, distilled water, 3 × 1 min (*see* **Note 4**).
3. Drain grids and incubate for 30 min at room temperature in drops of normal serum from the species of the donor of the secondary antibody, diluted to 1/30 in antiserum diluent (*see* **Note 5**).
4. Drain the normal serum lightly from the grids by touching the edge to fiber-free absorbent paper; place the grids directly into the primary antibody solution, at optimal dilution, which is determined experimentally (*see* **Note 6**).
5. Incubate at optimal dilution for 1 h at room temperature, or overnight at 0–4°C in a humidity chamber.
6. Wash grids thoroughly in 0.05 M Tris-HCl buffer, pH 7.4, Tris-I, 3 × 1 min (*see* **Note 7**).
7. Wash grids thoroughly in 0.05 M Tris-HCl buffer, pH 7.4, Tris-II, containing 0.1% BSA, 3 × 1 min.
8. Place grids in 0.05 M Tris-HCl buffer, pH 8.2, Tris-III, containing 1.0% BSA for 5–15 min.
9. Gold-labeled IgG must be centrifuged for 5 min at 700g immediately prior to use to remove aggregates.
10. Incubate grids in drops of gold-labeled secondary antibody, 1/20–1/30, diluted in Tris-III buffer, for 1 h at room temperature in a humidity chamber (*see* **Note 8**).
11. Wash very thoroughly in large quantities of Tris-II buffer, 3 × 1 min.
12. Wash very thoroughly in large quantities of Tris-I buffer, 3 × 1 min.
13. Wash very thoroughly in large quantities of double-distilled water, 3 × 1 min.

14. Counterstain the grids for conventional electron microscopy by immersing them in saturated methanolic uranyl acetate for 3–5 min, washing thoroughly, then placing them in filtered lead citrate solution for 4–10 min covered from the air.
15. Finally, wash grids thoroughly in double-distilled water.
16. View on the electron microscope operated at 80 kV.

3.2. Indirect ABC/Immunoperoxidase Method for Single Labeling Applications

Use nonosmicated tissue, because it is important to not have added any heavy metals (ABC = avidin, biotin complex).

1. Etch grid-mounted ultrathin sections in 10% H_2O_2 for 10–30 min at room temperature to permeabilize the resin. This will simultaneously block endogenous peroxidase activity in the tissue (*see* **Note 3**).
2. Wash thoroughly in microfiltered (0.2 mm pore size) distilled water, 3 × 1 min (*see* **Note 4**).
3. Drain grids and incubate for 30 min at room temperature in drops of normal serum from the donor of the biotinylated antibody (*see* **Note 5**).
4. Drain normal serum from the grids on to fiber-free absorbent paper and immerse them in the primary antibody at optimal dilution (*see* **Note 6**).
5. Incubate for 1 h at room temperature or overnight at 0–4°C in a humidity chamber.
6. Wash grids in 0.01 *M* standard PBS, pH 7.0–7.2, 3 × 1 min.
7. Incubate in highly diluted biotinylated antibody for 45 min (*see* **Note 9**).
8. Prepare the ABC or streptavidin-biotinylated peroxidase complex (streptABC), according to the maker's instructions, during the above incubation, at least 20 min before use and leave to react. The grids can be washed during this time.
9. Wash grids in 0.01 *M* PBS, pH 7.0–7.2, 3 × 1 min.
10. Incubate sections in the ABC complex for 1 h at room temperature (*see* **Note 10**).
11. Wash in 0.01 *M* PBS, pH 7.0–7.2, 3 × 1 min.
12. Immerse grids in the H_2O_2 peroxidase substrate/DAB solution for 3–7 min at room temperature (*see* **Subheading 2., item 6**).
13. Jet wash in filtered double-distilled water.
14. Postosmicate for 1.5 h in 1% OsO_4, or 30 min in 3% OsO_4 in the fume cupboard (*see* **Note 11**).
15. Jet wash.
16. View on the electron microscope operated at 60 kV to obtain greater contrast.

4. Notes

1. To determine optimal conditions, always process several grids simultaneously. We find six a good number to handle at the same time. This allows a range of four variables (of one item at a time) plus two controls that must be included every time. On the first occasion that a certain procedure is performed one has to determine the optimal conditions, e.g., time left in etching solution/dilution of

primary antibody. In each procedure change only one condition at a time, and when the optimal for that has been discovered move on to the next unknown. For example:

Run 1	Vary etching time	Primary antibody dilution 1:500
Grid 1	Negative control	
Grid 2	Etch 10 min	
Grid 3	Etch 15 min	
Grid 4	Etch 20 min	
Grid 5	Etch 30 min	
Grid 6	Positive control	

Let us say the best etching period turns out to be 15 min (Result: there was some labeling and the section was still in good physical condition), then:

Run 2	Vary primary antibody dilution	Etching time = 15 min
Grid 1	Negative control	
Grid 2	1:250	
Grid 3	1:500	
Grid 4	1:1000	
Grid 5	1:2000	
Grid 6	Positive control	

Here it will be discovered which dilution provides the best label with the lowest nonspecific background staining. All antibody incubations are carried out in multiwell microtest "Terasaki" plates; washing is done in individual drops of solution on a piece of fresh dental wax. The capacity of each well of the Terasaki plate is approx 25 µL—this allows you to be very economical regarding the quantity of expensive antibody used; in contrast, each drop of washing solution delivered from a syringe + microfilter is approx 50 µL, providing a good volume for rinsing.

2. A number of controls is desirable; on each occasion that the procedure is carried out, a positive control section must be included. This is tissue known to express the antigen being labeled; at the end it *must* be positively labeled, if it is not, it indicates that there has been an error in the procedure. At least one negative control must also be included every time. The purpose of negative controls is to ensure that no nonspecific labeling has taken place that would produce a false positive. The most basic of these is to substitute the primary antibody with buffer solution, usually PBS; any labeling appearing on this sample is clearly a false positive. Substituting the appropriate primary antibody with a different, inappropriate antibody or performing the primary incubation with a solution of the primary antibody already preabsorbed to purified antigen are further "fine-tuning" controls, which must provide a negative result.

3. Acrylic resins do not need to be etched. Antibodies are applied to tissue sections in aqueous solution, and the antibody molecules have no problem passing through a hydrophilic polymer.

Epoxy resins are hydrophobic, so they must be perforated to allow the aqueous solution to reach the tissue. Ideally, the more resin removed, the more tissue is exposed, therefore the better. However, the tissue section must remain intact, bearing in mind that an EM grid *is* a grid—if too much resin is removed the tissue will literally fall through the holes. The time that sections can be left in etching solution depends on the minutiae of conditions prevailing when the blocks were polymerized and it is impossible to predict more precisely than between 10 and 30 min on the initial occasion that a block is used. Thus, on the first attempt vary etching times of the four test grids—say 10, 15, 20, and 30 min (etch both control grids for 10 min until you have determined the optimal time experimentally). When you view the end result you will be able to detect which is most suitable. Note it for this block, and then use it always.

Choice of etching solution depends on whether the tissue has been osmicated: hydrogen peroxide for nonosmicated tissue, sodium metaperiodate for osmicated tissue. When H_2O_2 is used to etch, endogenous peroxidase activity is simultaneously blocked, when sodium metaperiodate is used to etch, if a peroxidase technique is to follow then endogenous peroxidase must be blocked in an additional step (0.3% H_2O_2, for 10 min) with a thorough water wash between solutions.

4. All buffers and washing solutions need to be microfiltered (0.2 mm pore size). Thorough rinsing of grids may either be carried out by individual jet-washing from a syringe fitted with a microfilter or, if many grids are to be washed, by depositing separate drops of solution on dental wax and moving the grids through them sequentially. For sections in epoxy resin (not those in acrylic resin—they come off), the dental wax might be placed on a magnetic stirrer that gently spins the metal grids inside their drops of solution; a problem is that this magnetizes the grids, and they tend to pass the magnetization onto forceps. Preparations must not be allowed to dry out at any stage in the procedure.

5. The normal serum incubation step is universal in immunolabeling procedures, and is taken to minimize nonspecific background staining. Sections are incubated in normal serum from the species that provides the visualizing antibody/conjugate. In this way, tissue epitopes that might be inappropriately recognized by the final layer antibody (when its turn comes) are previously bound. This incubation can be performed in 30 min (or less), but it does not damage the section in any way, so the period can be extended to fit in with laboratory routine—over lunch or overnight are both acceptable.

6. All antibodies are diluted in antibody diluent. If made freshly then discarded after use, sodium azide does not need to be added; this can help retain antigenicity. Monoclonal antibodies usually have to be used more concentrated than polyclonal antibodies, but one must pay attention to the amount of protein present—this is written on the bottle. As a rule of thumb, when determining the optimal dilution for the first time, for monoclonal primaries use a range from "straight-from-the-bottle" to 1:1000; and for polyclonal primaries try a range from 1:1000 to 1:5000.

The concentration that was successful at the light microscope level can be used as a guide, but on the one hand there are fewer epitopes present in the ultrathin section than in a 4-μm section (therefore perhaps indicating a more dilute solution), but because of the reduced antigenicity one would not want to miss any of them (so maybe a more concentrated solution should be used). Ultimately the optimal dilution is the one that provides the best "signal-to-noise ratio": the best label with the lowest background staining.

Incubating at low temperature overnight generally results in considerably less nonspecific activity and is always the procedure of choice. Be careful to cover the microtest plate—they come with close-fitting lids—thus providing the "humidity chamber" and protecting the specimens from drying out.

7. In the immunogold technique, washes between primary and secondary antibody steps are through sequential Tris buffers. Tris I is standard Tris buffer, Tris II has higher pH and added BSA, and the final Tris III has the highest pH and highest percentage of BSA. This decreasing acidity with increasing protein content stabilizes the immunogold conjugate. After the secondary incubation, the tissue is sequentially returned through the Trises and then washed in double-distilled water. The secondary antibody conjugate can be (and usually is) diluted in Tris III.

8. The easiest size gold grains to work with are 15 nm, when the ultimate grain density is very low, using smaller particles will improve the result. If despite all the described antidotes the final preparation has extremely high background staining, the cause is most likely crossreactivity between the secondary antibody conjugate and a native tissue epitope. To evade this, the species that donated the primary antibody (and thus the species that the secondary antibody recognizes) must be changed. For example, if initially one used primary antibody: rabbit antihuman antigen and secondary antibody: labeled goat antirabbit IgG, which gave rise to the excessive background, try something like primary antibody: guinea pig antihuman antigen and secondary antibody: labeled goat anti-guinea pig IgG.

9. Biotinylated secondary antibody is used at very low concentration to prevent nonspecific background staining.

10. Streptavidin (from *Streptococcus spp*) is commonly used in the complex in preference to avidin (from egg), but it has the same high affinity for biotin. The complex is constructed so that on each streptavidin molecule one site remains vacant to be bound to a biotin molecule already in place on the tissue. The further biotin binding sites are already taken up with biotin/peroxidase complex. This means that many peroxidase molecules are conducted to the site of each antigen, increasing the sensitivity of the technique.

11. There is no heavy metal treatment before postosmication of the DAB final reaction product. Initially the tissue is not osmicated; no uranyl acetate and no lead citrate counterstaining are carried out. This ensures that electron density observed in the final preparation is overwhelmingly the result of immunolabeling.

References

1. Polak, J. M. and Priestley, J. V. (eds.) (1992) *Electron Microscopic Immunocytochemistry. Principles and Practice,* Oxford Science Publications, Oxford University Press, Oxford, UK.
2. Faulk, W. P. and Taylor, G. M. (1971) An immunocolloid method for the electron microscope. *Immunochemistry* **8,** 1081–1083.
3. Sarraf, C. E., Ansari, T. W., Conway, P., Notay, M., Hill, S., and Alison, M. R. (1993) Bromodeoxyuridine-labelled apoptosis after treatment with antimetabolites in two murine tumours and small intestinal crypts. *Br. J. Cancer* **68,** 678–680.
4. Sarraf, C. E., Alison, M. R., Ansari, T. W., and Wright, N. A. (1995) Subcellular distribution of peptides associated with gastric mucosal healing and neoplasia. *Microsc. Res. Tech.* **31,** 234–247.
5. Poulsom, R., Chinery, R., Sarraf, C., Lalani, E.-N., Stamp, G., Elia, G., Wright, N. (1992) Trefoil peptide expression in intestinal adaptation and renewal. *Scand. J. Gasteroenterol.* **27(Suppl. 192),** 17–28.

Further Reading

Polak, J. M. and Van Noorden, S. (1986) *Immunocytochemistry Modern Methods and Applications,* 2nd ed., John Wright & Sons, Bristol, UK.
Polak, J. M. and Van Noorden, S. (1997) *Introduction to Immunocytochemistry,* 2nd ed., Microscopy Handbooks 37, BIOS Scientific Publishers, Oxford, UK.

VII

ANTIBODY ENGINEERING

36

PCR of the V Region

Rakesh Verma

1. Background

To engineer or manipulate antibody or Fv-based molecules, isolation of the V region of the antibodies is necessary. A number of strategies can be adopted for amplification; one such approach is to use subgroup-specific oligonucleotides for the amplification of the V-region genes. Small differences in the conserved regions of variable genes have allowed the division of murine V_H and V_L genes into subgroups and families, with the members of one family having more homology with each other than members of another family. Therefore, it is possible to categorize the variable genes of particular hybridoma, and there are fewer chances of amplifying V_L genes of myeloma partners of the hybridoma with the family-specific primers as compared to a set of highly degenerate primers. Therefore, many (up to six) different 5′ primers can be designed from the FR1 of the kappa chain using the Kabat database (1). Similarly, four different 5′ primers are usually designed for the heavy chain. The 3′ primers are designed from constant segments of the chains (2).

2. Materials

2.1. Extraction of mRNA

1. 10^5–10^6 hybridoma cells.
2. Diethylpyrocarbonate DEPC-treated 0.5- and 1.5-mL tubes.
3. mRNA extraction kit (if commercially available a mRNA purification kit is used), or
4. RNA Zol™ B.
5. Chloroform.
6. Isopropanol.
7. 75% ethanol.
8. DEPC-treated water.

From: *Methods in Molecular Medicine, Vol. 40: Diagnostic and Therapeutic Antibodies*
Edited by: A. J. T. George and C. E. Urch © Humana Press Inc., Totowa, NJ

2.2. Preparation of cDNA

1. mRNA.
2. Super reverse transcriptase.
3. 10X reverse transcriptase buffer.
4. 5 mM of each dNTP.
5. 0.1 M dithiothreitol (DTT).
6. RNAguard.
7. 20 pmole of forward primer, or
8. First-strand cDNA synthesis kit.

2.3. Amplification of V-Region Genes

1. cDNA.
2. 5 mM of each dNTP (only when the cDNA synthesis process does not give an appropriate final concentration of the dNTPs).
3. *Taq* polymerase.
4. 10X *Taq* polymerase reaction buffer.
5. MgCl$_2$ (1.5–2.5 mM final concentration, if the MgCl$_2$ is absent in the 10X PCR reaction buffer).
6. Distilled water.
7. 10–20 pmole of each primer.
8. Mineral oil.
9. A thermocycler.

3. Methods

3.1. Extraction of mRNA

Two methods of isolating mRNA from hybridoma cells are described in this section. Both methods are equally effective in extracting mRNA from the cells. The choice of method will depend on the availability of the reagents and the investigator's preference.

3.1.1. Method I

Messenger RNA (mRNA) can usually be extracted from 10^5–10^6 hybridoma cells either using commercially available kits, such as the QuickPrep micro mRNA purification kit (Pharmacia, St. Albans, UK) in accordance with the manufacturer's protocol or as described in **Subheading 3.1.2.** In this section the method of isolating mRNA using one such kit will be described.

1. Homogenize the cell pellets in 0.4 mL extraction buffer, which contains guanidinium thiocyanate and *N*-lauroyl sarcosine, and dilute in 2 vol (0.8 mL) elution buffer.
2. Centrifuge the mixture and transfer the clear cellular homogenate to oligo(dT)-cellulose.
3. Resuspend the oligo(dT)-cellulose in 0.3 mL low-salt buffer, transfer it to a microspin column, and elute the mRNA with an appropriate volume (100 µl) of prewarmed (65°C) elution buffer. Store the mRNA at –70°C.

Table 1
Subgroup-Specific Primers for Amplifying Variable Region Genes

Primer	DNA Strand
Light chain	
CκN1	CTG CTC ACT GGA TGG TGG GAA
VκL I/III	GAC ATT GTG ATG AC(CT) CA(AG) TCT
VκL-IV/VI	CAA A(AT)T GT(TG) CTC ACC CAG TCT
VκL-IIa	GAT GTT TG(TG) ATG ACC CAA ACT
VκL-IIb	GAT ATT GTG ATA ACC CAG G(AC)T
VκL-Va	GAC ATC (GC)AG ATG AC(CT) CAG TCT
VκL-Vb	GA(CT) ATT GTG (AC)TG AC(AC) CAG TCT
Heavy chain	
VH1FOR	TGA GGA GAC GGT GAC CGT GGT CCC TTG GCC CCA G
VhN1-I	CAG GTG CAG CT(GT) AC(AG) GAG TCA
VhN1-II	CAG GTC CA(GA) CTG CAG CAG (TC)CT
VhN1-III	GA(GA) GTG AAG CTG GTG GA(GA) TCT
VhN1-V	GAG GTT CAG CTT CAG CAG TCT

3.1.2. Method II

1. Wash the hybridoma cells twice in phosphate-buffered saline (PBS) before isolation of RNA.
2. Homogenize the cell pellet in 1.4 mL RNA Zol B (Biotecx Laboratories Inc., Houston, TX), which contains guanidinium thiocyanate and phenol.
3. Extract the RNA by adding 140 μL chloroform (BDH Laboratory Supplies, Poole, UK) to the homogenate.
4. Vortex the mixture and centrifuge at 12,000g for 15 min to partition it into two layers and the interphase.
5. Precipitate the RNA in the aqueous layer with an equal volume of isopropanol (Sigma, Poole, UK). Wash the white-yellow pellet of RNA in 75% ethanol.
6. Resuspend the RNA pellet in 100 μL DEPC (Sigma)-treated water.

3.2. Preparation of cDNA

3.2.1. Method I

1. Heat the mRNA at 65°C for 3 min, and then incubate on ice for 2 min.
2. Add super reverse transcriptase (50 U) (Northumbia Biological Ltd, Northumberland, UK) to the mRNA along with 5 μL 10X reverse transcriptase buffer (Northumbia Biological Ltd.), 5 μL dNTPs (5 m*M* of each dNTP) (Pharmacia), 5 μL of 0.1 *M* DTT (United States Biochemical Corporation [USB], Cleveland, OH), 2 μL RNAguard (Pharmacia), and 20 pmole of each forward primer (**Table 1**) (CκN1 for light chain and VH1FOR for heavy chain).
3. Incubate the reaction mixture at 42°C for 1 h.

3.2.2. Method II

1. Heat the RNA for 10 min at 65°C and then chill on ice. Heating the RNA disrupts regions of secondary structure that might have been formed. This method describes the use of a commercially available kit (First-Strand cDNA Synthesis kit [Pharmacia P-L Biochemicals]) to prepare cDNA.
2. Add 5 μL bulk first-strand cDNA reaction mix, 1 μL DTT (200 mM aqueous solution), and 1 μL NotI-d(T)$_{18}$ primer to 8 μL RNA. Bulk first-strand cDNA reaction mix contains the enzyme (Cloned FPLCpure® M-MuLV reverse transcriptase), RNA guard (porcine), RNase/DNase-free bovine serum albumin (BSA), and dNTPs (dATP, dCTP, dGTP, and dTTP) in aqueous buffer. Dilute the primer 1 in 25 (0.2 μg/reaction).
3. Incubate the mixture for 90 min at 37°C. The final first-strand cDNA reaction contains 45 mM Tris (pH 8.3), 68 mM KCl, 15 mM DTT, 9 mM MgCl$_2$, 0.08 mg/mL BSA, and 1.8 mM each dNTP.

3.3. Amplification of V Region Genes

In this section the use of subgroup-specific primers and the amounts of the reagents for 50 μl PCR reaction will be described.

1. To 5 μL of cDNA add 1 μL (5 mM) of each dNTP, 5 μL 10X buffer, 2.5 U Taq polymerase (Perkin Elmer Cetus, Beaconsfield, UK), and 20 pmoles of each primer and make up the volume with water.

    To amplify the variable domain of the kappa light chain (V_κ), the 3′ primer CκN1 and a panel (VκL-I/III, VκL-IV/VI, VκL-IIa, VκL-IIb, VκL-Va, VκL-Vb) of 5′ primers (**Table 1**) are used; similarly, the variable domain of the heavy chain (V_H) is amplified with 3′ primer VH1FOR and a panel (VhN I-I, VhN I-II, VhN I-III, VhN I-V) of 5′ primers (2) (**Table 1**).
2. Heat-cycle the reactions 30 times in a thermocycler using the following conditions: 30 s at 94°C, 30 s at 55–65°C, and 30 s at 72°C after a hot start at 94°C for 2 min. Check the PCR products by agarose gel electrophoresis.

3.4. General Discussion

3.4.1. mRNA

Polyadenylated mRNA makes up about 1–5% of total cellular RNA in most eukaryotic cells (3). The non-polyadenylated RNA molecules, such as ribosomal RNA or fragmented RNA genomes or certain RNA viruses, have to be prepared for cDNA synthesis by addition of a homopolymeric tail to their 3′ end. Most of the eukaryotic mRNAs have a poly(A) tail of 50–200 bases at their 3′ ends. Proper inhibitors of RNase have to be used during the process of RNA extraction to inactivate the extraneous RNase (from glassware, plasticware, hands, and so forth) and RNase released during the lysis of cell. DEPC treatment of microfuge tubes and glassware inactivates the RNase. All the solutions required for the extraction of mRNA should be prepared in DEPC-treated water. Traces of DEPC may modify the purine residues in RNA by carboxymethylation. The ability of RNA to form DNA:RNA and RNA:RNA hybrid is not seriously effected, unless large fractions of purines are carboxymethylated. Therefore, proper care should be taken to remove the excessive DEPC after treatment by autoclaving.

3.4.2. Optimization of the Amplification Conditions

The main factor that influences the quality of a PCR is the annealing that occurs between the primers and their complementary sequences in the target DNA. However, because of the high concentration of the primers, annealing with noncomplementary sequences may also occur and leads to nonspecific amplification of the products. These products are generated in competition with the specific product and reduce the yield of the latter.

Annealing is influenced by the temperature and the concentration of the cations, mainly of magnesium (Mg^{2+}) and potassium (K^+). Mg^{2+} and K^+, neutralize the negatively charged phosphate groups on the DNA and weaken the forces between the two strands facilitating the annealing between primer and DNA. K^+ is usually provided in the reaction by the PCR buffer, whereas Mg^{2+} is added separately and is used at a final concentration of 1.5–2.5 mM. However, higher concentrations of Mg^{2+} result in nonspecific annealing, since it stabilizes annealing without discriminating between specific and nonspecific base pairing.

The optimal annealing temperature is that temperature at which the primer binds specifically and with high stringency to the DNA sequence of interest. The annealing temperature depends on the melting temperature (T_m) of the primers and especially of the primer with the lowest T_m. In fact, the optimal annealing temperature may lie in a range of temperatures close to the theoretical T_m of the primers. The best way to optimize the annealing conditions is by performing the reaction at several temperatures.

3.4.3. Primers

The CDR1 is flanked by FR1 on its 5′ side and FR4 is on the 3′ side of CDR3. The sequences at the 3′ end of the V regions are fairly conserved and the residues at the 5′ end are semiconserved. There is slight variation in the conserved sequences of different immunoglobulins. On the basis of this variation V_H and V_L genes have been divided into families (1).

There are number of strategies for the PCR amplification of immunoglobulin V region genes. Initially degenerate oligonucleotide primers were described that were derived from relatively conserved sequences present at the 5′ and 3′

ends of the rearranged V region gene. The incorporation of nonspecific nucleotides during the PCR amplification, or inappropriate and inconsistent amplification may be a problem with degenerate primers. The alternative is to construct multiple unique primers for different families *(4)*. The panel of primers, which have been derived from the constant region just next to the 3' end of the J gene segments and signal peptide sequences, have been used to isolate different families of V region genes *(2,5)*.

In some cases the product can be amplified with more than one primer at a particular annealing temperature. This can probably be caused by the amplification of the aberrant κ chain with one of the primers. The myeloma fusion partner, such as NS-1, may have such aberrant κ chain, and it has been reported in the literature that hybridomas in which the myeloma fusion partner is derived from MOPC-21 parent line, such as P3, NS-1, 1-Ag4-1, and P3X63-Ag8.653 *(6)*, may express an aberrantly rearranged kappa light chain. These hybridomas encode for a nonfunctional light chain because of the aberrant rearrangement at the VJ recombination site. There is deletion of four nucleotides at the recombination site, which leads to inclusion of a translation termination codon at amino acid position 105 *(1)*. The levels of aberrant transcript may exceed the levels of productive light chain in these hybridomas *(2)*.

Therefore, a proper design of primers, a careful optimization of the amplification conditions, and a keen, ever-alert and suspicious eye to spot the aberrant PCR products are required to amplify the desired V region genes.

4. Notes

1. Guanidinium thiocyanate, in association with *N*-lauroyl sarcosine, acts to disrupt nucleoprotein complexes. Therefore, RNA is isolated free of protein complexes. In addition, guanidinium thiocyanate is an inhibitor of RNase and so helps in the isolation of intact RNA.
2. In the cellulose pellet the mRNAs are attached by hybridization to the 3'-polyA tails and retained under conditions of high salt concentration (washing with high-salt buffer). Dissociation from the oligo(dT)-cellulose occurs in conditions of low salt concentration (washing with low-salt buffer).
3. The RNA Zol B promotes the formation of complexes of RNA with guanidinium and water molecules after cell lysis.
4. The hydrophilic interactions between DNA and proteins are reduced, and removed from the aqueous phase, and enter the organic phase and interphase, whereas RNA remains in the aqueous phase.
5. The formation of double-stranded RNA:DNA heteroduplexes is catalyzed by Moloney Murine Leukemia Virus (M-MuLV) reverse transcriptase.
6. *Not*I-d(T)$_{18}$ is a bifunctional primer with the sequence 5'-d[AAC TGG AAG AAT TCG CGG CCG CAG GAA T$_{18}$]-3' consisting of a "tail" of 18 thymidines and a sequence containing a *Not*I restriction site.

References

1. Kabat, E. A., Wu, T. T., Perry, H. M., Gottesman, K. S., and Foeller, C. (1991) *Sequences of Proteins of Immunological Interest*. US Department of Health and Human Services, Bethesda, MD.
2. Nicholls, P. J., Johnson, V. G., Blanford, M. D., and Andrew, S. M. (1993) An improved method for generating single-chain antibodies from hybridomas. *J. Immunol. Methods* **165,** 81–91.
3. Sambrook, J., Fritsch, E. F., and Maniatis, T. (1989) *Molecular Cloning: A Laboratory Manual*. Cold Spring Harbor Laboratory Press, Cold Spring Harbor, NY.
4. Sastry, L., Alting-Mees, M., Huse, W. D., Short, J. M., Sorge, J. A., Hay, B. N., Janda, K. D., Benkovic, S. J., and Lerner, R. A. (1989) Cloning of the immunoglobulin repertoire in *Escherichia coli* for generation of monoclonal catalytic antibodies: construction of a heavy chain variable region-specific cDNA library. *Proc. Natl. Acad. Sci. USA* **86,** 5728–5732.
5. George, A. J. T., Titus, J. A., Jost, C. R., Kurucz, I., Andrew, S. M., Nicholls, P. J., Huston, J. S., and Segal, D. M. (1994) Redirection of T cell mediated cytotoxicity by a recombinant single-chain Fv molecule. *J. Immunol.* **152,** 1802–1811.
6. Carroll, W. L., Mendel, E., and Levy, S. (1988) Hybridoma fusion cell lines contain an aberrrant Kappa transcript. *Mol. Immunol.* **25,** 991–995.

37

Phage Display Technology

Protocols

Michael Johns and Donald B. Palmer

1. Introduction

Over the past few years, considerable effort has gone into genetic engineering and manipulation of antibody molecules. One consequence of this research has been the use of filamentous phage as a vehicle on which to display antibody fragments. It is possible to express a variety of molecules on the surface of phage, including peptides and antibody fragments. With regard to antibodies, libraries of both sFv and Fab fragments have been successfully cloned onto the surface of bacteriophages, usually via the N terminal of the gene III product, although expression on the gene VIII product has also been employed to isolate low-affinity antibodies.

A variety of different libraries of phage expressing randomly combined V_H and V_L chain genes have been created from different sources, e.g., mouse, human, and chicken. One of the most commonly used libraries is that of Nissim et al. (*1*), who has developed a semisynthetic phage library of $>10^8$ different specificities. The library has been made in vitro from 50 cloned human V_H gene segments, which have random nucleotide sequences encoding CDR3 lengths of 4–12 residues, combined with a single V_L. They have used the library to select a variety of sFv against 18 different antigens after four or five rounds of panning. The selected phages and sFv were used in western blotting and also for epitope mapping and staining of cells.

De Kruif et al. (*2*) have also constructed a semisynthetic sFv library using cloned human germline V_H genes and synthetic CDR3. However, in contrast to Nissim et al., they have used a 6–15 amino-acid CDR3 containing short

From: *Methods in Molecular Medicine, Vol. 40: Diagnostic and Therapeutic Antibodies*
Edited by: A. J. T. George and C. E. Urch © Humana Press Inc., Totowa, NJ

stretches of fully randomized amino acid residues flanked by regions of limited variability (selected on the frequency of amino acids in the CDR3 of natural antibodies). In doing so the authors reason that this will increase occurrence of phage displaying functionally useful fragments. They also attempted to increase variability by using seven different light chains from both λ and κ subclasses rather than λ3 alone, as Nissim et al. *(1)* used.

Griffiths et al. *(3)* have produced a Fab library of 6.5×10^{10} specificities using a combinatorial infection process that involves transforming bacteria with a library of heavy chains on a plasmid and then infecting the culture with a library of light chains on a phage and also a Cre recombinase on a separate phage. The Cre recombinase then uses lox P sites within the library vectors to randomly combine H and L chains (from the plasmid and phage vectors) on the same phage replicon within each bacterium. With the increased size of this library, the authors report antibody fragments of affinities >80-fold higher than those isolated from smaller libraries. A similar library in the sFv format has also been developed from the same V_H and V_L sublibraries and termed the griffin library. This offers greater potential with regard to selection of high-affinity sFv for use in many aspects of research.

The generation of phage display libraries has revolutionized screening of antibody V genes. Specific phage can be selected directly from a mixed pot by several rounds of selection with the library against a desired antigen followed by amplification of the bound phage in bacteria. It is possible to isolate rare phage from a complete mixture with as much as 1000-fold enrichment after one round of selection and a million-fold enrichment after two rounds. Several ways exist to select phage, including immobilization of the Ag on plastic and selection against cells *(4,5)*—both live and fixed.

The use of phage display libraries has allowed the isolation of a number of antibody fragments against a number of different antigens including closely related molecules and those that have proved difficult to raise antibodies against by conventional hybridoma technology. The following chapter details some commonly used methods for selection of specific phage from diverse libraries. However, it does not cover techniques on how to make a library which are outside the scope of this book and have been reviewed else where.

2. Materials

1. 0.45 μm sterile filters (Millipore, Bedford, MA).
2. Ampicillin (100 mg/mL stock), filter sterilize.
3. 20% Glucose (autoclaved).
4. Glycerol.
5. 1 *M* IPTG (aliquot and keep frozen).
6. Kanamycin (25 mg/mL stock), filter sterilize.

7. Marvel/PBS (M/PBS) dried milk powder in (PBS)—must be virtually fat free.
8. 100 mM NaHCO$_3$, pH 9.6.
9. Nunc Immunotubes (Life Technologies, Paisley, UK).
10. 20% polyethyleneglycol (PEG) 8000/2.5 M NaCl (To make 1 L melt 200 g PEG on its own in the microwave, allow to cool, make up NaCl in 500 mL distilled water, and when disolved mix with the cooled PEG and adjust the volume to 1 L. Autoclave.)
11. PBS, pH 7.4.
12. Phosphate buffered saline-Tween 20 (0.1%) (PBS/T).
13. 1,2-Phenylenediamine (OPD) (Dako, Denmark).
14. Rabbit anti M13 antibody (Sigma, Poole, UK).
15. 3,3',5,5'-Tetramethylbenzidine (TMB) (Sigma).
16. 1 M Tris-HCl, pH 7.4–9.0.
17. Top agarose: 0.7% agarose in media—Melt in the microwave and allow to cool to ~55°C before use.
18. 2X TY: 16 g bactotryptone, 10 g yeast extract, 5 g NaCl in 1 L.
19. TYE Agar: 15 g bactoagar, 8 g NaCl, 10 g bactotryptone, 5 g yeast extract in 1 L.
20. VCS-M13 or M13-KO7 helper phage: Strategene (Cambridge, UK).

In addition, certain reagents will be required that are specific to your library,

3. Methods

3.1. Growth and Selection of Phage Display Libraries

3.1.1. Growth of Phage Display Libraries

The details of how to grow your particular phage display library will be unique to each library and should be obtained from the supplier of the library. Furthermore, in some cases, the libraries come supplied as phage rather than bacterial stocks, in which case amplification is not necessary although making a secondary stock is essential. Again, details of how to make a secondary library should be available from the supplier of the library. This chapter is therefore going to begin assuming you have already amplified your particular library.

3.1.2. Preparation of Phage Particles

Having grown your phage library, it will be necessary to purify the phage particles. The most commonly used method is that of PEG precipitation. This is a simple, reliable, and relatively quick method that provides phage of suffi cient purity for most applications (*see* **Note 1**).

1. Following overnight culture of the library, remove the bacteria by centrifugation. Approximately 5000g for 20 min at 4°C is adequate.
2. Add 1/5 to 1/4 the vol ice-cold 20% PEG/2.5 M NaCl. Mix well and incubate for 1 h on ice.

3. Harvest the phage by centrifugation at approx 10,000–12,000*g* at 4°C for 30 min. Pour off the supernatant and aspirate off any remaining supernatant if necessary. Resuspend the pellet in 40 mL sterile distilled water.

4. Re precipitate the phage with 1/5 to 1/4 vol of ice-cold 20% PEG/2.5 *M* NaCl and incubate at 4°C for a minimum of 30 min.

5. Harvest the phage by centrifugation as above (**step 3**). Remove all supernatant and then briefly respin and aspirate off any remaining supernatant.

6. Resuspend the phage in either sterile distilled water or PBS. Approximately 1.5–2 mL should be sufficient.

7. Briefly centrifuge (approx 1 min) to remove any bacterial debris. Then filter-sterilize using a 0.45-μm filter.

8. Titer phage (*see* **Subheading 3.3.1.**).

9. Phage can be stored at 4°C for short periods of time. For selection procedures, it is best to use freshly prepared phage particles.

Note: Cleavage of the sFv alone from the surface of the phage is possible, resulting in a phage particle capable of infecting bacteria (e.g., TG1) (via gene III) but unable to bind specifically to an antigen. It is therefore important to use fresh preparations of phage wherever possible, particularly for selection procedures.

3.1.3. Selection of Phage Antibodies from Libraries

A variety of different methods have been developed for the selection of phage from diverse libraries. The majority are based on immobilization of a known antigen followed by several rounds of selection and amplification of the phage that bind the immobilized antigen. However, other, more intricate, methods have been developed recently, including selection against both fixed and live cells. I shall give a detailed basic protocol for selection of phage against immobilized antigen.

3.1.4. Selection Using Immobilized Antigen

1. Coat the antigen (10–100 μg/mL) onto a solid surface (e.g., Nunc immunotube) by incubation overnight at high pH. We use 100 m*M* NaHCO₃, pH 9.6; however, PBS, pH 7.4, can be used. The higher pH encourages more binding of the protein to the tube, but consideration must be given to the stability of the antigen at the higher pH. Coating can be carried out either at 4°C or room temperature; again, the choice depends on the stability of the antigen.

2. Wash the tube three times with PBS/T and then once with PBS.

3. Block the remaining sites on the immunotube by incubation with 2% *M*/PBS and fill the tube to the top. Incubate at 37°C for a minimum of 2 h.

4. Wash the tube three times with PBS/T and then once with PBS.

5. Add your purified phage (in sufficient number to exceed the size of your library, therefore ensuring representation of all the different specificities present) in 1%

M/PBS. Incubate at 4°C overnight, preferably with gentle rotation, then stand for 90 min at room temperature. Shorter incubation times can be used successfully at 37°C and may be desirable but dependent on the stability of your antigen.

6. Pour off and keep the phage. You may wish to add the phage to a second tube coated with a different antigen. Wash the tube twenty times with PBS/T and then once with PBS to remove non specifically bound phage (*see* **Note 2**).

7. Bound phage can then be eluted by adding 1.3 mL of either 100 m*M* triethylamine or 100 m*M* glycine, pH 2.8, to the immunotube. Incubate for 10 min on a rotator.

8. Collect the eluted phage and neutralize the elution solution using 200 µL 1 *M* Tris, pH 7.5. This is typically added in advance to separate tubes into which the eluted phage are pipeted in order to rapidly neutralize the elution buffer.

At this point the phage can be stored at 4°C or immediately added to bacteria for infection and subsequent rounds of selection. Typically 4–6 rounds of selection are carried out against any one antigen. The selection procedure should be monitored by ELISA (*see* **Subheading 3.2.1.**) after each round.

The above details a basic selection procedure for isolation of phage against immobilized antigen. However, a variety of more complex selection procedures have been developed, including selection against live cells known to express certain surface antigens (*4,5*).

3.1.5. Infection of Selected Phage Particles into Bacteria and Subsequent Amplification

At this stage the choice of bacteria to use will depend on the vector your library has been cloned into. You must choose a strain capable of infection by phage (F′ positive) and also production of complete phage particles expressing sFv on their surface. The pHEN1 vector used by a number of groups (e.g., Nissim et al. *[11]*) is a phagemid (*see* Chapter 4) that has been designed with an amber stop codon between gene III and the sFv, allowing expression of the sFv on the surface of phage in sup E⁺ bacteria (*Escherichia coli* TG1) while permitting expression of soluble sFv alone in sup E⁻ bacteria (*E. coli* HB2151 or SF110). In contrast, other libraries, such as the Barbas library (*6*), do not use such a system and require subcloning of the sFv gene in order to get expression of the sFv alone. Be careful. Regardless of the strain of bacteria used, however, the method remains the same.

1. Add 9 mL of bacteria (grown until OD at 600 nm is 0.5, then incubated without shaking for 20 min) to 1 mL of the neutralized eluted phage in a universal (keep the remaining 0.5 mL eluted phage for sFv expression, if required). If you are continuing directly from the stage above, you can add 4 mL of the bacteria to the immunotube to rescue any residual phage.

2. Incubate for 20–30 min at 37°C to allow for infection.
3. If necessary, pool the bacteria from **step 2** and do the following two steps sequentially:
   a. Take 100 µL from the pooled bacteria for serial dilutions ($10^{-1}–10^{-9}$) to assess the number of selected phage particles and acquire single colonies for ELISA assay (*see* **Subheading 3.2.1.**). The bacteria should be plated on agar plates supplemented with the appropriate antibiotic and grown overnight at 37°C. It should also be noted that libraries under control of the *lacZ* promoter should be grown in the presence of 1% glucose to ensure no phage are produced at this stage.
   b. Spin the infected bacteria at 3000–5000*g* for 10 min. Resuspend the bacteria in 1 mL of 2X TY and plate on a 22 × 22 cm agar plate supplemented with the appropriate antibiotic and glucose if necessary. Incubate overnight at 37°C.
4. Add 2–5 ml 2X TY to the bioassay dish, loosen the cells with a glass spreader, and collect in a tube.
5. Add glycerol to a final concentration of 15% to the bacterial suspension and snap freeze/store at –70°C.
6. The selected library can then been grown again for subsequent rounds of selection.

3.2. Monitoring Selection of Phage Particles Expressing sFv

Following each round of selection, it is necessary to determine whether phage specific for your antigen have been selected. The simplest and most commonly used method for this is the phage ELISA. This allows rapid and sensitive detection of any clones that bind specifically to your chosen antigen. It should also be noted that other methods do exist, including the use of DNA fingerprint analysis using, for example, *BstN*1. At later stages of selection, DNA sequencing can be used. However, neither of the latter two methods indicate whether the selected clones bind your antigen; they merely reflect how many different clones exist in your selected population.

3.2.1. Phage ELISA

3.2.1.1. Rescue of Phage Particles for ELISA

1. Pick 96 separate colonies and inoculate into separate wells of a 96-well plate containing 100 µL bacterial medium and appropriate antibiotics. Typically, colonies from one of the plates used to titer the phage are used for this purpose.
2. Incubate overnight with shaking at 37°C.
3. Take a small innoculum from each well of this plate into the corresponding well of a second 96-well plate containing 150 µL of medium/well. Incubate this second plate for 1 h at 37°C. In the meantime, add glycerol to each well of the original 96-well plate to give a final concentration of 15% glycerol and then freeze the plate for future use.
4. Add 10^9 helper phage/mL to each well of the plate. This is usually done by making a stock solution of helper phage in medium and aliquoting this into each well.

5. Incubate at 37°C for 45 min without shaking followed by 1 h at 37°C with shaking.
6. Centrifuge the plate at 1500g for 20 min at 20°C. Remove all supernatant.
7. Resuspend the pellet in 200 µL of bacterial medium containing the appropriate antibiotics. Note that at this stage those libraries under the control of the *lacZ* promoter should be grown in the absence of glucose. Furthermore, at this stage, it is usually necessary to grow the bacteria in the presence of two antibiotics in order to select those bacteria infected with both phagemid vector and helper phage.
8. Grow overnight at 30°C. The lower temperature is necessary to produce phage particles expressing the sFv on their surface.
9. On the following day, spin the plate as in **step 6** and use 50 µL of the supernatant in the ELISA (*see* **Subheading 3.2.1.2.**).

3.2.1.2. ELISA

1. Coat an ELISA plate with antigen and then block the remaining sites on the plate with 4% *M*/PBS (*see* Chapter 30 for details of ELISA).
2. Wash the plate three times with PBS/0.1% Tween.
3. Add 50 µL 4% *M*/PBS to each well followed by 50 µL supernatant from each well of the above culture plate. Mix and leave at room temperature for 2 h.
4. Wash wells three times with PBS/T and then twice with PBS.
5. Add 100 µL of primary antibody at appropriate dilution in 1% *M*/PBS. For phage ELISA, we use rabbit anti-M13 as the primary antibody. Incubate for 1 h at room temperature.
6. Wash the plate 3 times with PBS/T and then twice with PBS.
7. Add 100 µL of the secondary antibody at an appropriate dilution in 1% *M*/PBS. We use swine anti-rabbit peroxidase. Incubate for 1 h at room temperature.
8. Wash the plate four times with PBS/T and then twice with PBS.
9. Develop ELISA with 100 µL of an appropriate chromogenic substrate (e.g., OPD or TMB). Stop the reaction according to the manufacturer's recommendations.
10. Read on plate reader at the correct wavelength for your substrate. Determine which wells are positive. Positive wells are usually detected at the third or fourth round of selection (*see* **Note 3**).

3.3. Supplementary Protocols

3.3.1. Titering of Phage Particles

There are two different ways to titer phage preps: by plaque-forming units and by transducing units. Both these methods are described below.

3.3.1.1. TITRATION OF PHAGE PARTICLES BY PLAQUE-FORMING UNITS

1. Grow the host cell to mid log phase in a suitable medium and then leave them for 20 min at 37°C without shaking. Bacteria must be F′ positive to permit infection.
2. Prepare the appropriate amount of soft agar. Keep in a waterbath at 50°C, until ready to use.

3. Make 10-fold serial dilutions of the phage to be quantified (be sure to make enough dilutions to properly dilute out the phage). Change the tip between each dilution to reduce the carryover from one dilution to the next.
4. Aliquot 10 µL of each phage dilution into a separate universal tube and then add 400 µL bacterial cells. Leave for 20 min at 37°C.
5. Pour 3–4 mL soft agar into each tube of phage/bacteria, immediately pour the mixture onto an agar plate (without antibiotics), and swirl to cover the plate.
6. Grow overnight at 37°C or until plaques are formed.

3.3.1.2. Titration of Phage Particles by Transducing Units

1. Grow the host cell to mid log phase in a suitable medium and then leave them for 20 min at 37°C without shaking. Bacteria must be F' positive to permit infection.
2. Make 10-fold serial dilutions of the phage to be quantified (be sure to make enough dilutions to properly dilute out the phage).
3. Aliquot 10 µL of each phage dilution into a separate Eppendorf tube and then add 100 µL bacterial cells. Leave for 20 min at 37°C.
4. Spread the infected bacteria on the appropriate selection medium and grow at 37°C overnight.

3.3.2. Production of Helper Phage

It is possible to buy VCS-M13 or M13-K07 commercially. However, they are simple to produce and it is often more economical to grow them yourself. The following protocol is appropriate for both strains, either of which can be used for all the above protocols.

1. Infect 500 µL *E. coli* TGI (OD 0.5) with 10 µL serial dilutions of helper phage in universals and incubate at 37°C without shaking for 20 min (dilutions between 10^{-6} and 10^{-10} should allow you to identify separate plaques within a lawn of bacteria). Add 5 mL molten top agarose (50°C) and pour onto agar plates. Allow to set and incubate overnight at 37°C.
2. Select a small individual plaque and infect into 3–4 mL of an exponentially growing culture of TG1. Grow for about 2 h shaking at 37°C.
3. Inoculate into 500 µL 2X TY in a 2-L flask and grow for 1 h at 37°C. Add kanamycin (25 mg/mL in water) to a final concentration of 50–70 µg/mL. Grow for a further 8–16 h at 37°C.
4. Prepare phage particles as described in **Subheading 3.1.2.**

4. Notes

1. Precipitation of phage should be obvious. The solution will get cloudy almost immediately after the addition of PEG/NaCl. The precipitation will increase with incubation. One hour is the recommended minimum for the first precipitation. Longer incubation periods cause no damage to the phage-sFv. Precipitation is more rapid the second time and is also more obvious.

   At **step 5** of **Subheading 3.1.2.**, it is extremely important to remove all the PEG/NaCl. Its can effect subsequent application. If the presence of PEG is believed to be a problem in subsequent applications, density centrifugation can be used to remove all PEG present in the phage preparation.

Phage-sFv can be stored at −20 or −80°C without significant loss in infectivity. However, care should be taken to ensure such phage still express sFv on their surface. It is possible that although phage are still infectious, the sFv has been lost from the surface. With myc-tagged libraries, cloned into M13 derivatives, a simple sandwich ELISA can be performed to assess the sFv status of the phage particles. 9E10 antibody can be used to capture the phage-sFv via the myc tag and rabbit anti-M13 can be used to detect bound phage.

2. One of the most important aspects of phage selection is to wash the selection tubes thoroughly before the elution of the specifically bound phage sFv. Poor or inadequate washing will severely reduce the selection potential.

3. When doing phage ELISAs, a number of controls are necessary to ensure specific binding is being assessed. First, primary and secondary antibodies must be assessed for crossreactivity to your antigen in the absence of phage. You must also ensure your phage are binding specifically to the antigen on the plate. A number of phage have been found to stick nonspecifically to any antigen coated on an ELISA plate. Therefore, the use of a second plate coated with an irrelevant antigen is a necessary control.

It is possible to perform this ELISA using sFv. However, this is far more time-consuming and owing to the monovalency of sFv can prove difficult to obtain positive results. The sFv ELISA should only be used for clones that have previously shown up positive using a phage ELISA approach. If you wish to perform an sFv ELISA, the protocol is the same, except sFv are usually detected by the presence of a tag either C or N terminal of the molecule. Different libraries use different tags and therefore the primary and secondary antibodies to be used are dependent on the library you choose to use.

Again, controls are extremely important and the use of an irrelevant antigen coated onto a second plate is appropriate. Furthermore, before deciding to use a particular sFv in further experiments, the monovalency of the sFv preparation should be checked, i.e., it is necessary to ensure the sFv being produced is 30 kDa in size and has not formed a noncovalent aggregate during preparation. This is a common problem, particularly if the sFv has been purified from a culture supernatant by a process involving acidic elution from a column, e.g., antigen column. The easiest way to check this is by size exclusion chromatography. A 30-kDa band on an SDS-PAGE gel does not exclude the possibility that the sFv have formed noncovalent aggregates. Clearly an aggregated rather than monomeric protein could have extremely diverse effects in some assays.

References

1. Nissim, A., Hoogenboom, H. R., Tomlinson, I. M., Flynn, G., Midgley, C., Lane, D., and Winter, G. (1994) Antibody fragments from a "single pot" phage display library as immunological reagents. *EMBO J.* **13,** 692–698.

2. De Kruif, J., Terstappen, L., Boel, E., and Logtenberg, T. (1995) Selection and application of human single chain Fv antibody fragments from a semi synthetic phage antibody display library with designed CDR3 regions. *J. Mol. Biol.* **248,** 97–105.

3. Griffiths, A. D., Williams, S. C., Hartley, O., Tomlinson, I. M., Waterhouse, P., Crosby, W. L., Kontermann, R. E., Jones, P. T., Low, N. M., Allison, T. J., et al. (1994) Isolation of high affinity human antibodies directly from large synthetic repertoires. *EMBO J.* **13,** 3245–3260.

4. de Kruif, J., Terstappen, L., Boel, E., and Logtenberg, T. (1995) Rapid selection of cell subpopulation-specific human monoclonal antibodies from a synthetic phage antibody library. *Proc. Natl. Acad. Sci USA* **92,** 3938–3942.

5. Palmer, D. B., George, A. J. T., and Ritter, M. A. (1997) Selection of antibodies to cell surface determinants on mouse thymic epithelial cells using a phage display library. *Immunology* **91,** 473–478.

6. Barbas, C. F., 3rd, Bain, J. D., Hoekstra, D. M., and Lerner, R. A. (1992) Semi synthetic combinatorial antibody libraries: a chemical solution to the diversity problem. *Proc. Natl. Acad. Sci. USA* **89,** 4457–4461.

Index

framework regions, 39
Fv, 3, 35, 38, 39, 325
heavy chain, 1, 6, 8
hypervariable regions, *see*
    Complementarity determining
    regions
light chain, 1, 6, 8
Antigen expression, 70, 71
    antigenic variation, 169
Antigen presentation
    antigen-presenting cells 108, 109
        dendritic cells, 148
        macrophages, 100
        passenger lymphocytes, 146–148,
            150
    costimulation blockade, 100, 108-
        110
    CD80, 86, 28, CTLA4, CD40 see
        Cell surface molecules
Apopotosis, 71, 87, 89, 90, 92 104
Autoimmune disease, 66, 69, 99–110,
    249
    autoimmune cytopenia, 258
    Crohn's disease, 120, 128, 132, 182
    diabetes mellitus type 1, 100
    multiple sclerosis, 100, 106, 258
    psoriasis, 106
    rheumatoid arthritis, 100, 103, 106,
        115–133, 182, 187, 257
    scleroderma, 258
    systemic lupus erythematosis (SLE),
        106
    uveitis, 258
    vasculitis, 154–255, 256

B

β2 microglobulin, *see* Cell surface
    molecules
Biosensor, 59, 363–372, 382, 387, 388
Bispecific antibodies, 18, 19, 44, 77,
    94, 188, 333–339
    diabodies, *see* Antibody engineering

Blood–brain barrier, 157, 168, 169, 249

C

CAMPATH-1, *see also* Antibody
    specificity, CD52, 243–262
    structure CD52,
        259, 260
Cancer, *see* Neoplastic disease
Cardiovascular disease
    myocardial infarct, 186
    thrombosis, 180, 181
Cell surface molecules
    β2 microglobulin, 150–152
    CD28, 100, 108, 109
    CD3, 100, 107, 149
    CD4, 33, 43, 100, 106
    CD40, 92, 100, 108
    CD45, 71
    CD8, 33, 149
    CD80 & 86, 100, 108
    CTLA4 (CD152), 68, 100,
        108, 109
    ICAM-1 129, 149, 150
    LFA-1, 149
    LFA-3, 149, 150
    VCAM-1, 129, 130
Cost, 170
Cytokines and chemokines, 100
    GM-CSF, 43, 117, 119, 130
    IL1 receptor antagonist,
        119, 129
    IL1, 43, 115-117, 119, 129, 131,
        132, 159, 163, 165, 166
    IL10, 115, 116, 119, 121,
        136, 259
    IL11, 136
    IL2, 117
    IL4, 116, 117, 121, 136
    IL6, 117, 119, 124, 127, 129, 136,
        159, 163, 165, 166
    IL8, 119, 129, 130
    Interferon-γ, 80, 100, 115, 117, 259